Theoretical Alternatives to the Psychiatric Model of Mental Disorder Labeling

Contemporary Frameworks, Taxonomies, and Models

Edited by

Arnoldo Cantú, Eric Maisel and Chuck Ruby

Theoretical Alternatives to the Psychiatric Model of Mental Disorder Labeling is the fourth Volume of the Ethics International Press *Critical Psychology and Critical Psychiatry Series.*

Theoretical Alternatives to the Psychiatric Model of Mental Disorder Labeling: Contemporary Frameworks, Taxonomies, and Models

Edited by Arnoldo Cantú, Eric Maisel and Chuck Ruby

This book first published 2024

Ethics International Press Ltd, UK

British Library Cataloguing in Publication Data

A catalogue record for this book is available from the British Library

Print Book ISBN: 978-1-80441-276-3

eBook ISBN: 978-1-80441-277-0

To my parents, Maria and Pedro,
whose unconditional and immeasurable love
have made me the person I am today.
-AC

Contents

Editor's Introduction

Arnoldo Cantú

We live in a divisive and polarizing time in which it is becoming increasingly important for people to be able to speak their minds and contribute to our "epistemic commons" (i.e., the "stock of evidence, ideas, and perspectives that are alive for a given community"[1]) lest we fall prey to the *spiral of silence*—that is, how comfortable and willing an individual feels in voicing (or, more concerningly, not) a particular view or opinion may be associated with how popular or unacceptable that thought is perceived to be.[2]

Now more than ever—especially in the field of mental health with its predominant and controversial biomedical model used for labeling and "treating" human suffering—we need to embody and exert a sort of "cognitive liberty"[3] to satiate our collective hunger for wanting to voice (and hear) differing views, opinions, and perspectives about addressing complex social problems.

The World Health Organization (WHO) recently produced a reported in October of 2023 entitled "Mental health, human rights and legislation: guidance and practice"[4] that some are suggesting is *more* than advocacy for a paradigm shift in the field of mental health.[5] Relatedly, just a few years ago in 2017, United Nations Special Rapporteur, Dainius Pūras, pointedly stated that "there is unequivocal evidence that the dominance of and the overreliance upon the biomedical paradigm, including the front-line

---

[1] Joshi, H. (2021). *Why it's OK to speak your mind*. Routledge. p. xvi

[2] Noelle-Neumann, E. (1974). The spiral of silence a theory of public opinion. *Journal of Communication*, 24(2), 43–51. https://doi.org/10.1111/j.1460-2466.1974.tb00367.x

[3] https://www.madinamerica.com/2019/07/cognitive-liberty-principle-rally-behind/

[4] https://www.who.int/publications/i/item/9789240080737

[5] https://www.madinamerica.com/2023/11/the-who-and-the-united-nations-let-freedom-ring-for-the-mad/

and excessive use of psychotropic medicines, is a failure."[6] He added
that the biomedical model is an "obstacle" that neglects "the importance
of context, relationships and other important social and underlying
determinants of mental health."[7]

This volume is an attempt at that—at contributing to our epistemic
commons as it pertains to the field of mental health and considering how
associated disciplines (e.g., psychiatry, clinical psychology, social work,
counseling) play a role in contributing to a paradigm shift. As the title
suggests, this book consists of differing philosophical views, models,
taxonomies, frameworks, and perspectives across the globe for viewing
and supporting those experiencing suffering and distress.

It is my hope that these alternatives can, hopefully, further help the reader
move away from viewing "mental health problems" through the
traditional biomedical model lens, and consider more humanistic, nonmedicalized, and non-pathological ways for helping people. We are *all*
weary travelers roaming this earth—trying to make sense and meaning of
it all—with our common humanity binding us together. It is only fair for
us to help bring one another up—not disempower each other through
questionable labels and models—when we are already suffering.

Disclaimer: *If you or anyone you know is taking a prescriptive psychiatric
medication for any reason deemed appropriate by the prescribing physician,
alteration or discontinuation of the drug(s) is not recommended by any of the
information provided by the reading material found in this volume, Similarly, the
content in this book should not be interpreted, directly or indirectly, as suggestions
for any other current support (e.g., psychotherapy, counseling) to be abruptly
discontinued without discussion with your healthcare provider.*

---

[6] https://www.ohchr.org/en/statements/2017/09/statement-mr-dainius-puras-special-
rapporteur-right-everyone-enjoyment-highest
[7] Ibid.

Setting the Stage

The Foundational Flaw of the DSM

Chuck Ruby

Abstract: *The DSM is seriously flawed and, therefore, isn't a legitimate professional tool. It is a collection of moral pronouncements about appropriate ways of living and not a diagnostic guide that identifies and classifies illnesses. As such, it has been used over the years under the pretext of advancing mental health to oppress people who do not conform to certain desired behaviors and experiences. In essence, it extends the reach of the criminal justice system to enforce desired conduct, but it does so without the protections of due process of law. Furthermore, it provides no basis for helping people who are in the throes of emotional distress. We would be far better off abandoning the attempt of squeezing the square peg of human suffering into the round hole of medical nosology.*

Moral Disorders

The *Diagnostic and Statistical Manual of Mental Disorders* (DSM) is a compendium of human experiences and behaviors that have been deemed abnormal by psychiatric fiat. They are called mental *dis*orders because they deviate from sanctioned mental orders, but they are presented as illnesses or diseases of the mind. Such a capricious distinction between mental normality and abnormality, and the illogical leap from deviation to illness and disease, places in doubt the legitimacy of the manual and the categories within it, especially when using it under the guise of the assessment and care of one's health.

It is important to emphasize that all attempts to distinguish between mental normality and abnormality (order vs. disorder) are necessarily based on everchanging moral value judgments about the appropriateness of human thoughts, emotions, and conduct.[1] Classifying these purported forms of abnormality into different categories is not a clinical or medical task, but an

---

[1] Unfortunately for a large portion of the population subjected to the *DSM*, these moral value judgments grew from a European, White, male, Judeo-Christian perspective.

administrative one primarily for the purpose of communicating about them with others. This can occur in the larger interest of coercing people into more convenient (i.e., "normal/ordered") ways of being. It is not a process of identifying and classifying illnesses, diseases, or "dysfunction[s] in the individual"[2] as is claimed by the *DSM* and commonly believed within psychiatry, clinical psychology, and other allied clinical professions.

Physical and chemical processes of the body do, in fact, have abnormal ways of functioning from a *biological viability standpoint*. Those dysfunctions directly threaten ongoing biological capacity and life, and that is why they are assessed and treated with medical science. As with all fields of science, this is independent of moral values of those who identify and classify the abnormalities. Most importantly, the choice to remedy or ignore these physical and chemical dysfunctions is a decision made by the affected individual, not the physician. This is in line with the humanistic principles of informed consent and self-determination.

On the other hand, the only way to judge dysfunction (i.e., "abnormality/ disorder") of human experiences and behaviors is from a *moral standpoint* – that which an observer considers good or bad, right or wrong, too much or too little, appropriate or inappropriate. The etymological origin of the term supports this assertion as the prefix in *dys*function means "…destroying the *good* sense of a word or increasing its *bad* sense…."[3] [italics added for emphasis]. So, a mental dysfunction would be claimed based on a lack of good thoughts, feelings, and actions and a surplus of bad ones. But how do we determine if those things are good or bad? This moral foundation is also revealed in the fact that, contrary to when physical and chemical dysfunctions occur, people who are labeled mentally disordered are often forced or cajoled into treatment "for their own good." They are not afforded the right of informed consent and self-determination or to seek out help at their own choosing and for their own reasons. In short, they are not permitted to determine what they desire or what is good or bad for themselves.

---

[2] American Psychiatric Association. (2013). *The Diagnostic and Statistical Manual of Mental Disorders* (5th *Edition*). Washington, DC: American Psychiatric Association, p. 20.
[3] https://www.etymonline.com.

This moral quagmire is accentuated by the failure of the psychiatric community to provide robust evidence for the claim that mental disorders are the result of "dysfunction in the individual." In fact, if physical and chemical dysfunctions were ever discovered as the cause of what had been deemed a mental disorder, the problem would no longer fall within that domain. As examples, the lethargy of low thyroid functioning, the delirium of urinary tract infections, and the mood changes of Lyme disease are not symptoms of mental disorders; they are symptoms of *physical and chemical process dysfunctions*. These bodily defects are the critical targets of treatment. Ignoring the defect and merely treating the symptoms can be lethal. The point is that mental disorders *cannot* have a bodily dysfunction as the cause because if they did, it would be oxymoronic – they wouldn't be mental disorders. Instead, they would be physical disorders and the target of medical specialties like neurology, endocrinology, and oncology— not psychiatry.

With mental disorders, only the so-called symptoms can be treated. This means disrupting the central nervous system with chemicals, electricity, or surgery with the intention of interfering with *normal* brain functioning for the sole purpose of preventing the unwanted experiences and behaviors from happening, or to wheedle a person to stop behaving and thinking as they do. Thus, psychiatric treatment doesn't correct, cure, or medicate a defect that is responsible for symptoms since no such defect exists. It merely dampens or eliminates the so-called symptoms. This is especially problematic since the above forms of psychiatric treatment obscure personal meaning—meaning that sprouts forth from our experiences. Remove or numb the experiences and you remove or numb the meaning, potentially resulting in a pointless life.

There are nagging questions that result from the foregoing discussion. How do we identify bad or inappropriate thinking? Does it have to be very different from what other people think? Different from which people? How much different? Must thoughts cause social and interpersonal problems? Or is it sufficient that they only result in an internal sense of distress that no one else would notice? What about the reverse? What if others deem the thoughts bad and troublesome but the thinker does not? How attentive should a child be during boring classroom instruction? Which beliefs are good, and which are delusions?

This predicament applies to behaviors as well. Is it bad to take drugs? Does it depend on whether the substance is illegal or prescribed? How much of a quantity would it take to reach the appropriate-inappropriate threshold? How about other problematic behaviors? Is it bad when a person exhibits road rage? Is violent crime a sign of dysfunction in the individual or just a criminal choice and failure to inhibit urges? When someone is in despair, how long can they stay in bed and isolate from others before it is considered inappropriate?

This also applies to emotions. What are bad emotions? Are despair and fear bad? Or is it only inappropriate when no one else is feeling those things? What level of emotional distress is inappropriate? Is it bad to hold a grudge against a spouse for something they said that was hurtful? Does it matter how long the resentment lasts? What are valid reasons for feeling shame? How much excitement or pride is too much? Are emotions inappropriate only when they lead to problematic actions?

We have no authoritative basis for answering these questions, and this means we have no authoritative basis for using the *DSM*. They are not medical questions or matters of literal health and illness that can be studied through laboratory analysis of human functioning. Instead, when it comes to the orthodox assessment and treatment of people struggling with life problems, clinicians use their own personal moral values or the mental health industry's ambiguous conventional wisdom contained in *DSM* diagnostic guidelines. It comes down to how *should* a person think, how *should* a person act, and how *should* a person feel.

Historical Examples

Despite the fundamental moral basis of determining mental and behavioral abnormality, psychiatry has identified numerous types over the years, passing them off as bona fide illnesses and subjecting them to medical forms of treatment. The following are just a few illuminating examples.

In the early 19th century, slaves who had the urge to run away from their masters were said to be suffering from the mental disorder *drapetomania*. Those who resisted working for their masters were said to suffer from *dysaesthesia aethiopica*.[4] Whereas these were considered legitimate psychiatric diagnoses then, it is now obvious to us they were wholly based in the morality of the times when ideas of racial inferiority were commonplace, and resisting the institution of slavery was considered a bad thing.

Another example is autism. In her book, *Asperger's Children: The Origins of Autism in Nazi Vienna*,[5] historian Edith Sheffer explained that scientists in 1930s Germany wanted to identify children who were socially reticent—in particular, those who were disinterested in joining the Hitler Youth. They enlisted the help of pediatrician Hans Asperger to study the problem. Building on earlier 20th century concepts of autism[6] as something akin to schizophrenia, where inner life dominates over the outer world, Asperger eventually came up with a category for these children called *autistic psycho-pathology*. This culminated in dozens of them being euthanized because they were not interested in joining social groups, which was considered a mental abnormality. But this was nothing more than a moral judgment about the appropriateness of their interests and disinterests.

Further examples live on in more modern times. Homosexuality was classified as a mental disorder until 1973 when the American Psychiatric Association (APA) polled its members during the annual convention and found a majority of them *believed* it shouldn't be considered a mental disorder anymore. Out of nearly 10,000 members in attendance, 61% voted to remove it from the *DSM*.[7] Alarmingly, almost 40% were still committed

[4] Cartwright, S. (1851). Diseases and Peculiarities of the Negro Race. *DeBow's Review, 11*.
[5] Sheffer, E. (2018). *Asperger's Children: The Origins of Autism in Nazi Vienna*. New York: W. W. Norton & Company.
[6] The term autism was coined in 1911 by the German psychiatrist Eugene Bleuler as explained in Evans, B. (2013). How autism became autism: The radical transformation of a central concept of child development in Britain. *History of the Human Sciences, 26(3)*, 3-31. http://doi: 10.1177/0952695113484320. The ideas of autism at this pre-Nazi time were still, nonetheless, based on moral judgments about how much inner life should dominate over the outer world.
[7] Burton, N. (2015, September). When homosexuality stopped being a mental disorder: Not until 1987 did homosexuality completely fall out of the DSM. *Psychology Today*.

to the idea that it was a mental/behavioral abnormality. In contrast to other medical specialties, voting on the reality of mental disorders is not uncommon in psychiatry—it just isn't as blatant as this example. More typically, mental disorders are discussed and negotiated in committee meetings behind closed doors where committee members use their moral values (and financial interests) in determining what is and what isn't a mental abnormality.

In her book, *They Say You're Crazy: How the World's Most Powerful Psychiatrists Decide Who's Normal*, psychologist Paula Caplan, Ph.D. reviewed the case of masochistic personality disorder, which was eventually abandoned in the 1980s after activists argued it was discriminatory against women – it was.[8] The category was intended to describe people who appear to allow themselves to be abused in relationships. To quell the activists' protests, the name was changed to self-defeating personality disorder to remove the negative connotation of the term masochistic. An incident during the negotiations over this proposed category further demonstrates its moral, not scientific or medical, foundation. During a committee meeting about the proposed symptoms, a committee member noted that one of them applied to her, and so the chair removed it from the list.[9] The committee was trying to decide how much mistreatment a person should tolerate in a relationship—and how much was too much.

As another example, Asperger's disorder (named after the pediatrician from Nazi Germany above) was eliminated as a diagnostic category during the 2013 revision of the *DSM*. It was removed because a large study demonstrated "there was great variation in how BEC [best-estimate clinical] diagnoses within the autism spectrum (i.e., autistic disorder, PDD-

---

Retrieved from: https://www.psychologytoday.com/us/blog/hide-and-seek/201509/when-homosexuality-stopped-being-mental-disorder.

[8] Caplan, P. (1995). *They Say You're Crazy: How the World's Most Powerful Psychiatrists Decide Who's Normal*. Boston, MA: Addison-Wesley. This same information was also reported later in Kutchins, H. & Kirk, S. (1997). *Making Us Crazy: DSM: The Psychiatric Bible and the Creation of Mental Disorders*. New York: Free Press.

[9] Ibid, p. 91.

NOS, and Asperger syndrome) were assigned to individual children."[10] In other words, well-trained clinicians couldn't agree on what it was, even when using specific diagnostic criteria in the *DSM*. This suggests that diagnostic decisions about Asperger's disorder were substantially based on clinicians' individual ideas of the inappropriateness of certain behaviors and experiences. But it wasn't just Asperger's disorder that was eliminated. All three diagnoses above (autistic disorder, PDD-NOS, and Asperger syndrome) were eliminated and combined into a new category label – autism spectrum disorder (ASD). This is nothing more than a semantic sleight of hand and, more problematically, there is still only minimal agreement about what the new category ASD is, suggesting a continuation of personal moral criteria used in diagnosing it.[11]

One last illustrative example of morality at play in determining mental abnormality was in May 2019 when the World Health Organization's (WHO) legislative body ratified a proposal to reclassify gender incongruence (also called gender dysphoria and commonly known as transgender) in the *International Classification of Diseases* (ICD) so it would no longer be considered a mental disorder.[12] Like the issue earlier with homosexuality, this is a clear example of how political pressure and changes in moral views—not science—dictate whether or not something is considered inappropriate and, thus, a mental abnormality. The advocates of this change claimed it "...was taken out from the mental health disorders because we had a better understanding that this wasn't actually a mental

---

[10] Lord, C., Petkova, E., Hus V., Gan, W., Lu, F., Martin, D., Ousley, O., Guy, L., Bernier, R., Gerdts, J., Algermissen, M., Whitaker, A., Sutcliffe, J., Warren, Z., Klin, A., Saulnier, C., Hanson, E., Hundley, R., Piggot, J., Fombonne, E., Steiman, M....Risi, S. (2012). A Multisite Study of the Clinical Diagnosis of Different Autism Spectrum Disorders. *Archives of General Psychiatry, 69(3)*, 306–313. doi:10.1001/archgenpsychiatry.2011.148.
[11] Rice, C., Carpenter, L., Morrier, M., Lord, C., DiRienzo, M., Boan, A., Skowyra, C., Fusco, A., Baio, J. Esler, A., Zahorodny, W., Hobson, N., Mars, A., Thurm, A., Bishop, S., & Wiggins, L. (2022). Defining in detail and evaluating reliability of *DSM-5* criteria for autism spectrum disorder (ASD) among children. *Journal of Autism and Developmental Disorders, 52(12)*, 5308–5320. doi:10.1007/s10803-021-05377-y.
[12] Human Rights Watch. (2019, May). New health guidelines propel transgender rights: World Health Organization removes 'Gender Identity Disorder" diagnosis. Retrieved from: https://www.hrw.org/news/2019/05/27/new-health-guidelines-propel-transgender-rights.

health condition and leaving it there was causing stigma."[13] What this translates to is they removed it as a mental disorder because they no longer thought it was a deviation from normal experiences and behavior; in other words, it was no longer inappropriate.

These are noteworthy illustrations of the moral basis of mental disorder diagnoses. The same criticism applies to all other mental disorder categories in the *DSM*.[14] They are descriptive category labels for different kinds of human experiences and behaviors that are considered inappropriate by those in power, yet they are camouflaged as internal dysfunction to be addressed with a medically-minded approach. This evolution of mental disorder diagnoses has been an ongoing process of medicalizing moral injunctions.

The Psychiatric Bible

The orthodox mental health industry ignores the moral basis of mental disorder and insists on creating an ever-increasing array of categories in the *DSM*. The *DSM* is mockingly by some, yet reverently by others, called the "psychiatric bible." Whereas I think this nickname is appropriate as the manual is a collection of moral pronouncements, the name also, unfortunately, implies some kind of legitimacy. In its opening pages, it starts with this puzzling disclaimer: "Although DSM-5 remains a categorical classification of separate disorders, we recognize that mental disorders do not always fit completely within the boundaries of a single disorder."[15] It is alarming that the manual admits at the outset that its guidelines do not define separate disorders. The categories have such

---

[13] Ravitz, J. (2019, May). Transgender people are not mentally ill, the WHO decrees. CNN. Retrieved from: https://www.cnn.com/2019/05/28/health/who-transgender-reclassified-not-mental-disorder/index.html.

[14] This excludes diagnoses in the *DSM* that describe real biological pathology and associated mental symptoms (e.g., major and mild neurocognitive disorder due to diseases such as Alzheimer's disease and HIV infection, substance withdrawal, and substance/medication induced mental disorders).

[15] American Psychiatric Association. (2013). *The Diagnostic and Statistical Manual of Mental Disorders (5th Edition)*. Washington, DC: American Psychiatric Association, p. xli.

blurred boundary lines that they substantially overlap with each other, and they are so inclusive as to define almost any human problem.

But, arguably, the most confusing thing about the *DSM* is the official definition it gives for mental disorder, at last count numbering in the hundreds:

> A mental disorder is a syndrome characterized by *clinically significant* disturbance in an individual's cognition, emotion regulation, or behavior that reflects a *dysfunction in* the psychological, biological, or developmental processes underlying mental functioning. Mental disorders are usually associated with *significant distress* in social, occupational, or other important activities. An *expectable or culturally approved* response to a *common* stressor or loss, such as the death of a loved one, is not a mental disorder. *Socially deviant behavior* (e.g., political, religious, or sexual) *and conflicts* that are primarily between the individual and society are not mental disorders unless the deviance or conflict results from a *dysfunction in* the individual, as described above.[16] [italics added for emphasis].

I remember the first time I read this definition. I felt like I was watching a shell game, desperately trying to keep my eye on the pea. Consider how the italicized terms above make it impossible to settle on a firm operational definition of the construct, and, thus, to decide whether something is a mental disorder. The only way to interpret these terms is to use moral value judgments about what constitutes clinical significance and distress, dysfunction, expectations, cultural norms, commonness, social deviance, and conflicts. These morality-laden terms and phrases also show up in each diagnostic category's criteria as well.

The last sentence in the definition is particularly troublesome. It claims, "socially deviant behavior (e.g., political, religious, or sexual) and conflicts that are primarily between the individual and society" are not mental disorders. But since everything in the *DSM* is based on moral judgments about what behaviors and experiences are inappropriate enough to be

---

[16] American Psychiatric Association. (2013). *The Diagnostic and Statistical Manual of Mental Disorders (5ᵗʰ Edition)*. Washington, DC: American Psychiatric Association, p. 20.

considered disordered, they are necessarily some kind of deviant behavior or conflict with societal (moral) norms. So, this caveat would dictate nothing in the manual is a mental disorder. However, immediately after this proviso, it claims these deviant behaviors and conflicts are mental disorders if they arise from a dysfunction in the individual. But this is exactly what the definition says they are in the first place, making the absurd argument that a mental disorder is not a mental disorder unless it is a mental disorder!

Research on the *DSM* exposes this poor foundation. In scientific terms, the *DSM* is neither reliable nor valid. First, it has poor *reliability*.[17] Reliability is when an assessment tool provides the same results regardless of who uses it or how many times it is used to assess one person for the same problem. Ideally, we want an assessment tool to be consistent in its conclusions and not be biased by the evaluator's personal values. The *DSM* fails in this regard, as reflected in the previously noted lack of expert consensus regarding autism and in the manual's own admission that it doesn't identify distinct problems. They are not different kinds of discrete dysfunctions in the individual.[18] Second, the *DSM* has poor *validity*. Validity is when an instrument identifies the thing it says it is identifying. As has been mentioned already, the thing it says it is identifying is not really a dysfunction in the individual.

Because of these reliability and validity problems, the *DSM* has received severe criticism, even from top mainstream authorities in the field. The Task Force Chair of one of the editions, Allen Frances, M.D., exclaimed: "There is no definition of mental disorder. It's bullshit. I mean you just can't

---

[17] Cooper, R. (2014). How reliable is the DSM-5? Blog entry at Mad in America. Retrieved from: https://www.madinamerica.com/2014/09/how-reliable-is-the-dsm-5/; Kirk, S. & Kutchins, H. (1992). *The Selling of DSM: The Rhetoric of Science in Psychiatry*. New Brunswick, NJ: Aldine Transaction.; Regier D. A., Narrow W.; Clarks D.; Kraemer H.; Kuramoto S.; Kuhl E.; & Kupfer D. (2013). DSM-5 field trials in the United States and Canada, Part II: Test-retest reliability of selected categorical diagnoses. *American Journal of Psychiatry, 170*, 59-70. https://doi:10.1176/appi.ajp.2012.12070999.
[18] Allsop, K.; Read, J.; Corcoran, R.; & Kinderman, P. (2019). Heterogeneity in psychiatric diagnostic classification. *Psychiatric Research, 279*, 15-22. https://doi.org/10.1016/j.psychres.2019.07.005.

define it."[19] He later discouraged professionals from buying and using the *DSM*. He said the *DSM* was so "dangerous in its product that many mental health professionals may choose not to use it…. My advice - don't buy DSM 5, don't use it, don't teach it."[20] Two Directors of the National Institute of Mental Health (NIMH) have also denounced the *DSM*. Steven Hyman, M.D. (1996-2001), said the *DSM* was "totally wrong," "an absolute scientific nightmare," "a fool's errand," that it had "wasted human capital and industry funds,"[21] and contained "widely accepted but fictive diagnostic categories…."[22] Hyman's successor, Thomas Insel, M.D. (2002-2015), said the *DSM*'s "weakness is its lack of validity" and its categories are "based on a consensus…not any objective laboratory measure."[23] Because of these serious problems, the NIMH has abandoned the *DSM* for research purposes, yet bizarrely suggested that it continue to be used by practitioners.[24]

Some mental health member organizations also registered their complaints about the *DSM*. The British Psychological Society (BPS), representing over 70,000 members, declared that the diagnoses were based on social norms, subjective value judgments, and had no confirmatory evidence of biological causation (dysfunction in the individual).[25] The Society for

[19] Frances, A. (2010, December). Inside the battle to define mental illness. *Wired*. Retrieved from https://www.wired.com/2010/12/ff_dsmv/.

[20] Frances, A. (2013, July). Should social workers use the DSM-5. *SWHELPER*. Retrieved from: https://www.socialworkhelper.com/2013/06/07/should-social-workers-use-dsm-5/.

[21] Hyman, S. (2013, May). Psychiatry Framework Seeks to Reform Diagnostic Doctrine. *Nature*. Retrieved at https://www.nature.com/news/psychiatry-framework-seeks-to-reform-diagnostic-doctrine-1.12972.

[22] Casey, B.; Craddock, N.; Cuthbert, B.; Hyman, S.; Lee, F.; & Ressler, K. (2013). DSM-5 and RDoC: progress in psychiatry research? *Nature Reviews Neuroscience, 14(11)*, 810-814. https://doi:10.1038/nrn3621.

[23] Insel, T. (2013, April). Post by Former NIMH Director Thomas Insel: Transforming Diagnosis. Retrieved at https://www.nimh.nih.gov/about/directors/thomas-insel/blog/2013/transforming-diagnosis.shtml.

[24] American Psychological Association. (2013). NIMH funding to shift away from DSM categories. Retrieved from: https://www.apa.org/monitor/2013/07-08/nimh#:~:text=Instead%2C%20the%20institute%20is%20developing,%22abandonment%22%20of%20the%20DSM.

[25] British Psychological Society. (2011). Response to the American Psychiatric Association: DSM-5 Development. Retrieved from: http://whatcausesmentalillness.com/images/110630britishpsychologicalassnresponse2dsm-5.pdf.

Humanistic Psychology (SHP) (Division 32 of the American Psychological Association) drafted an open letter in opposition to the *DSM* because of these problems. The petition eventually received over 15,000 endorsements from individuals and more than 50 organizations, including 16 other divisions of the American Psychological Association. Members from the American Counseling Association (ACA) also submitted a petition to address these very same problems.[26]

Despite this uproar from within professional circles, the American Psychiatric Association, who publishes the *DSM*, refuses to address this serious problem with the foundation of the orthodox psychiatric belief system. Other major mental health member organizations in the United States have likewise ignored it.[27] As a prime example of this intransigence, it was only after two years of repeated urging that the Chief of Professional Practice of the American Psychological Association finally responded in 2019 to a request for ethical guidance about the *DSM*, saying "I can appreciate that this is an important issue to you, and I hope that I can be of service by offering clarity and a conclusion. The APA will not be making a comment on this issue now, nor in the foreseeable future."[28] This is an unacceptable response from an organization that has the responsibility to address ethical issues facing its members.

This is not just an academic question. On the contrary, the *DSM* can be harmful to the people who are labeled with its dubious diagnoses. First, it can damage one's sense of identity, worth, and power. This is especially true if the person believes the diagnosis reflects an innate personal defect

---

[26] Robbins, B.; Kamens, S.; & Elkins, D. (2017). DSM reform efforts by the Society for Humanistic Psychology. *Journal of Humanistic Psychology*, 1-23. https://doi.org/10.1177/0022167817698617.

[27] International Society for Ethical Psychology and Psychiatry. (2017). ISEPP Demands Ethical Guidance on the DSM: In the Face of an Ethical Double Bind, ISEPP Petitions Leading Professional Mental Health Member Organizations. *PRNewswire*. Retrieved from: https://www.prnewswire.com/news-releases/english-releases/isepp-demands-ethical-guidance-on-the-dsm-300504497.html.

[28] Personal email communication with Dr. Jaren L. Skillings, Ph.D., ABPP, Chief of Professional Practice, American Psychological Association, September 26, 2019.

in functioning, just like how the *DSM* says it is a "dysfunction in the individual."

Second, having a diagnosis can affect how other people interact with the person. Not only do laypeople tend to keep their distance from someone who has been diagnosed mentally disordered, many professionals' perceptions are negatively affected as well. In other words, many professionals view and treat people based on the *DSM* label they've been assigned, not necessarily based on their actions or stated desires. A classic study showed just how powerful this effect can be.[29]

Third, *DSM* diagnoses (even the relatively "minor" ones) in a person's record can also jeopardize many rights and privileges. These include employment suitability, security clearances, military service, health and life insurance eligibility, parenting and adoption rights, and parole and probation actions. As our private lives are increasingly subjected to the prying eyes of government and industry, will we see a *DSM* label being the basis for denying other things like housing and financial eligibility and acceptance at colleges and universities? It seems they are as harmful as criminal conviction records. Given the moral basis for how people are branded with them, this is not surprising. They are little more than derogatory moral judgments of people who face very common and understandable human struggles.

Moral Categories Run Amuck

Despite having this overabundance of mental disorder diagnoses in the *DSM*, just three categories would be sufficient: *Up, Down,* and *All-Around.*

---

[29] Rosenhan, D. (1973). On being sane in insane places. *Science, 179 (4070)*, 250-258. This study was critiqued in Cahalan, S. (2019). *The Great Pretender: The Undercover Mission that Changed Our Understanding of Madness.* New York, NY: Grand Central Publishing. In it, Cahalan expresses great concern about some of the study's results possibly being fabricated. However, in a recent interview with *Psychiatric Times*, she said: "I still think that the idea of seeing a patient, not just a diagnostic label, is an extremely valuable lesson. I also believe that his [Rosenhan's] statements about being primed to see certain behaviors as pathological in certain contexts and perfectly normal in others is something that all doctors should be aware of. Those parts of the paper, I believe, still have value." Aftab, A. (2020, February). 50 shades of misdiagnosis. *Psychiatric Times*. Retrieved from: https://www.psychiatrictimes.com/qas/50-shades-misdiagnosis.

People who are very excitable or obsessed are Up; those who are in the depths of despair are Down; and those who are very confused, disoriented, and disconnected are All-Around.[30] Although these are somewhat lighthearted categories, they do accurately describe the most basic forms of human distress and subcategorizing them any further has little value. But how did the number of mental disorder categories grow so much?

In 1812, Benjamin Rush, who was considered the father of American psychiatry, classified only two types of mental and behavioral problems: "They have been divided, 1, into such as act, *directly* upon the body; and, 2, such as act *indirectly* upon the body, through the medium of the mind" [italics in the original].[31] Examples of the first category were brain lesions, tumors, epilepsy, exposure to toxic substances, and excessive consumption of alcohol. Some examples of the second category were intense study, rapid shifting of attention from one topic to another, extensive and constant imagination, excessive memorization, and intense emotions. It seems clear from our vantage point that Rush's first category consisted of physical (neurological) diseases, not mental disorders. On the other hand, the second category formed the forerunner of the present-day mental disorder construct.

Twenty-eight years later, in line with Rush's second category, there was only one category officially tracked by the U.S. census.[32] This was idiocy/insanity. Forty years after that, the census differentiated among seven different categories that could be grouped into the Up, Down, and All-Around distinctions. These were mania, monomania, dipsomania, melancholia, paresis, dementia, and epilepsy. Mania, monomania, and dipsomania would correspond to the Up category. The latter two of them are obsessions with something: a fixed idea and alcohol, respectively.

---

[30] Even these three categories suffer from reliability problems. This is because human experiences are multifactorial. It is far too simplistic to claim a person only suffers from one of these. In reality, we are all suffering from all three of these, with the intensity on a continuum, at any point in our lives.

[31] Rush, B. (1812). *Medical Inquiries and Observations Upon the Diseases of the Mind.* Philadelphia: Kimber & Richardson. Retrieved from: https://archive.org/details/2569037R.nlm.nih.gov, p. 30.

[32] American Psychiatric Association. (2018). DSM History. Retrieved from: https://www.psychiatry.org/psychiatrists/practice/dsm/history-of-the-dsm.

Melancholia corresponds to Down. Paresis, dementia, and epilepsy belong to the medical specialty of neurology (as did Rush's first category above), and it doesn't make sense to include them as mental disorders. Still, the symptoms of these last three would be classified as psychosis, and so would fall within the All-Around category.

Later in the 19th century, psychiatrist Emil Kraepelin (1856-1926) presented two categories, again aligned with Up, Down, and All-Around. He differentiated between *dementia praecox* (All-Around) and *manic-depression* (Up and Down).[33] Over the subsequent decades after Rush, Kraepelin, and others, there were efforts to subdivide these basic mental disorder categories into a multitude of more specific types of inappropriateness, but they were disguised as matters for medical assessment and care.

In *Cultures of Healing: Correcting the Image of American Mental Health Care*,[34] philosopher and psychotherapist Robert Fancher described how in the late 19th and early 20th centuries, in addition to expanding the categories of mental disorder, there was also a significant transition in psychiatry's focus. It shifted from remotely located rural asylums to urban-based hospitals that were centers of general medical care, the latter whose various medical specialties had far better scientific reputations than asylum psychiatrists who relied mostly on confinement, isolation, chains, and straitjackets to treat (subdue) people.

Psychiatry also expanded its influence at this time by targeting additional forms of mental abnormalities. These were mild to moderate forms of distress that were not as devastating as the more severe situations common in the asylums, and they could be handled in outpatient as well as short-term inpatient settings. These developments allowed psychiatry to join the ranks of other, more respected, medical specialties, thus setting the stage for diagnostic expansion. However, this apparent elevation of the profession to the level of other medical specialties, such as neurology and

---

[33] Hoff, P. (2015). The Kraepelinian tradition. *Dialogues in Clinical Neuroscience, 17(1)*, 31- 41.
[34] Fancher, R. (1995). *Cultures of Healing: Correcting the Image of American Mental Health Care*.
New York: W. H. Freeman/Times Books/Henry Holt & Co.

ophthalmology, was only a medical disguise as psychiatry's raison d'être continued to be the moral judgment of people and their conduct.

The *DSM* did not arrive on the scene until the mid-20ᵗʰ century, but, since then, it has been the scaffolding used to drastically expand the number of diagnoses. The first *DSM* was published in 1952. Over the subsequent 70 years, it has undergone seven revisions. During that time, it grew into a hefty tome, increasing from its original 132 pages to 1,120 pages in *DSM-5-TR*, which was published in 2022.

The number of mental disorder diagnoses also increased, but the American Psychiatric Association doesn't provide an official tally. One source reported that the 2013 *DSM-5* had 541 separate categories.[35] However, the actual number is debatable depending on how one counts its categories, subcategories, and specifiers. The *DSM-5* has 22 main categories. If all midlevel subtypes of the main categories are counted, there are 193 separate diagnoses, not counting 72 additional "unspecified" and "other specified" categories. Each midlevel category has at least one these, such as "unspecified depressive disorder" and "other specified anxiety disorder," that identify problems as mental disorders even when they don't meet the full *DSM* criteria. It is very telling that more than one out of four *DSM* categories has such ambiguous rules for diagnosing. It leaves much of the decision up to the diagnostician's personal moral values.

Yet, despite this explosion of apparent diagnostic specificity, subdividing human problems any further than Up, Down, and All-Around has little value other than to create the illusion that the *DSM* is a medical catalogue facilitating precise understanding and diagnoses of several distinct kinds of mental disorders and, thus, more (putative) fine-tuned and effective treatment.

Treating the Name?

Advocates of conventional psychiatry believe that getting the correct mental disorder diagnosis is essential in determining how to help the

---

[35] Blashfield, R.; Keeley, J.; Flanagan, E.; & Miles, S. (2014). The cycle of classification: The DSM-I through DSM-5. *Annual Review of Clinical Psychology, 10*, 25-51.

person. Whereas it is important to pay attention to and understand the specifics of their problems, and then to address those problems and not others, many professionals spend a lot of time parsing criteria and fretting about which diagnosis is the correct one. This makes it appear as if they haven't heard the news about the *DSM*'s unreliability and invalidity or the *DSM's* own admission that "mental disorders do not always fit completely within the boundaries of a single disorder," as mentioned earlier. Quibbling over the correct *DSM* diagnosis is like debating whether a person's behaviors and interests make them a Capricorn or Aquarius without knowing their birth date.

A mental disorder diagnosis is irrelevant for purposes of helping since it doesn't point to a dysfunction in the individual that can be treated. This is especially evident when we consider the fact that there are a limited number of interventions available to psychiatrists and psychotherapists. Psychiatrists typically prescribe drugs that have generally inebriating effects or, in the more serious of cases, they might administer electric shock to the brain or perform surgery to disable certain brain functions.

Describing psychiatric drugs as antidepressants, antianxiety, antipsychotic, and mood stabilizers is more of a marketing tactic than a true description of their chemical properties or effects. Prescribing one over another is mostly a trial-and-error process, not one dictated by precise medical rules or how each chemical affects the brain. This is in stark contrast to real medical problems such as diabetes, where insulin is prescribed to lower dangerous levels of blood sugar. There are no drugs tailored for a particular disorder, notwithstanding what the advertisements claim, and how some psychiatrists and patients will anecdotally swear that certain drugs work better than others with certain types of problems.

This lack of psychiatric chemical specificity is further revealed in the fact that drugs in one class are frequently used for problems in another class. For instance, antidepressants are used for anxiety, antipsychotics are used with depression, antianxiety and stimulant drugs are used for depression, and anticonvulsant and blood pressure drugs are used for psychiatric reasons. This lack of chemical specificity is also why antidepressants can cause suicidal thoughts and depression while antianxiety drugs can cause agitation and anxiety. Which drug works the best is based mostly on what each person taking the drug feels, not the drug's chemical properties or what the drug is advertised to do.

This same problem with the imprecision of psychiatric drugs applies to electric shock treatment and surgery as well. They don't target specific brain dysfunctions. Instead, electric shock is a "Hail Mary" attempt to reset the person's experiential world and "wipe the slate clean" while psychosurgery intentionally damages brain areas that are involved in the development of distress and behaviors so that the distress and behaviors are no longer possible.

Along similar lines as psychiatric drugs, electric shock, and psychosurgery, psychotherapy is not based on the diagnostic names given to the person. It is based on an understanding of the specific problems the person is complaining about. Basically, this kind of work is a process of exploring and helping people to better understand their life problems and to identify possible solutions. It is not a process of the precise application of a treatment protocol that targets specific symptoms of a dysfunction in the individual or the dysfunction itself. How could it be if the diagnostic criteria themselves (which contain the symptoms) are so unreliable and invalid?

The *DSM* is flawed at its foundation. It falsely presents a multitude of mental disorder categories as the effects of dysfunctions in the individual similar to how the symptoms of diabetes are the effects of an insulin dysfunction in the individual. However, at closer examination from a scientific and critically reasoned perspective —not a clinical lore perspective (which is currently the perspective of orthodox psychiatry)— there are no theorized or verified dysfunctions in people that cause "mental disorder." At best, the morally-derived dysfunctions and the mental disorder symptom clusters are one and the same. At worst, each *DSM* category is merely a moral injunction about the appropriateness of behaviors and experiences. Either way, the scientific value of the *DSM* is nil. Instead, it has taken on only an administrative and bureaucratic position within the conventional mental health system and removing it (as is warranted) poses a significant existential threat to that system.

The Alternatives

Do We Need a New Taxonomy?

Richard Hallam

Abstract: *The classification of human problems in the field demarcated as 'mental health' is presented as just one expression of the transformation of help and advice-giving, traditionally part of friendship, into professional services that have to justify what is on offer, advertise their services, and subject themselves to ethical and legal regulation. As a commercial service or one that government health departments are keen to streamline at minimum cost, there has been a trend towards "McDonaldization," that is, reducing the product to standardized components, simplifying the description of problems, aiming for predictability and control of service-provision, and quantifying outcome with minimal effort. The classification of 'mental health' problems therefore has to be understood as reflecting a much wider process, which will vary according to whether this is e-therapy, trimmed-down state provision, extended one-to-one psychotherapy, or an open-ended group drop-in session providing free-support. A case is made for avoiding taxonomic preconceptions, in line with the author's advocacy, in various publications, of a process of individual case-formulation, arguing that alternatives are likely to be a false economy and lead to burn-out in the personnel providing them.*

I will state my belief at the outset that seeking advice and help from others has always been a feature of socialising in human societies and that we should be careful to preserve it in forms that are, as far as possible, free from commercial interests and government policy. Life rarely runs smoothly for individuals, families, or communities—and since time immemorial people have worked together to find their way through difficulties.

I will focus here on one-to-one helping which, for around a century, has created opportunities for an increasing number of professionals to offer their paid-for services. In general, these professionals have been well-trained, subjected themselves to supervision, and have abided by good ethical standards. Quite apart from informal helping, societies have always made a space for these specialised roles which includes shaman and priest.

Help-seekers buy into a convincing rationale which means that advertising and salesmanship are always part of the enterprise. Potential clients seek out suppliers who have the right credentials and a good reputation. In practice, satisfaction with the outcome is frequently luck-of-the-draw. Advertising is necessarily formulaic, and the product can only be properly evaluated when translated into practice.

The process of seeking "certified guidance" in the last millennium of western culture can be traced back to religious practices. John Myrc, in the 15C, produced a kind of self-help handbook for parish priests with examples of how to deal with issues that commonly arose during confession (Hallam, 2015). In the background lay all the doctrines of the Catholic Church.

In the often-unstated premises of current expertise lie shared assumptions about "mental health," taxonomies of psychiatric disorders, and psychological models of "dysfunction." Unless the potential client is extremely sophisticated, all of this is taken on trust and not even questioned.

The title of this book, *Theoretical Alternatives to the Psychiatric Model of Mental Disorder Labeling: Contemporary Frameworks, Taxonomies, and Models*, implies that new frameworks are needed. Alternatives in the plural also implies that we should be suspicious of any single model of help or the substitution of a psychological taxonomy for a medical one. The concept of a "mental health problem" is a historically recent fabrication that fails to mean anything much at all, and we should be wary of a new terminology that is equally vacuous.

A request for help can be prompted by so many different reasons with so many contributary causes (relating to ingrained habits, ignorance, somatic disorder, existential dilemmas, overwork, past trauma, rigidity of belief, family breakdown, etc.) that it makes little sense to lump them together into one overarching category. It is for this reason that I advocate a process of *individual case formulation* before proceeding on to suggest potential solutions (Hallam, 2013), a process in which problem formulation is a disciplined form of abductive reasoning pursued in partnership with a client that strives to arrive at the most likely explanation for a problem.

In general, it aims to analyse blocks to change in order to free up individual choice. Abduction does not exclude fitting a client into a taxonomic category—whether medical, psychiatric, or psychological—but this kind of pigeonholing rarely contributes more than one small piece of evidence in the overall picture. It is difficult to "sell" an open-ended approach of this nature in a sector that has become increasingly commodified and associated with narrow (chiefly medical) causal assumptions.

Nevertheless, open-endedness is, I suggest, a feature of the historical roots of help-seeking which I consider to lie in friendship. The ethical and practice guidelines for the helping professions illustrate the strong influence of this legacy (Hallam, 2015). A key point about advice from a friend is that it is not supposed to be tainted by personal advantage or manipulation. Professional groups are strictly regulated in an attempt to ensure that their motives are "pure" while everyone is also happy to accept that they are paid for their services.

The history of discourses on friendship are enlightening. In his collected essays, Francis Bacon (1625) singles out the psychological effects of relating to a sympathetic person and points out the benefits of dialogue. He finds it strange that even the very powerful rate friendship so highly that they will put themselves at risk and inconvenience. They are required to "raise" subjects or servants into "companions" and "almost equals."

He says that the Roman name for these people was *Participes Curarum* or partners in care. He regards these relationships as beneficial because they help to remove the "darkness and confusion of thoughts." He thinks it is better to tell your thoughts to a statue than to suppress them. He also emphasises that personal thoughts are a product of habit and emotional investments, and that the freedom of speech and frankness of a friend are a remedy against this.

A friend can help in practical ways, too, acting as an advocate and becoming almost an extension of oneself. Montaigne (1580), in his essays, expressed similar thoughts but placed greater emphasis on brutal honesty from his friends. In the words of Oscar Wilde a few centuries later, a friend "is one who stabs you in the front" (quoted in Grayling, 2013, p. 10).

Modern helping relationships have been formalised in a way that acknowledges a debt to friendship in the sense that therapy is not seen as a straightforward commercial transaction on a par with dentistry, hairdressing, or massage. The very personal nature of the relationship is recognised and its boundaries strictly regulated. Clients usually understand this. They know that a sexual relationship is out of bounds, that gift-exchange is not expected, and that a therapist will decline to work with one of their own family members or friends in order to avoid bias.

The Commodification of Advice and Help

Understood within the bounds of friendship, ordinary help-seeking is an extremely open-ended and unregulated practice. Its conversion into a commodity is justified by the argument that traditional practices are intuitive, subjective, and often illogical. In other words, it is thought that the provision of help needs to be rationalised.

To make it credible, it lays claim to a rationale (scientific, philosophical, technical, etc.) or at least it refers to a proven record of success ("evidence-based practice"). In the current era, when personal problems are modelled on "ill-health," methods of evaluating an "intervention" mimic their equivalent in medicine. This appeal to proven efficacy is essential for purposes of advertising and to ward off any legal challenge that a technique might cause harm.

When a traditional social practice is rationalised, a set of logically consistent rules is substituted for what was formerly done in a rather messy way. Ritzer (1993) refers to this process as McDonaldization. This amounts to:

1. Breaking down a task into its smallest constituent components.
2. Finding the single most efficient method for their completion.
3. Aiming for predictability and control over the whole process.

4.   Quantifying performance in order to measure outcome.

Helping services also require centralised control of training, administration, and ethical regulation (i.e., governmental, professional, and commercial). The product has to be streamlined so that the required skills are easily taught. It is necessary to ensure that workers are committed and do not suffer burnout.

Regarding the efficacy of contemporary helping services, it would be surprising if a century of research had not resulted in some progress, and I certainly do not wish to underestimate technical advances in bringing about personal change. For psychiatry, these have been, principally (and passing quickly over leucotomy), medications to influence the brain directly. For a non-medical technical therapist, the removal or amelioration of a "disorder" is the chief criterion of success. In order to satisfy commodification, its measurement has to be simple and quick.

Organisations concerned with mental health (e.g., in connection with medical insurance or the law) rely heavily on taxonomies, such as DSM-5, which offer (mostly) clear descriptive definitions without implying an aetiology. Rating scales and questionnaires have been constructed that reflect official taxonomies, usually client-completed because it saves time. These measures also satisfy the requirement of problem definition. The resolution of a problem is inferred from a low (or lower) score.

A standard theoretical conceptualisation is developed for each so-called disorder (to yield "disorder-specific models") and research is conducted into manualised techniques that can reliably demonstrate change in outcome measures within a standard period of time. To cut costs further, the least amount of training is provided for the workers who apply the technology. Quality control is monitored on a regular basis, within clients, across clinics, and, in the case of the UK, through national statistics.

Rationalisation is not necessarily all bad and my attempt to analyse and conceptualise the process of case formulation is an example. Moreover, people seeking help should be given a rational explanation for what is on offer. One question posed by this book is whether it is worth trying to develop taxonomies that disengage from a medical concept of psychological health—for instance, one that relates to well-being, authenticity, or something else. However, if all personal problems are intrinsically multidimensional and cannot be fitted into a single taxonomic category, any new proposal could turn into a bed of Procrustes.

Perhaps there is a systematic way of narrowing down types of human problem, but after fifty years of working as a therapist I have not yet discovered one. The best first question still seems to be "What is your problem?" The answer is often that the help-seeker has only a vague idea and has come to find out what it is. Sometimes, a person will not tell you what they think their problem is until they have built up sufficient trust in you as a therapist. Even so, as a starter, a checklist of possible problems is not without its uses.

Moreover, a help-provider cannot be expected to be competent in every type of problem or method and will want to specialise (e.g., working with children rather than adults). Specialisation usually leads to greater skill and knowing what to look out for. If a taxonomy is needed for social, administrative, or legal purposes, one can fairly easily be constructed to serve these pragmatic purposes, much as the DSM is used. The danger of a taxonomy is to believe that its disorder categories point to some sort of underlying essence, a common problem with the DSM.

The Unintended Consequences of Commodification

Criticism of traditional forms of helping can be countered by pointing out that they are not as irrational as might seem. Moreover, if commodification means following a manual, it can degrade the product and potentially lead to worker burn-out when conducted inhumanely. Hochschild (1983) distinguished between "emotion work" that is undertaken in private life from emotion work that is done in a job and traded for a wage. In whatever setting it is employed, emotion work can be trying.

For a paid help-giver, the interpersonal strategies of daily life (short of violence or calling the police) can be helpful when working with an intransigent client. When the adult nature of helping cannot be sustained (for instance, with people who do not follow advice, live chaotic lives, or fail to attend appointments) the help-provider falls back on tried and tested strategies.

According to Linehan (1993, p. 296), a therapist suspends their spontaneous emotional reaction and manages the situation by role-playing a helpful response. Although this could be viewed as a mechanical technique to handle stressful emotion work, it would not be unfamiliar to a mother dealing with a three-year old displaying a temper tantrum. In Linehan's words, "the therapist first develops a strong positive relationship and then uses it to 'blackmail' the patient into making targeted, but excruciatingly difficult, changes in her behavior."

In brief, commodified helping still depends heavily on familiar forms of emotion work. This can, of course, lead to burnout, as in daily life. Commodified techniques can eventually become dehumanising when they lose sight of traditional norms of friendship and familiar ways to relate socially. Another common effect of becoming the consumer of a product is that more and more of the service provided devolves onto the help-seeker. One example is the customer of a bank having to do all the tedious transactional work on their mobile phone, leading to the local branch of a bank, with face-to-face interaction, being closed down. One justification for "e-therapy" and also video communication mediated online, is to reduce costs and "streamline" the service.

These technical advances have both pros and cons—and could be understood as a new form of self-help (Hallam, 2015, pp. 113-122). However, when the manner in which a problem is framed is determined by the help-provider, who also decides how its successful resolution is measured, the service provided is equivalent to a McDonald's hamburger. Rationalisation then has a dehumanising effect. For instance, this can be seen in the policy of health insurance companies to only reimburse for a problem if the right slot can be found for it in a psychiatric taxonomy.

There are also detrimental consequences of rationalising helping as "evidence-based practice." The research and development stages are rarely a good model for the dissemination (field application) stage. Participants for research are highly selected. Practising help-providers cannot be so choosy and have to deal with complex, multiple, psychological, health, and socio-economic problems. Different methodologies and practices are rational in an applied context. In any case, another objection to a "disorder-specific model" is that the nature of the "disorder" is not necessarily obvious at the outset. It also changes over time and circumstances.

In the new rationalised methods, therapy is broken down into its smallest constituents and the single most efficient method for completing them is devised. The aim is to make the whole process predictable and controllable. It is monitored for quality by measuring performance on each component task. An applied science/technological approach is therefore rather prosaic, aiming to achieve a worthwhile effect in the most efficient way possible. For certain types of problem, this style might have something to recommend it.

However, it does not encourage an open-ended examination of the way a client is leading his or her life, nor is it an attempt to deal with a client's conflicts, confusion, or alienation. Psychological change is not simply a matter of preferring one thing, or state of being, over another. Simply engaging in the *process* of making a change can carry with it a message about *how* to live, quite apart from the specific "goods" it is designed to yield (Smith, 2009).

In pragmatic fashion, the goals of commodified help are clearly set out and "improvement" is unambiguously defined. Help-seekers are typically assigned a psychiatric diagnosis and improvement is understood as a reduction in the number of so-called symptoms. This is not the only way of classifying a problem when adopting a technical approach because it is not beyond the wit of researchers to produce alternative definitions of problems and their resolution.

Commodified help need not be dehumanising, but this depends on how a service is set up. The commitment to a help-seeker is usually more than the offer of a technical fix. It may include an honest and empathic assessment of a person's life circumstances that goes beyond the officially designated problem. However, if the service is strictly time-limited and adopts inflexible procedures, it is likely to be a substandard response and a false economy.

As perceived by agencies that provide such services, the lack of clear-cut outcome measures is an unsatisfactory state of affairs. They would prefer a guaranteed result with a price tag attached, even if they know they are not offering an optimal service. Commercial enterprises are suspicious of vague rationales, unverified claims to expertise, and uncertain promises of relief. Even the customers of a technical service may come to believe that the "removal" of their personal problem is like the extraction of a painful tooth.

NHS Talking Therapies for Anxiety and Depression: A Case Example of McDonaldization

This service, formally known as IAPT (Improving Access to Psychological Therapies), was introduced in 2008. It is part of the British National Health Service (NHS) and free to people registered with a general practitioner. A person is able to self-refer. In some areas, provision of the service has been contracted out to private companies or charities. IAPT now caters to over 1 million people each year, with around half of them receiving a course of therapy.

This is offered at two levels of "intensity": "high" and "low" (the latter delivered by "personal wellbeing practitioners"). At first glance, this sounds like a worthwhile initiative. Following a brief initial assessment, eligibility is determined by scores on three questionnaires, one for symptoms of depressed mood (9 questions scored 0-3), one for anxiety symptoms (7 questions scored 0-3), and a work and social adjustment scale (5 questions scored 0-8). As befits a health service, it is completely sold on a medical view of distress—in other words, that people seek help because they have a "disorder."

If a person scores above a certain threshold on the questionnaires, they become a "case." Sixty-seven per cent of people who receive two or more sessions are said to "show reliable and substantial reductions in their anxiety/depression," meaning that their scores on questionnaires have reduced (NHS Digital, 2022). If after therapy the scores reduce below a certain threshold (which is currently true of 50.2%), the person has been "cured."

The average number of sessions is currently 7.9. A government department, NHS Digital, releases monthly statistics and seems to be very proud of them. A long-term plan is to expand the service so that 1.9 million people are seen each year by 2024. That represents around a quarter of the latest psychiatric prevalence figures for "depression/anxiety" (Clark, 2019). The service has been extended to children and other types of problem reported by so-called "clinical groups."

Clark (2018) points out that when first proposed, it was argued that "access to psychological therapies would have no net cost" because "the savings to the health service would exceed that amount, [the cost per episode of care] as would the savings to the Treasury (in increased tax revenues and reduced benefit payments for people returning to work)." I am not aware of further cost/benefit analyses but if they showed a net cost, the implication could be that the funding would be cut.

Clark maintains that a "person-centred assessment . . . identifies the key problems that require treatment (problem descriptors), clarifies patients' goals, assesses risk, and agrees a course of treatment." Unfortunately, this information does not appear to have been gathered in a way that can be reported or analysed. It would be interesting to know why consumers of the service have become anxious or depressed, what their goals are, and why 49.8% do not obtain significant relief.

If this were known, social measures could perhaps be directed towards whatever is causing these mood states to arise. As "disorders," they are perhaps viewed as unfortunate and unpreventable afflictions like the common cold. A small clue lies in data showing that people who live in deprived areas are more likely to seek help but less likely to respond to what is offered.

I leave it up to the reader to form their own opinion of this public service as I am allergic to phrases on NHS websites such as "adequate dose of treatment." As the fabled Irishman is supposed to have said, "If you want to get to Cork, I wouldn't start from here," which I consider a sign of wisdom rather than rustic obscurantism. My objections to medicalisation are set out in *Abolishing the Concept of Mental Illness* (Hallam, 2018).

I concur with one critic of IAPT who argues that the failure of the programme "is obscured by the smoke and mirrors of its statistical evidence" (Atkinson, 2014). Another critic simply doesn't believe the evidence (Scott, 2018). The burn-out experienced by IAPT workers has been widely reported (e.g., Owen et al., 2021; Wheatley, 2023) and the whole project has been the subject of a book-length critique (Jackson and Rizq, 2019).

The claim for success of the service is that the results match the outcomes achieved by academic researchers upon which the methods of help are based. These studies compare an active therapy with no-treatment or a placebo intervention that is not expected to help. Remarkably, there appear to be few if any direct research comparisons between the IAPT service and an alternative. One that compared an IAPT digital intervention (e-therapy) with a waiting-list control found that 46.4% of the former "recovered" compared to 16.7% of the latter (Richards et al., 2020).

However, to be placed on a waiting list expecting future help is unlikely to change anything at all and 16.7% sounds impressive. An effective alternative would need to have some face credibility. Who knows, perhaps expectant help-seekers given some self-help material and told to discuss their problems amongst themselves in a group setting would outperform e-therapy. An advocate of e-therapy would probably counter this suggestion by declaring that the cost of providing a meeting room and the inconvenience of participants having to travel there would nullify any gains.

Commodification: The Next Step

The example of IAPT, with its readymade digital tools, has inspired entrepreneurial start-up services elsewhere. Here is Quenza's (US) sales pitch[1]:

> Ready to improve your clients' wellbeing with your own custom solutions? To start sharing unique, personalized treatments today, don 't forget to try out Quenza. Our all-in-one blended care software gives you all the features and tools you need to create and share online stepped care solutions with your clients, so you can help them enhance their wellbeing and mental health for the long run.

Perhaps the current stage of rationalisation will fade into insignificance with the arrival of artificial intelligence (AI) which holds out the promise of eliminating the need for a real professional altogether. In a book entitled *The Future of the Professions: How Technology Will Transform the Work of Human Experts* (2015), Susskind and Susskind argue that old-fashioned, inefficient, and unnecessarily exclusive, inscrutable, and expensive services could be replaced by dedicated software and machines.

I think it unlikely that the legal profession will buy into this opportunity, but it is well advanced in "mental health" (Giansanti, 2023). But like courtroom battles, a person's face-to-face encounter with an expert who is trying to change the way she or he thinks or behaves are replete with stratagems, cut-and-thrust exchanges, challenges, and retreats—not to mention debate around rather insoluble dilemmas that concern how to live. It is only when problems are reduced to disorders with known parameters and with "proven treatment solutions" that AI sounds feasible.

Susskind and Susskind have in mind the simulation of empathy, which is already well within the capacity of AI robots. As they claim:

> It is entirely conceivable that systems will eventually be better than people in gauging the mood of human beings. More, by using advanced speech synthesis (ensuring a kindly voice perhaps),

---

[1] https://quenza.com/features/

drawing on a large database of triggers and appropriate responses (a collection of *mots justes*), and by reference to users' psychological and emotional profiles, it is foreseeable that machines will be equipped to respond to their users in a manner that would *appear* to be *more* empathetic than a human being. (Susskind and Susskind, 2015: 252)

However, the appearance of empathy is not enough. When a help-seeker is at a loss to define what their problem is, it might take some time for AI to figure out where to begin. Moreover, problems involve other people with their own priorities, and the help-seeker may be locked into irresolvable conflicts with members of their own social circle.

The medicalisation of problems can individualise them in a totally unrealistic way as if your "depression" just belongs to you or your faulty neurochemicals. Open-ended dialogue, either face-to-face or in groups, is still the best way to reconcile interpersonal differences and move on. This can be accomplished in a variety of ways (see Hallam, 2018, pp. 151-156).

As an aid to self-help currently offered through books, apps, and e-therapy, AI may yet prove invaluable as an inexpensive option when governments or individuals cannot afford face-to-face alternatives. However, rule-based chatbots that cannot generate novel responses are a poor substitute (Abd-Alrazaq et al., 2019). An AI simulation of a therapist would need to be trained on samples of actual therapy sessions conducted by therapists rated as experts in their field. Perhaps a variety of AI therapists could be trained in different schools of thought, even ones adhering to pre-selected moral principles.

However, there are practical obstacles and ethical objections to this development. Given the confidential nature of therapy, people would be reluctant to supply training samples. Anonymity would have to be guaranteed during development of the software as well as when a client engaged an AI therapist. Given the suspicion that personal data may not be safe even when encrypted, the risks might be perceived as outweighing the benefits.

Moreover, real therapists are regulated by their professional body and by the law, meaning they must take action when a client poses a threat to themself or to others. Inevitably, a small minority of clients using AI would take their own life or contemplate/inflict violence. There is a possibility of litigation against suppliers of the software, enforcing a legal examination of the advice provided or even of the unanticipated effect of a certain line of questioning. An AI therapist would have to foresee this possibility and flag it up to the client and/or a nominated confidante or real professional who could intervene.

This would be a hit-and-miss safeguard that is unlikely to stand up in court. In the UK, a lawyer or the government health-professions regulator can demand that therapy session notes be released, even if these are mere musings on a possible diagnosis. In one example, the therapist's hypothesis was regarded as defamatory and he was struck off, ending his career (Hallam, 2023). One author advises therapists to restrict their recorded information to the bare facts (Jenkins, 2017) and to destroy the rest after it has been used in supervision.

Perhaps a feasible alternative to an AI therapist would be something like the simulation of an open-ended philosophical dialogue about why, say, the user thought or believed something or was trying to justify acting in a certain way. In this case, AI would not be an attempt to cure a problem or to suggest a solution but merely give the user something to ponder over. Certain topics, such as suicidal thinking, abuse, or trauma could be proscribed. It could prove useful as an adjunct to self-help. The Japanese already have a Buddha Bot, so why shouldn't we have a Beck Bot?

Conclusion

This chapter has taken an historical approach to help-seeking, arguing that it has long been an integral part of social life. Forms of help-seeking that rely on dialogue, especially in group settings, have been practiced for many decades, sometimes with an explicitly non-medical/non-psychiatric philosophy (Hallam, 2018, pp. 103-23). These groups may or may not be led by a professional with therapy expertise.

Some specialisation with regard to type of problem is likely to be necessary so that group members can be linked to useful self-help materials. This chapter has severely criticised commodified forms of helping, despite streams of research that claim to support its "effectiveness" suggesting, instead, that seemingly identical problems have nuanced differences and pose moral/existential challenges of an idiographic nature. This is an impediment to the development of new taxonomies apart from ones that serve pragmatic or bureaucratic purposes.

Psychological problems need to be understood and formulated, and one of the advantages of one-to-one helping is time to follow systematic procedures for identifying key issues and solutions.

References

Abd-Alrazaq, AA, Alajlani, M, Alalwan, A et al. (2019) An overview of the features of chatbots in mental health: A scoping review. *International Journal of Medical Informatics*, 132. 103978. https://doi.org/10.1016/j.ijmedinf.2019.103978

Atkinson, P. (2014) *The sorry state of NHS provision of psychological therapy.* https://freepsychotherapynetwork.com/2014/03/09/the-sorry-story-of-state-provision-of-psychological-therapy/

Clark, D. M. (2018) Realising the mass public benefit of evidence-based psychological therapies: The IAPT program. *Annual Review of Clinical Psychology.* 14: 159–183. doi:10.1146/annurev-clinpsy-050817-084833.

Clark, D. M. (2019) *IAPT at 10: Achievements and challenges.* NHS England. https://www.england.nhs.uk/blog/iapt-at-10-achievements-and-challenges/).

Giansanti, D. (2023) The chatbots are invading us: A map point on the evolution, applications, opportunities, and emerging problems in the health domain. *Life*, 13, 1130. https://doi.org/10.3390 /life13051130

Grayling, A. C. (2013) *Friendship*. New Have, CT: Yale University Press.

Hallam, R. (2013) *Individual Case Formulation*. Oxford: Academic Press

Hallam, R. (2015) *The therapy relationship: A special kind of friendship*. London: Karnac.

Hallam, R. (2018) *Abolishing the concept of mental illness*. London: Routledge.

Hallam, R. (2023) The end of 'therapy' as we know it? *The Psychologist* (letters), July/August, 78-79. https://www.bps.org.uk/psychologist/end-therapy-we-know-it

Hochschild, A. R. (1983) *The managed heart: Commercialization of human feeling*. Berkeley: University of California Press.

Jackson, C. and Rizq, R., (Eds) (2019) *The Industrialisation of care: Counselling psychotherapy and the impact of IAPT*. Monmouth: PCCS Books.

Jenkins, P. (2017) Record-keeping and the law. *Private Practice*, BACP, Summer. https://www.bacp.co.uk/bacp-journals/private-practice/summer-2017/record-keeping-and-the-law/

Linehan, M. (1993) *Cognitive-behavioral treatment of borderline personality disorder*. New York: Guilford.

NHS Digital (2022) *Psychological therapies annual report on the use of IAPT services*, 2021-22. https://digital.nhs.uk/data-and-information/publications/statistical/psychological-therapies-annual-reports-on-the-use-of-iapt-services/annual-report-2021-22

Owen, J., Crouch-Read, L., Smith, M., and Fisher, P. (2021) Stress and burnout in Improving Access to Psychological Therapies (IAPT) trainees: a systematic review. *The Cognitive Behaviour Therapist*, 14, e20, 1-18. doi:10.1017/S1754470X21000179

Richards, D., Enrique, A., Eilert, N. *et al.* (2020) A pragmatic randomized waitlist-controlled effectiveness and cost-effectiveness trial of digital interventions for depression and anxiety. *npj Digital Medicine*. 3, 85. https://doi.org/10.1038/s41746-020-0293-8

Scott, M.J. (2020) Improving access to psychological therapies (IAPT) - The need for radical reform. *Journal of Health Psychology*. 23(9), 1136-1147. https://doi.org/10.1177/1359105318755264

Smith, K. R. (2009). Psychotherapy as applied science or moral praxis? The limitations of empirically supported treatment. *Journal of Theoretical and Philosophical Psychology*. 29:34-46.

Susskind, R. and Susskind, D. (2015) *The future of the professions: How technology will transform the work of human experts.* Oxford: Oxford University Press.

Wheatley, K. (2023) Working NEAR the brink. *The Psychologist*, March. https://www.bps.org.uk/psychologist/working-near-brink

Challenges Facing Alternatives to the DSM

Jonathan D. Raskin

Abstract: *Although many psychologists are dissatisfied with the Diagnostic and Statistical Manual of Mental Disorders (DSM), emerging alternative diagnostic schemes seeking to supplant it face significant obstacles. Psychologists' theoretical values favor developing a diverse set of theoretically grounded psychosocial ways to diagnose and conceptualize mental distress. However, these values conflict with psychologists' practical need (especially in the U.S.) for a universally used diagnostic system that facilitates collection of third-party payments. The DSM and its close sibling, the International Classification of Diseases (ICD), serve this practical purpose well despite being theoretically out-of-step with psychologists' psychosocial worldview. This conflict is unlikely to be resolved any time soon, which means that the hegemony of the DSM and ICD will likely continue. Consequently, diagnostic alternatives might need to settle for supplementing rather than replacing them.*

Challenges Facing Alternatives to DSM

As anyone who works in the field of mental health knows, the American Psychiatric Association's Diagnostic and Statistical Manual of Mental Disorders (DSM) is the seminal manual for diagnosing mental distress (American Psychiatric Association, 2022). Research over the past 50 years finds that roughly 90% or more of practicing psychologists use it, albeit not very enthusiastically (Miller et al., 1981; Raskin et al., 2022; Raskin & Gayle, 2016; Smith & Kraft, 1983).

The data suggests psychologists have been hungry for an alternative to the DSM since at least the early 1980s. However, despite consistently indicating a desire for alternatives, psychologists continue to overwhelmingly use the DSM. What gives?

Theoretical Values vs. Practical Demands in Conceptualizing Mental Distress

Psychologists' forced marriage to the DSM stems in part from an often-unarticulated tension between theoretical values and practical demands that complicates clinical work. Theoretically, most psychologists tend to conceptualize clients through psychosocial lenses. Regardless of whether they emphasize early relationship patterns, cognitive distortions, behavioral conditioning, conditions of worth, family dynamics, or social inequality (to name a few possibilities), psychologists generally privilege *psychological* and *social* factors in understanding mental distress.

The form and quality of people's relationships, what happens to them in life, what they learn from it, and how they make sense of it take center stage in psychosocial approaches, which then rely on various forms of conversation and interpersonal interaction between client and therapist to alleviate client upset. Psychological therapies do not forbid using medical model diagnostic terms such as those in the DSM but neither do they require it. This is because each psychological perspective contains a built-in theory of mental distress and how to alleviate it. Psychotherapies differ in the kinds of client-therapist interactions they encourage, but they all take for granted that such interactions are key ingredients in initiating client change.

Unfortunately, the lack of theoretical need for medical model diagnostic categories does not override practical reasons why psychologists overwhelmingly use the DSM. There are powerful outside pressures that conflict with psychologists' psychosocial orientation: "The money, skills, and networks that the American Psychiatric Association has built up over time mean that it now has a huge advantage over other organizations that might attempt to produce similar classifications of mental disorder" (Cooper, 2019, p. 379). To get reimbursed for their services by third-party payers, psychologists must use the DSM or its sibling, the mental disorders section of the World Health Organization's *International Classification of Diseases* (World Health Organization, 2022). In fact, in the U.S. the Health Insurance Portability and Accountability Act requires ICD diagnostic codes (which DSM borrows) for all insurance claims (Cooper, 2019).

The hegemony of the DSM and the ICD places an administrative demand on psychologists that has nothing to do with how they conceptualize client concerns. A psychodynamic therapist who assesses and diagnoses clients by gathering data on early child-parent relationships and current transference patterns may feel no compunction to use the DSM or the ICD—except as a requirement for getting paid. The same goes for a cognitive therapist who diagnoses cognitive distortions and irrational beliefs, a humanistic therapist who assesses client incongruence, a feminist therapist who evaluates the psychological impact of gender norms and practices, and so on.

None of these therapists' theoretical conceptualizations necessitate incorporating DSM diagnosis. It is the practical demands of the healthcare system that push them to do so. This is backed up by research on psychologist attitudes toward DSM, which finds that the desire to get paid is the most common reason psychologists cite for using the manual (Miller et al., 1981; Raskin et al., 2022; Raskin & Gayle, 2016). Psychologists do not primarily use the DSM because it fits with their orientation or is indispensable to their clinical understanding. They mainly use it for bureaucratic purposes.

One Alternative or Many?

Given that psychologists view the DSM as a practical necessity more than anything else, it is not surprising that they also report being open to DSM alternatives (Miller et al., 1981; Raskin et al., 2022; Raskin & Gayle, 2016). Unfortunately, most psychologists are largely unfamiliar with non-DSM and non-ICD diagnostic options and, from a highly practical standpoint, say that they would likely only use them if accepted by insurance companies for third party billing (Miller et al., 1981; Raskin et al., 2022; Raskin & Gayle, 2016; Smith & Kraft, 1983). This makes sense given the need for psychologists to get paid but poses significant challenges to alternative diagnostic systems.

Alternatives such as the Hierarchical Taxonomy of Psychopathology (HiTOP) (Conway et al., 2022; Kotov et al., 2018), the *Psychodynamic Diagnostic Manual* (PDM) (Lingiardi & McWilliams, 2017), and the Power

Threat Meaning Framework (PTMF) (Johnstone et al., 2018) will only gain so much influence on their merits alone. Without something akin to the almighty diagnostic codes that grease the wheels of third-party payments, they can at best only expect to supplement (rather than replace) the DSM and the ICD among psychologists who accept health insurance.

This disincentivizes psychologists from learning about or receiving training in alternatives such as HiTOP, PDM, and PTMF. It is difficult to imagine busy professionals investing the time to master new diagnostic schemes without an economic motivation for doing so. Psychologists might not like the DSM, but they also might not like keeping up with research and training on multiple diagnostic systems—especially ones unable to get them paid.

This is why, in a previous article on diagnostic alternatives, I emphasized practical concerns when outlining things that psychologists could do to develop a more psychologically-oriented alternative to the DSM and the ICD's medical model (Raskin, 2019). My three recommendations were:

a) Devise a diagnostic approach not bound to a specific theoretical orientation but that emphasizes conversational, relational, and behavioral therapeutic interventions.

b) In creating such a system, include all relevant professions and constituencies among the helping professions that focus on alleviating mental distress—including insurance companies and consumers of services.

c) Make sure that whatever system is developed, it allows psychologists to code concerns so that insurers can process claims while also allowing for research on therapy effectiveness.

In retrospect, I think I was naïve in presuming that a single diagnostic alternative system was a viable option. My recommendations were met with skepticism because they attended to practical considerations (getting psychologists paid) rather than theoretical ones. Yes, diagnostic systems often serve "administrative purposes as much as serving clinical purposes" (Strong, 2019, p. 394). However, in doing so they reify our understandings and limit imagination by privileging particular viewpoints (Strong, 2019)—even when those viewpoints stress the psychosocial.

Further, by trying to devise a practical system that all psychologists could use, we propagate the same problems as the DSM and the ICD—namely, diagnostic schemes whose generality is administratively useful but theoretically incoherent: "Ad hoc combinations of incompatible languages inevitably result in a linguistic quagmire that is almost impossible to disentangle" (Efran & Cohen, 2019, p. 387).

Thus, retaining theoretical coherence likely necessitates the encouragement of myriad diagnostic systems, each internally grounded in a particular set of assumptions. This is essentially the current situation. HiTOP, PDM, and PTMF are all theoretically cogent and distinct schemes for assessing client difficulties—and they are not the only options.

The Research Domain Criteria (RDoC) initiative (Cuthbert, 2022), Jeffrey Rubin's proposed classification of "mental health concerns" (Rubin, 2018), and Karl Tomm's classification of interpersonal patterns (IPscope) (Chang et al., 2020) offer other examples of theoretically coherent (but non-reimbursable) diagnostic approaches in various stages of development and implementation. However, trying to balance the need for diversity of theoretical approaches with the need for a universal way to handle insurance payments leaves us right back where we started. What can be done?

Recommendations

Alternatives to the DSM face an uphill battle. They are unlikely to be widely adopted because they cannot legally be used for insurance payments (at least in the U.S.). The next best option might be for clinicians to advocate incorporating non-DSM approaches into other forms of reimbursement. There is nothing prohibiting the use of non-DSM/ICD diagnosis in third-party payments from life insurance companies, college and university counseling centers, and other domains where services are offered outside a health insurance setting—although implementation seems unlikely, even with the extensive advocacy and effort it would require (Cooper, 2019).

Another possibility would be for supporters of diagnostic alternatives to push health insurance companies to cover Z codes—diagnostic codes in the DSM and the ICD that describe situational circumstances (such as trauma, abuse, economic and relational difficulties, etc.) that do not necessarily rise to the level of diagnosable mental disorder (Cooper, 2019). This might not enhance the appeal or increase the use of non-DSM diagnostic approaches such as HiTOP or PDM, but it would potentially feel more consistent with the psychosocial emphasis embraced by most psychotherapists. Ultimately, conflicting theory versus practice demands may require less-than-perfect solutions for psychologists seeking alternatives to DSM and ICD. And that, in the end, is a challenge unto itself.

References

American Psychiatric Association. (2022). *Diagnostic and statistical manual of mental disorders* (5th ed., text revision). https://doi.org/10.1176/appi.books.9780890425787

Chang, J., Sesma Vazquez, M., Cheang, K. M., McIntosh, S., & Tomm, K. (2020). The IPscope: Applications to couple and family therapy supervision. *Journal of Family Psychotherapy, 31*(3–4), 114–140. https://doi.org/10.1080/08975353.2020.1809916

Conway, C. C., Forbes, M. K., South, S. C., & HiTOP Consortium. (2022). A Hierarchical Taxonomy of Psychopathology (HiTOP) primer for mental health researchers. *Clinical Psychological Science, 10*(2), 236–258. https://doi.org/10.1177%2F21677026211017834

Cooper, R. (2019). Commentary on Jonathan Raskin's "What might an alternative to the *DSM* suitable for psychotherapists look like?" *Journal of Humanistic Psychology, 59*(3), 376–384. https://doi.org/10.1177/0022167818793751

Cuthbert, B. N. (2022). Research Domain Criteria (RDoC): Progress and potential. *Current Directions in Psychological Science, 31*(2), 107–114. https://doi.org/10.1177/09637214211051363

Efran, J. S., & Cohen, J. N. (2019). Not so fast: A response to Raskin. *Journal of Humanistic Psychology, 59*(3), 385–391. https://doi.org/10.1177/0022167818777600

Johnstone, L., Boyle, M., (with Cromby, J., Dillon, J., Harper, D., Kinderman, P., Longden, E., Pilgrim, D., & Read, J. (2018). *The Power Threat Meaning Framework: Towards the identification of patterns in emotional distress, unusual experiences and troubled or troubling behaviour, as an alternative to functional psychiatric diagnosis.* British Psychological Society.

Kotov, R., Krueger, R. F., & Watson, D. (2018). A paradigm shift in psychiatric classification: The Hierarchical Taxonomy Of Psychopathology (HiTOP). *World Psychiatry, 17*(1), 24–25. https://doi.org/10.1002/wps.20478

Lingiardi, V., & McWilliams, N. (2017). *Psychodynamic diagnostic manual* (2nd ed.). The Guilford Press.

Miller, L. S., Bergstrom, D. A., Cross, H. J., & Grube, J. W. (1981). Opinions and use of the DSM system by practicing psychologists. *Professional Psychology, 12*(3), 385–390. https://doi.org/10.1037/0735-7028.12.3.385

Raskin, J. D. (2019). What might an alternative to the *DSM* suitable for psychotherapists look like? *Journal of Humanistic Psychology, 59*(3), 368–375. https://doi.org/10.1177/0022167818761919

Raskin, J. D., & Gayle, M. C. (2016). *DSM-5*: Do psychologists really want an alternative? *Journal of Humanistic Psychology, 56*(5), 439–456. https://doi.org/10.1177/0022167815577897

Raskin, J. D., Maynard, D., & Gayle, M. C. (2022). Psychologist attitudes toward DSM-5 and its alternatives. *Professional Psychology: Research and Practice, 53*(6), 553–563. https://doi.org/10.1037/pro0000480

Rubin, J. (2018). The classification and statistical manual of mental health concerns: A proposed practical scientific alternative to the dsm and icd. *Journal of Humanistic Psychology, 58*(1), 93–114. https://doi.org/10.1177/0022167817718079

Smith, D., & Kraft, W. A. (1983). DSM-III: Do psychologists really want an alternative? *American Psychologist, 38*(7), 777–785. https://doi.org/10.1037/0003-066X.38.7.777

Strong, T. (2019). Reconciling conversational handles with scientific and administrative classifications? A response to Jon Raskin. *Journal of*

Humanistic Psychology, 59(3), 392–400.
https://doi.org/10.1177/0022167818777655

World Health Organization. (2022). *International statistical classification of diseases and related health problems* (11th ed.). https://icd.who.int/

Developing Alternatives to the DSM: The Challenge of Overcoming 'Lock-In'

Rachel Cooper

Abstract: *The Diagnostic and Statistical Manual of Mental Disorders is a classification system that is currently much used, but not much loved. There have been many attempts to develop alternatives to the DSM, but it has proved very difficult for alternative classifications to achieve uptake. In this chapter I argue that the DSM is now difficult to replace because the classification has become 'locked-in'. In the same sort of way that it has proved hard for typists to move on from QWERTY keyboards, though this layout is likely suboptimal, it has become hard for mental health systems to move on from the DSM. I finish with some suggestions as to how lock-in might be overcome, focussing particularly on the challenges faced by those who aim to produce an alternative classification that might be employed for clinical and administrative purposes.*

Acknowledgement: This chapter incorporates portions of text from Rachel Cooper (2015). Why is the Diagnostic and Statistical Manual of Mental Disorders so hard to revise? Path-dependence and "lock-in" in classification. *Studies in History and Philosophy of Science Part C: Studies in History and Philosophy of Biological and Biomedical Sciences, 51,* 1-10.

Introduction

The Diagnostic and Statistical Manual of Mental Disorders currently provides a common language for mental health research, policy and care. However, surveys of mental health professionals regularly find that although the classification is widely used, it is not much loved. Many non-psychiatrists would prefer some alternative classification to be developed. In a recent survey of psychologists, Raskin and colleagues (2022) found that 90% use the DSM-5, mainly due to the requirements of insurance reimbursement, but that many would prefer some alternative.

Similar results have been found for decades. Psychologists have been unenthusiastic users of the DSM ever since the days of DSM-II (APA, 1968; Miller et al., 1981; Raskin & Gayle, 2016; Gayle & Raskin, 2017). Social workers similarly often use the DSM while longing for an alternative (Kutchins & Kirk, 1988; Frazer et al., 2009; Hitchens & Becker, 2014).

The fact that many mental health professionals report using the DSM but are unhappy with its basic assumptions raises questions: Why has it proved difficult to develop an alternative to the DSM? And, how might one go about developing an alternative classification that could be employed for clinical and administrative purposes? For the most part this chapter is pessimistic. I start with a reminder of the long history of failed attempts to overhaul the DSM. I argue that it is now extremely difficult to change practices of mental health classification because the DSM has become 'locked-in'.

In the same sort of way that it has proved hard for typists to move on from QWERTY keyboards, though this layout is likely suboptimal, it has become hard for mental health systems to move on from the DSM. On a more optimistic note, I finish by considering how it is that the locked-in status of the DSM might potentially one day be overcome.

Attempts to overhaul the DSM have a long history

Although currently widely used, the DSM has become important relatively recently (Cooper, 2005; Decker, 2013; Shorter, 2013). The earliest edition of the DSM, published in 1952 was slim, cheap, and little read. The DSM only came to be widely used in the United States in the 1970s and came to global prominence only following publication of DSM-III in 1980.

Almost as soon as the DSM system came to dominance, psychologists started to attempt to develop an alternative. In 1977, the American Psychological Association set up a "Task Force on Descriptive Behavioural Classification" charged with developing an alternative to the DSM (Board of Directors Minutes, June 24-25, 1977). The Task Force was created because the American Psychological Association was becoming concerned that the American Psychiatric Association controlled the DSM and that DSM diagnoses were coming to be required by insurance companies.

Voicing concerns that continue to resonate today, the Task Force worried that the DSM was "a disease-based model inappropriately used to describe problems of living" (Task Force on Descriptive Behavioural Classification, 1977, p. 1). Proposals were put forward to create a new, better alternative to the DSM, but after just a year, the Task Force was disbanded. The Board of Directors of the American Psychological Association decided that the plans of the Task Force were unrealistic in scope and that the likelihood of outside funding was slight (Board of Directors Minutes, December 1-2, 1978, p. 11).

More recently, the American Psychiatric Association itself has become unhappy with the DSM classification – but it has also found it difficult to bring about radical changes. The most recent edition of the DSM, the DSM-5-TR (2022), is only a 'Text Revision'; that is only the surrounding text, and not the sets of diagnostic criteria themselves, were revised in this edition.[1] It is thus no surprise that the DSM-5-TR and DSM-5 are highly similar. The similarities between the DSM-5 (2013) and its predecessor, the DSM-IV (1993), are more noteworthy. The American Psychiatric Association initially planned for these two editions to be very different, but ultimately failed to bring about major change.

The revision process that led up to the DSM-5 began in 1999 with an initial conference, later published as *A Research Agenda for DSM-V* (the Latin numerals only changed later) (Kupfer et al., 2002). *A Research Agenda* began by detailing problems with the DSM series. Chapters noted that high co-morbidity rates, and the slow progress of research projects which sought the biological mechanisms underpinning disorders, suggested that DSM categories likely lacked validity. The *Research Agenda* envisioned that a "paradigm shift" would be required (Kupfer et al., 2002, p. xix) and suggested that the DSM-5 should move towards more biologically-based and more dimensional approaches to classifying psychopathology.

The American Psychiatric Association invested huge amounts of work and money into producing the DSM-5. The total process involved thousands of experts, took over twelve years, and cost $25 million (Frances, 2013, p. 175).

---

[1] Although a few sets of diagnostic criteria were revised to correct errors, and a new diagnosis 'Prolonged Grief Disorder' was added.

In the end, however, and despite huge efforts at revision, the published DSM-5 differed very little from its predecessor. Although the committees revising the DSM started out with ambitions for radical changes, over time, one-by-one, the more radical suggestions for overhaul were dropped. In his final evaluation, David Kupfer, who chaired the Task Force to revise the DSM-5, described it as "an aggressive, conservative document"; in his view the committees were aggressive in their pursuit of revision, but conservative in their decisions in the end (Levine, 2013).

In its finally published form, the DSM-5 differs from its predecessor much less than originally envisaged; a few disorders have been added, a few disorders have been removed, and diagnostic criteria have been tweaked here and there. The failure to radically revise the DSM demonstrates that the American Psychiatric Association now struggles to revise its own classification. In the next section I examine why it is that the DSM has proved so difficult to change.

Why is the DSM now so hard to change? Lock-in and classification

In *Sorting Things Out* (2000), Geoffrey Bowker and Susan Star argue that classifications can be thought of as part of the information infrastructure of science and have features in common with material infrastructure, like electricity supply networks. They suggest that as with material technologies, it is possible for "path dependent" development to cause a sub-optimal classification to become "locked-in" and hard to replace (Bowker and Star, 2000, p. 14).

The QWERTY keyboard layout offers the classic example of path dependence leading to a suboptimal technology becoming locked-in (David, 1985). In the days of mechanical typewriters, the QWERTY layout was designed to reduce the chances of keys jamming together; the design minimises the frequency with which physically adjacent keys are used one after the other. Modern keyboards no longer jam, and so it may well be the case that a different layout would now be preferable. However, the costs of shifting from one layout to another are too great for QWERTY to now be displaced. Everyone finds it easier to type on keyboards that have a familiar layout, and so everyone buys QWERTY keyboards. Despite being sub-optimal, the QWERTY design has become locked-in.

As the QWERTY case illustrates, certain technologies are path dependent, and can become locked-in to suboptimal design. The phenomenon arises as follows: At an initial time, a particular technology comes to be adopted either because it has some temporary advantage over competitors or through chance factors. The technology is such that success breeds success, such that, at some later point, the adopted technology becomes very hard to dislodge.

Path dependence, potentially leading to lock-in, can occur whenever a technology is such that positive feedback mechanisms ensure that its greater use brings ever greater returns. The QWERTY keyboard layout manifests path dependence because the more used typists become to working with a particular layout, the harder and harder it becomes to change. I suggest that, like the QWERTY keyboard, the DSM has become locked-in. With each successive edition, the DSM has become more and more widely adopted, and it is now very difficult to develop a serious competitor.

In the late 1970s, when work started on DSM-III, few people were interested in classification in mental health (Decker, 2013). The lack of general interest enabled a small group of like-minded researchers to gain control of the revisionary process. These researchers, dubbed the "neo-Kraepelians" by Blashfield (1984), shared a particular outlook. They believed that diagnosis and classification mattered, that diagnostic criteria should be operationalised to achieve reliability, and that mental disorders would prove to be biologically-based medical disorders. The neo-Kraepelinians were left free to develop the DSM-III as they thought best.

Subsequent to publication, the success of the DSM-III took most by surprise (Decker, 2013). Crucially, the classification launched at a time when it was becoming the norm for mental health services to be paid for by insurance and for insurers to demand a diagnosis. While insurance for mental health care was rare in the US when the DSM-I was published in 1952, coverage gradually increased throughout the sixties and seventies, and had become widespread by 1980 (Cooper, 2005, pp. 127-132). The DSM contains the codes used to fill in insurance forms.

These codes are drawn from the version of the ICD (the classification of disorders published by the WHO) that is used in the US. Although these codes can be obtained without buying the DSM, the DSM contains them in a user-friendly format and most mental health professionals in the US access the codes via the DSM. This is the main reason that mental health professionals of all types (not just psychiatrists, but also psychologists, social workers, and counsellors) buy and use the DSM (Miller et al., 1981; Kutchins & Kirk, 1988; Frazer et al., 2002).

During the same period, the testing, regulation, and marketing of psychoactive drugs came to see them as directed at specific disorders as opposed to symptoms (Cooper, 2005, pp. 112-118; Shorter, 2013, p. 13). Researchers came to use DSM-III diagnostic criteria to pick out subject populations for research; the FDA demanded the use of DSM categories in drug trials; and advertising started to employ the idea that psychoactive drugs treat specific conditions. Such activities helped legitimise the notion that the descriptions included in the DSM-III were scientifically respectable and referred to real disorders. The net result was that the DSM-III classification came to be much more widely used and more respected than its predecessors. The successes of the DSM-III though have had a downside. The classification has become locked-in and is now very difficult to revise.

DSM categories are now employed in most mental health research. This means that when it comes to revising the classification, there is a substantial body of work available that can inform considerations as to whether particular DSM categories should be revised. The available research is directed at DSM categories, and thus evidence becomes available to guide tweaking DSM-categories. Studies may well show that an extra symptom should be added to the diagnostic criteria for a particular disorder, that a diagnosis could usefully be split into subtypes, or that two diagnoses should be merged together. However, finding research that might inform shifting to a radically different type of classification system is more difficult. Almost everyone uses the DSM, and so the research base for alternatives tends to be weak.

In addition, as the DSM has become ever more important, it has become tied to networks of other classifications and bureaucratic structures. The complex links between the DSM and systems for insurance reimbursement are especially noteworthy. It is important for American Psychiatric Association revenues that the codes included in the DSM be acceptable to insurance providers because the main reason that clinicians buy the DSM is for the codes. However, making the DSM insurance-friendly is a complex undertaking. The US is bound by international treaty to use a version of the ICD, the classification produced by the World Health Organisation, for official medical coding. The US Health Insurance Portability and Accountability Act (HIPAA) (1996) also requires the use of ICD codes. As such, the DSM needs to maintain compatibility with the ICD so that it contains codes that are acceptable to insurance companies.

In order to maintain compatibility with the ICD, when changing the DSM, the American Psychiatric Association consults with the WHO. The users and purposes of the ICD differ from those of the DSM (Reed, 2010). As such, there is no guarantee that changes that would promote the interests of the American Psychiatric Association will also satisfy the needs of the WHO. Although used around the world, the DSM is primarily directed at clinicians and researchers working in the US. In contrast, the ICD is specifically designed for international use. The ICD comes in various versions. While the most complex is intended for use by researchers, two simplifications of this are produced: one for specialist clinicians and one for use in primary care settings. Crucially, all three versions of the ICD are intended to be compatible and the WHO is committed to ensuring that the primary care version is suitable for use by non-specialist clinicians working in developing countries. This commitment constrains the possibilities for revising the ICD.

The need to maintain compatibility with the ICD, and to maintain acceptability by the insurance industry, creates complex constraints on the ways in which the DSM can be revised. Furthermore, the ICD-insurance-industry network is not the only network in which the DSM is embedded. In the US, DSM categories have been adopted by numerous government organisations. The DSM affects everything from the ways in which school children with special needs receive services to the laws governing the detention of sex offenders. Any revision can thus have huge ramifications. The difficulties involved in foreseeing possible consequences and negotiating with various stakeholders make it very difficult for substantial revisions to be made.

We can see that rather than lock-in being merely a contingent, and unfortunate, side-effect of success, lock-in will always be a risk when a classification comes to be widely used. As the classification came to be used by more and more communities, it became embedded in more and more systems, and became harder and harder to revise. As users became ever more familiar with the DSM system conceiving of shifting to anything radically different became more and more difficult.

How might lock-in be overcome

The DSM is currently locked-in, but this may change in the future. Lock-in is a time-specific and agent-relative phenomenon. Changes that the American Psychiatric Association was unable to make to the DSM-5 may turn out to be possible for some later edition of the DSM, or for some other new classification of mental disorders, possibly produced by another organisation.

How can lock-in be overcome? In the literature on the lock-in of technologies, a number of methods are commonly suggested: First, a central authority (for example, a government) may dictate a switch to a new system (Cowan & Hultén, 1996). This method of overcoming lock-in is best illustrated by those cases where a country switches from driving on one side of the road to the other. No individual driver could decide to make the switch, but the government has the power to make sure that everyone adopts the new standards.

Second, it may be possible to overcome lock-in via creating a niche market (Cowan & Hultén, 1996); if some smallish number of users of a technology are sufficiently isolated, then it may be possible to convert them to a new system even if most continue in the old ways. Edison's first electric lighting system, for example, was installed on a steamship – a niche isolated from the then dominant systems of urban gas lighting (Utterback, 1994).

Third, on occasion, lock-in has been overcome because users so dislike the idea of being locked-in that they employ heroic measures to shift to a new technology. Thus, the German municipality of Munich recently moved from Windows to Linux, in large part for political reasons (Dobusch, 2008).

Fourth, some crisis may render continuing with the status quo untenable. Cowan and Gunby (1996) discuss how the development of pest resistance has forced a switch away from the previously locked-in practices of heavy pesticide use in various types of agriculture. Each of these methods can only be employed when the time and circumstances are right. The levers of change - legislative clout, niches, grassroots resistance, crises – tend to be in short supply. The reason that lock-in is time- and agent-relative is because only certain agents, at certain times, have access to the means necessary for overcoming lock-in.

Developments are currently underway that may one day come to challenge the dominance of the DSM system. Today, various groups continue to propose ambitious projects that aim to present an alternative to the DSM. Recent years have seen the development of the Psychodynamic Diagnostic Manual 2 (PDM-2) (Lingiardi & McWilliams, 2017), the Hierarchical Taxonomy of Psychopathology (HiTOP) (Kotov et al., 2017), the Power Threat Meaning Framework (PTMF) (Johnstone & Boyle, 2018), and the Research Domain Criteria (RDoC) research initiative (NIMH, n.d.).

Of these initiatives, the RDoC project is the most advanced. The US National Institute of Mental Health developed the RDoC as a radically different approach to classification. The Research Domain Criteria project (RDoC) aims "to define basic dimensions of functioning (such as fear circuitry or working memory) to be studied across multiple units of analysis, from genes to neural circuits to behaviors, cutting across disorders as traditionally defined" (NIMH, n.d.). The system relies far more on dimensions and is more biologically-focussed than the DSM. Notably, the system is aimed only at researchers and is not intended for clinical or administrative use. The intention is that instead of researchers studying groups of patients diagnosed with say, schizophrenia or PTSD, using RDoC they will study groups suffering from problems with, say, impulse control or emotional lability.

We can see the RDoC project as aiming to break the hold of the DSM on psychiatric classification via utilising a number of the strategies that have been used to successfully overcome lock-in in other settings. First, insofar as RDoC only aims to be used by researchers, it can be understood as being aimed at a niche market. Second, as a major grant giver the NIMH is a "central authority," at least as far as US researchers are concerned. The NIMH can require grant applicants to employ RDoC and thus force use of the system (Insel, 2013; Pickersgill, 2019). In its first decade, NIMH funding resulted in over 1000 research papers that made use of RDoC (Morris et al., 2022). It remains, though, early days for the RDoC. Whether RDoC will succeed longer term and become more widely used by researchers remains to be seen.

In any case, while the RDoC has come to be used by some researchers, it should be emphasised that the RDoC system is unsuitable for everyday use by clinicians and administrators. Those who would develop alternatives to the DSM for clinical and administrative use face additional challenges. Clinicians primarily use the DSM for securing payment. As such, any group seeking an alternative to the DSM for use by regular clinicians must solve the economic and administrative obstacles to developing a different classification.

A major issue is that the Health Insurance Portability and Accountability Act (1996) mandates that health insurers use ICD codes. The version of the ICD currently employed in the US, ICD-10-CM, includes two types of code that, in principle, could be used by mental health services. Best known are the codes for DSM-style diagnoses. However, the ICD also contains non-disorder 'Z-codes' which include codes for a range of life issues, such as 'Burnout', 'Social role conflict', and 'Antisocial behaviour'. Historically, insurers in the United States have refused to reimburse for Z-codes. Still, if it were possible to convince some funders to reimburse for Z-codes, these codes might potentially be employed to enable the use of a classification that focussed on life problems rather than on mental disorders.

Another option would be to seek out niches that are unconstrained by the Health Insurance Portability and Accountability Act. The act applies only to health insurance. In some settings, mental health care may be funded in other ways, for example, counselling provided for university students or by Employee Assistance Programs (EAP). Bereavement counselling also offers an obvious example and is sometimes covered by life insurance. Such settings constitute special 'niches' in which there may be no need to use the DSM and where radically different forms of diagnosis, or no diagnoses at all, might be employed.

I acknowledge that my suggestions here are modest. The DSM is currently 'locked-in' and will be hard to replace. Insofar as mental health professionals currently employ the DSM largely for insurance purposes, the key problem to be addressed by those seeking an alternative is to make it compatible with the needs of the funders of mental health services.

References

Archive Resources
I consulted the archives of the American Psychological Association (held at the American Psychological Association offices in Washington, DC, and the Library of Congress) in 1997. Folder and Box locations were correct at this date.

Sources Cited in American Psychological Association Library
Board of Directors Minutes, June 24-25, 1977, in Folder "Board of Directors Minutes, 1974, 1975, 1976, 1977, 1978."

Board of Directors Minutes, December 1-2, 1978, in Folder "Board of Directors Minutes, 1974, 1975, 1976, 1977, 1978."

Sources Cited in Library of Congress, American Psychological Association Materials
Task Force on Descriptive Behavioural Classification, July 1977, Progress Report in Box 2087627, Board of Professional Affairs

Standard References
American Psychiatric Association. (1952). *Diagnostic and statistical manual: mental disorders.* Washington, D.C.: American Psychiatric Association.

American Psychiatric Association. (1968). *Diagnostic and statistical manual of mental disorders. (2nd edition).* Washington, D.C.: American Psychiatric Association.

American Psychiatric Association. (1980). *Diagnostic and statistical manual of mental disorders. (3rd edition).* Washington, D.C.: American Psychiatric Association.

American Psychiatric Association. (1994). *Diagnostic and statistical manual of mental disorders. (Fourth edition).* Washington, D.C.: American Psychiatric Association.

American Psychiatric Association. (2013). *Diagnostic and statistical manual of mental disorders. (Fifth edition).* Washington, D.C.: American Psychiatric Association.

American Psychiatric Association. (2022). *Diagnostic and statistical manual of mental disorders. (Fifth edition – Text Revision).* Washington, D.C.: American Psychiatric Association.

Blashfield, R. (1984). *The Classification of psychopathology: Neo-Kraepelinian and quantitative approaches.* New York: Plenum Publishing Corporation.

Bowker, G. & Star S. (2000). *Sorting things out.* Cambridge, Massachusetts: MIT Press.

Cooper, R. (2005). *Classifying madness: a philosophical examination of the diagnostic and statistical manual of mental disorders.* Dordrecht: Springer.

Cowan, R. & Gunby, P. (1996). Sprayed to death: path dependence, lock-in and pest control strategies. *The Economic Journal, 106*: 521-542.

Cowan, R. & Hultén, S. (1996). Escaping lock-in: The case of the electric vehicle. *Technological Forecasting and Social Change, 53*, 61-79.

David, P. (1985). Clio and the economics of QWERTY. *American Economic Review, 75*, 332-337.

Decker, H. (2013). *The making of DSM-III.* New York: Oxford University Press.

Dobusch, L. (2008). Migration discourse structures: Escaping Microsoft's desktop path. In B. Russo, E. Damiani, S. Hissam, B. Lundell. G. Succi (Eds.) *Open Source Development, Communities and Quality.* (pp. 223-235). Boston: Springer.

Frances, A. (2013). *Saving normal.* New York: Harper Collins.

Frazer P., Westhuis D., Daley J. G., & Phillips I. (2009). How clinical social workers are using the *DSM-IV*: A national study. *Social Work in Mental Health, 7*, 325-339.

Gayle M. C. & Raskin J. D. (2017). *DSM-5*: Do counselors really want an alternative? *Journal of Humanistic Psychology, 57*, 650-666

Hitchens K. & Becker D. (2014). Social work and the DSM: A qualitative examination of opinions. *Social Work in Mental Health, 12*, 303-329.

Insel, T. (2013). *Director's blog: Transforming diagnosis*. April 29 2013. Available at https://psychrights.org/2013/130429NIMHTransformingDiagnosis.htm

Johnstone, L. & Boyle, M. (2018). *The power threat meaning frame-work: Towards the identification of patterns in emotional distress, unusual experiences and troubled or troubling behaviour, as an alternative to functional psychiatric diagnosis* (with J. Cromby, J. Dillon, D. Harper, P. Kinderman, E. Longden, D. Pilgrim, & J. Read). London, United Kingdom: British Psychological Society. Retrieved from http://www.bps.org.uk/PTM-Main

Kotov, R., Krueger, R. F., Watson, D., Achenbach, T. M., Althoff, R. R., Bagby, R. M., Brown, T. A., Carpenter, W. T., Caspi, A., Clark, L. A., Eaton, N. R., Forbes, M. K., Forbush, K. T., Goldberg, D., Hasin, D., Hyman, S. E., Ivanova, M. Y., Lynam, D. R., Markon, K., . . . Zimmerman, M. (2017). The Hierarchical Taxonomy of Psychopathology (HiTOP): A dimensional alternative to traditional nosologies. *Journal of Abnormal Psychology, 126*(4), 454–477. https://doi.org/10.1037/abn0000258

Kupfer, D., First, M., & Regier D. (2002). Introduction. In D. Kupfer, M. First & D. Regier (Eds.) *A Research Agenda for DSM-V*. Washington, DC: American Psychiatric Association. Pp. xv-xxiii

Kutchins, H. & Kirk, S. A. (1988). The business of diagnosis: DSM-III and clinical social work. *Social Work, 33*: 215-220.

Levine, M. (2013). Pitt prof oversees psychiatric guide revision. *University Times. 45*, no page. Available at http://www.utimes.pitt.edu/?p=23893.

Lingiardi, V. & McWilliams, N. (Eds.). (2017). *Psychodynamic diagnostic manual (2nd ed.)*. New York, NY: Guilford Press

Miller, L., Bergstrom, D., Cross, H., & Grube, J. (1981). Opinions and use of the DSM system by practicing psychologists. *Professional Psychology, 12*, 385- 390.

Morris, S.E., Sanislow, C.A., Pacheco, J. *et al.* Revisiting the seven pillars of RDoC. *BMC Med* **20**, 220 (2022). https://doi.org/10.1186/s12916-022-02414-0

NIMH. (n.d.). Research domain criteria. Available at http://www.nimh.nih.gov/research-priorities/rdoc/index.shtml

Pickersgill, M. (2019). Psychiatry and the sociology of novelty: Negotiating the US national institute of mental health "research domain criteria" (RDoC). *Science, Technology, & Human Values, 44*(4), 612-633.

Raskin J. D. & Gayle M. C. (2016). DSM-5: Do psychologists really want an alternative? *Journal of Humanistic Psychology,* 56, 439-456.

Raskin, J. D., Maynard, D., & Gayle, M. C. (2022). Psychologist attitudes toward DSM-5 and its alternatives. *Professional Psychology: Research and Practice, 53*(6), 553.

Reed, G. (2010). Toward ICD-11: Improving the clinical utility of WHO's International Classification of Mental Disorders. *Professional Psychology: Research and Practice, 41*: 457-464.

Shorter, E. (2013). The history of DSM. In J. Paris and J. Phillips (Eds.) *Making the DSM-5* (pp. 3-19). New York: Springer.

Utterback, J. (1996). *Mastering the dynamics of innovation.* Harvard Business Press.

Diagnosing Psychiatry's Failure: The Need for a Post-Positivist Psychiatry

Niall McLaren

Abstract: *This chapter considers the current state of theorising in psychiatry and how we got here. There are currently only two accepted models of mental disorder, the "biomedical," and the "biopsychosocial." The former is reductionist while the latter is a dualist-interactionist model. However, as a matter of established fact, neither of these exists as anything more than a name. Psychiatry is operating without scientific warrant. Psychiatry's rejection of a psychological component in mental disorder stems from its embrace of the principles of positivism, which were formalised in 1929. It is argued that these principles condemn psychiatry to intellectual sterility, and that, in order to advance beyond the descriptive phase in the development of a science, it needs to move to a post-positivist stage where mental life is established as real and causally-significant.*

Introduction: Psychiatry as the positivist views it

Anybody working in a scientific field is fully aware of the need to maintain the highest standards of objectivity about our work. In the clinic, laboratory or in the field, we must always avoid subjectivity, sentiment, anthropomorphism and all other hints of emotional involvement. We can see this clearly in behaviorist psychology, which talked of people as "organisms"—though it's the same in all the life sciences, including the technology known as medicine. However, remarkably few people are aware of how this ethos arose, how it is justified, and the extent of its influence.

Just over a hundred years ago, the French philosopher Henri Bergson (1859-1941) published a book translated in English as *Creative Evolution*. He proposed that living matter is animated by an *élan vitale* or Vital Force that isn't present in non-living matter, and that this directs evolution. The criticism was swift: nobody could see or isolate his "force" and it didn't actually explain anything.

In Vienna at about the same time, Sigmund Freud, a neurologist-turned-psychiatrist, was developing a complex theory of mind that he believed could explain mental disorder and a whole lot more. While for outsiders it was practically impossible to understand, it gained support in psychiatry and spread to the major Western countries, especially the US where it was enormously influential. Gradually, it became more and more complicated, and Freud's followers split into squabbling tribes. Criticism was slower coming but it amounted to the same thing: "You talk about interpreting dreams or of drives that nobody can see or measure, so how do you know you're right?"

This demand for justification became the driving force in twentieth century science: How do you know you're right? How can we distinguish between meaningful statements and plain fantasy? However, the movement didn't start in science—it began with the French philosopher, Auguste Comte (1798-1857). Comte, a complex character, is regarded as the father of sociology. He wanted to write a scientific account of human society based in his perception of societies evolving through set stages.

The first he named the theological stage in which everything revolves around the idea of the divinity as creator and judge. Absolute power rests with a conservative priesthood that compels everybody to believe the same set of supernatural beliefs. Magic dominates life but, as a society matures, it moves to the second or metaphysical stage. In this, citizens question all their forefathers' beliefs and try build a rational society based in the notion of natural but non-divine universal rights. The third and final stage he termed the scientific or positive stage, in which all social and other problems are solved by rational enquiry with no preconceptions. With this came the concept of a pure, empirical science free of metaphysical content.

By the end of the nineteenth century, events were moving quickly, especially in physics and chemistry, with biology catching up rapidly due to the work of Helmholtz, of Pasteur, and of Darwin. In 1878, Wilhelm Wundt (1832-1920), one of Helmholtz's students, opened the first dedicated psychological laboratory in Leipzig. His goal was to put psychology on the same footing as the other natural sciences.

Just thirty-five years later in a paper entitled "Psychology as the behaviorist views it," an American psychologist, John B Watson (1878-1958), declared that psychology as the study of the mind was going nowhere. Psychology, he thundered, needed to free itself of such idle considerations by building a new science of behaviorism on the solid evidence of observable behavior. Nothing else could provide the scientific certainty needed; he thought it would take a few years. With that proclamation, psychology had set its course for the century.

Meanwhile, also in Vienna, a group of mathematicians, physicists and logicians had formed a society dedicated to the work of the physicist and philosopher, Ernst Mach (1838-1916). They were committed to his idea that science and philosophy had to eliminate all unobservables from their fields of study. Science must be built only on what can be seen or measured. Philosophy itself had to undergo some fairly radical pruning until all that was left was what they called logical analysis. Religious and undefined metaphysical notions had no place in their hard-headed view of the world.

In 1929, a smaller group who called themselves the Vienna Circle published a manifesto which is generally taken as the coming-of-age of the movement now known as positivism [1]. It was dedicated to the physicist and philosopher Moritz Schlick (1882-1936) who was instrumental in organising the group and has been called "the father of positivism." It outlined their intention to set science, mathematics, philosophy, and all other fields of rational enquiry on a new course. Biology, psychology, and sociology are briefly mentioned as part of their program of empirical investigation of the universe according to their very strict logic.

Their goal was to build a unified system of science on reliable knowledge which, to them, meant knowledge derived from sense data alone. A great deal of their motivation was anti-religious, so they had no time for metaphysical musing: "Neatness and clarity are striven for, and dark distances and unfathomable depths rejected. In science there are no 'depths'; there is surface everywhere ..." [1, p 9]. They firmly believed that the old ways of trying to *reason* how the world must be were going nowhere, while their methods, exemplified in the rapid progress in physics—and *only* their methods—would forge ahead:

> Everything is accessible to man; and man is the measure of all things ... The scientific world-conception knows no unsolvable riddle. Clarification of the traditional philosophical problems leads us partly to unmask them as pseudo-problems, and partly to transform them into empirical problems and thereby subject them to the judgment of experimental science. The task of philosophical work lies in this clarification of problems and assertions, not in the propounding of special 'philosophical' pronouncements. The method of this clarification is that of *logical analysis* of it ... [1, p 9; their emphasis].

When it came to practice, the method of science was reductionism: the idea that to understand something was to understand what it was made of, how it was made, and how it functioned as a processor of matter and energy. Formally, reductionism says that the behavior and properties of a higher order entity are fully explained by the behavior and properties of the lower order entities of which it is composed.

While the concepts embraced by positivism were not new, they essentially redefined and justified the direction of many fields of science, including biology, economics, history, linguistics, psychology, philosophy, and, of course, medicine:

> We have characterised *the scientific world-conception* essentially by *two features. First* it is *empiricist* and *positivist*: there is knowledge only from experience which rests on what is immediately given. This sets the limits for the content of legitimate science. *Second,* the scientific world-conception is marked by application of a certain method, namely *logical analysis*. The aim of scientific effort is to reach the goal, unified science, by applying logical analysis to the empirical material. Since the meaning of every statement of science must be statable by reduction to a statement about the given, likewise the meaning of any concept, whatever branch of science it may belong

to, must be statable by step-wise reduction to other concepts, down to the concepts of the lowest level which refer directly to the given [1, p 12; their emphasis].

This radicalism became the guiding light of twentieth century science and rationality. No, it was much more than a guiding light—it was the searing sun that dispelled the cloying tendrils of ignorance and prejudice drifting in the darkness of religiosity. A faith, in other words. A central part of that faith was to eradicate any and all traces of spiritualism including, naturally enough, human mental life.

In no time, positivism became the foundation of science, mathematics, engineering, philosophy, and logic—so basic, indeed, that most students were not actually taught it. Today, few people working in fields cast entirely in the positivist framework would even know about it. As a medical student in the 1960s, as a trainee psychiatrist (resident) in the 1970s, and as a philosophy student in the 1980s, I was never taught anything about it.

It was not that it became part of the furniture—positivism was the very air we breathed, and nothing has changed. There was only ever one form of rationality, and that was the form specified by the Vienna Circle in the 1920s. People who lived and worked before the Age of Positivism were groping in the dark; nice people, for sure, but only we moderns have a solid grip on the universe.

The next year, Moritz Schlick published a brief essay on what he saw as "the turning point" of philosophy [2]. Echoing Wittgentstein's opinion that "anything that can be said at all can be said clearly, and what we cannot talk about we must pass over in silence," Schlick shoved philosophy in a new direction:

There are consequently no questions which are in principle unanswerable, no problems which are in principle insoluble. What have been considered such up to now are not genuine questions, but meaningless sequences of words. To be sure, they look like questions from the outside, since they seem to satisfy the customary rules of grammar, but in truth they consist of empty sounds, because they transgress the profound inner rules of logical syntax discovered by the new analysis ... There is, in addition to it, no domain of "philosophical" truths. Philosophy is not a system of statements; it is not a science. But what is it then? Well, certainly not a science, but nevertheless something so significant and important that it may henceforth, as before, be honored as the Queen of the Sciences. For it is nowhere written that the Queen of the Sciences must itself be a science [2].

This has been called the "linguistic turn" in philosophy, away from formulating metaphysical structures in some undefined space to a process of careful analysis of language itself, later known as ordinary language or analytic philosophy. Somewhat surprisingly, early positivists were sympathetic to Freud's psychology. As late as 1949, in his classic monograph *The Concept of Mind*, philosopher Gilbert Ryle (1900-1976) referred to Freud as "psychology's one man of genius" [3, p 305].

Under this stringent influence, biology eagerly rid itself of all considerations of sentiment, prejudice, hope and so on: in other words, of all humanity. Because their training was thoroughly biological, physicians accepted without demur what was actually an ultra-radicalist policy. Without the distraction of searches for the invisible *élan vitale* and other metaphysical notions, the life sciences powered ahead, their success constantly reinforcing the idea that positivism was the correct policy.

Recasting itself as "applied bioscience," medicine transformed daily life for the masses but, while physicians occupied an exalted position in society, not everybody was happy. Instead of the caring family doctor, we had enormous hospitals working as production lines staffed by "clinical consultants" and "biomedical technicians." By the 1970s, even physicians themselves were starting to realise something was missing [4] but medicine as clinical bioscience was on a roll.

Meanwhile, back in the mental hospital, things were changing. There had always been a wing of psychiatry that saw mental illness as just an unusual sort of brain illness, but psychiatry had never been able to make up its mind [5]. Was mental disorder all physical or, as the Freudians claimed, was it psychological? Over the years, there had been an armistice of sorts in their endless squabbles with mental hospitals hewing closely to a biological line while private practice indulged the vastly more interesting (and rewarding) vision of mental disorder as a primary psychological disturbance. However, under the hammerings of positivist philosophy, Freud's profoundly metaphysical psychiatry gradually fell into disrepute.

In 1980, when a totally new and biologically-oriented version of the American Psychiatric Association's Diagnostic and Statistical Manual (DSM) was launched, positivists proudly took control of the last medical specialty to resist them (see, for example, [6]). The goal of the new DSM was to classify each mental disorder as a category of disease in itself with no overlap with other mental conditions. And that was it.

In the struggle to become free of "... meaningless sequences of words ... (that) look like questions from the outside ...", psychiatry eliminated all traces of emotion, leaving only a hostile anti-dualism. Uninvolved in their patients' turmoil, detached and dispassionate, psychiatrists became, in their words, "clinical neuroscientists." Using the same tools pathologists use to study bacteria, psychiatrists studied the physical brain for the causes of mental disorder. To paraphrase the Vienna Circle:

> "Neatness and clarity are striven for, and dark distances and unfathomable depths of mind rejected. In psychiatry, there are no 'depths'; there is surface everywhere ... The scientific psychiatry knows no unsolvable riddle. Clarification of the traditional psychiatric problems leads us partly to unmask them as pseudo-problems, and partly to transform them into empirical problems and thereby subject them to the judgment of experimental science."

And that, in one brief paragraph, is the entire ethos (n: the distinguishing character, sentiment, moral nature, or guiding beliefs of a person, group, or institution) of modern psychiatry: "Don't give us all this moral and mental stuff. If we can't see it on a scan, it doesn't exist. Onward, ever upward!" It is, however, a rare psychiatrist who recognises this as ideology because, as positivism applied to human mental life, that's what it is [7].

Fewer still would know that nobody has ever shown that this is the correct move. Steeped in reductionist biology since early high school, with no knowledge of the history of philosophy and surrounded by people who think alike, mainstream psychiatrists accept that theirs is the only conceivable approach to mental disorder. Like all ideologues, their self-perception is grounded in the idea that they cannot be wrong. By definition, critics are not reasonable—they are hostile actors.

Skeptics may ask "But how do you know you're right? How can you distinguish between meaningful scientific statements and pseudoscience, or even fantasy?" To ask such a question of a committed biological psychiatrist is to invite a contemptuous dismissal: "How can we possibly be wrong?" they demand. "Our science of mental disorder has no metaphysical assumptions. Our evidence consists of reproducible data only."

Unfortunately for them, that is itself a metaphysical assumption driving psychiatry further down an uncharted path, a point dedicated biological psychiatrists will never accept: "Please don't interrupt the interview with your emotional problems. My role as psychiatrist is to make a diagnosis and prescribe treatment." Whether they are correct is wholly a question of philosophy. Very few mainstream psychiatrists are familiar with such matters.

The state of theorising in psychiatry: Biological psychiatry

A positivist account of mental disorder absolutely excludes things such as demonic possession, astrological influences, spells and enchantments, lack of faith, and so on. We are left with a range of possible explanations:

a) Mental disorder is a matter of individual biology; except where they act as trigger events to expose an inherent pathology, life events are irrelevant to the precipitation and maintenance of mental disorder

b) Mental disorder is a matter of individual psychology; brain factors are irrelevant except where they expose inherent psychological instabilities

c) Mental disorder is a matter of social pathology; individuals suffer,
    but the causes and potential remedies are entirely within the social
    structure
d) All of the above in various forms
e) There is no such thing as mental disorder; so-called mental patients
    are involved in an elaborate game of deception with their equally
    complicit psychiatrists (This is the view of the late Thomas Szasz; I
    mention it for completeness but won't discuss it further [8].)

The dominant model today is a) *Mental disorder is just a special form of brain
disorder*. This is not new and can take various forms. Probably the oldest
would be the notion that there is something that we can add to or subtract
from the diet that will cure all sorts of ailments and woes. While this has a
certain uncluttered appeal, there is no evidence that, in healthy humans
eating a balanced diet, food has anything to do with mental disorder.

We could mention various types of infections but, again, this has been
extensively explored in the past (as in "the search for the elusive
schizococcus") and has little or no research interest at present. More
recently, there has been some interest in forms of inflammation as "the
cause" of mental disorder, which has more to do with the availability of the
technology than any real chance it will prove productive.

Modern biological psychiatry is firmly in the reductionist camp, meaning a
full explanation of the individual's brain will give a full account of any
mental disorders with no questions unanswered. By biology, we mean the
individual's native biological state—essentially, the genetic endowment.
We can see the scope of this claim in the views of historian and naturalistic
philosopher, Richard Carrier:

> ... everything can be reduced to matter and energy in space and time:
> quarks and other sub-atomic particles and their behaviors are all that
> there is, out of which everything without exception is made. And this
> fits with the fact that society can be reduced to humans, and humans
> can be reduced to cells, and cells can be reduced to chemical systems,
> which can be reduced in turn to sub-atomic particles. So therefore
> societies can be reduced to sub-atomic particles. The natural

corollary of this view is that the sciences follow the same pattern: sociology can be reduced to psychology, psychology to biology, biology to chemistry, and chemistry to physics. So, theoretically, all of sociology and psychology can be described entirely by physics [9, S.III.5.5].

Elsewhere, Carrier qualifies this by saying that the arrangement and performance of a physical structure also count, but physicalism's naive reductionist view drives biological psychiatry. A generation ago, the influential American psychiatrist, Samuel Guze (1923-2000), asked whether there is any other kind of psychiatry besides the biological, adding: "...there is no such thing as a psychiatry which is too biological" [10].

His view remains at the very heart of psychiatry today. David Kupfer, chairman of the DSM-5 Committee stated bluntly: "Psychiatric disorders are brain disorders ... Psychiatric disorders *are* medical disorders" [11] (his emphasis). Similarly, Thomas Insel, former director of the US NIMH, which disburses the great bulk of psychiatric research money in the US, ca. $1.5bln each year, had no doubts: "First, the RDoC framework conceptualises mental illnesses as brain disorders... Second, (it) assumes that the dysfunction in neural circuits can be identified with the tools of (ordinary) neuroscience..." [12].

This didn't come out of the blue. Insel, who trained in neurophysiology and built his reputation on his research on small rodents called voles, had often made similar claims:

> The good news is that we now have the tools to enable a new science of mental disorders... this science will revolutionize the diagnosis and treatment of mental illness and... transform psychiatry, ultimately realigning it with neurology and potentially creating a new discipline of clinical neuroscience... [13]

> Mental disorders are brain disorders ... By Congressional proclamation, the 1990s were designated the 'Decade of the Brain'... that decade marked an end to a three-century division between mind and brain. Increasingly, the most complex aspects of the mind were being addressed through studies of neural activity ... the focus on

mental activity as neural activity has widened to include a focus on mental disorders as neural disorders [14].

In 1984, Nancy Andreasen, former editor-in-chief of the *American Journal of Psychiatry*, recipient of the National Medal of Science and a host of other awards and honours, published her views in a book entitled *The Broken Brain: The biological revolution in psychiatry*: "Psychiatry is moving from the study of the "troubled mind" to the "broken brain" ... the biological revolution in psychiatry has already occurred" [15, pviii]. This credo is repeated throughout the book:

> The person who wants to discover the causes of major mental illnesses... must proceed from a medical model and assume they are diseases (p 151-52) ... Mental illness is truly a nervous breakdown – a breakdown that occurs when the nerves of the brain have an injury so severe that their own internal healing capacities cannot repair it (p 219) ... The various forms of mental illness are due to many different types of brain abnormalities, including the loss of nerve cells and excesses and deficits in chemical transmission between neurons... (p 221).

The psychiatric geneticist Kenneth Kendler has made similar claims. He believes mental disorders are real and of essentially of the same nature as "classical physical-medical disorders," thus explicable in biological terms [16]. He sees psychiatry as "a legitimate biomedical discipline," its scientific status not in doubt, but psychiatric disorders are "probably inherently multifactorial" which creates problems in understanding "the pathophysiologies of major mental health disorders."

Psychiatrists are not alone in this view. After a long career studying the cellular basis of memory, Nobel Prize-winning neurophysiologist Eric Kandel published two books, including a collection of his papers [17] and his autobiography [18]. He explicitly stated in both that biological reductionism will answer the problems of mind and of psychiatry. The first lines in his autobiography spell this precisely:

> Understanding the human mind in biological terms has emerged as the central challenge for science in the twenty-first century. We want

to understand the biological nature of perception, learning, memory, thought, consciousness, and the limits of free will [18].

It should be clear he was not saying "understand the biological mechanisms of consciousness etc." Throughout his career, Kandel was sympathetic to Freudian psychoanalysis and was sure that what he called "radical reductionism" could provide a solid basis to this theory. He saw no limits to the capacity of biology to explain human behavior. Such statements are liberally scattered throughout both these works:

> ... my insistence that ... biology can transform psychoanalysis into a scientifically grounded discipline [17, pxxi] ... in the near future, neurobiology will address a matter of more general and fundamental importance: the biology of human mental processes... Psychology and psychiatry can illuminate and define for biology the mental functions that need to be studied if we are to have a meaningful and sophisticated understanding of the biology of the human mind [17, p 7] ... to understand behavior, one had to apply to it the same type of radical reductionist approach that had proved so effective in other areas of biology [18, p 236] ... the underlying precept of the new science of mind is that *all* mental processes are biological ... Therefore, any disorder or alteration of those processes must also have a biological basis [18, p 336, his emphasis].

Philosopher Paul Thagard is equally clear as to the nature of mental disorder:

> Psychiatry assumes that mental disorders are as biologically objective as diseases like infections and cancers ... Neuroscience is beginning to provide the biological basis for the view that mental illnesses are just as objectively real as infections, cancers, and other diseases ... Attacks on the objectivity of mental illness will become even more ridiculous if mental illnesses can be effectively classified on the basis of the causal mechanisms that produce them, if these causal mechanisms provide detailed pathways from genetic and environmental conditions to mental symptoms, and if biological understanding paves the way for improved therapies. I expect that

advances in theoretical and experimental neuroscience will satisfy all these requirements [19].

Given all these authorities, we have to ask whether they are correct. Thomas Insel may have had some doubts, but only after he had left NIMH for the greener pastures of Silicon Valley. In an interview, he said:

> I spent 13 years at NIMH really pushing on the neuroscience and genetics of mental disorders, and when I look back on that, I realise that while I think I succeeded at getting lots of really cool papers published by cool scientists at fairly large costs - I think $20 billion - I don't think we moved the needle in reducing suicide, reducing hospitalisations, improving recovery for the tens of millions of people who have mental illness. I hold myself accountable for that [20].

He might, but it won't bring back the money, it won't change any lives, and his concerns about the reality of mental disorder haven't affected psychiatry or slowed the flood of funds toward biological research. Since psychiatrists show no awareness that their chosen program amounts to an ideology of mental disorder and not a science, it behoves us to ask the critical question for them: Is it true that mental disorder can be reduced to brain disorder?

By the dictates of positivism, any questions remaining after reduction to the physical substance of the brain "... are not genuine questions, but meaningless sequences of words ... they look like questions ... but in truth they consist of empty sounds ..." [2]. So far, so neat and satisfyingly clinical, so where is the problem?

The first problem is straightforward: At no stage in human history has any psychiatrist, or psychologist, or neuroscientist, or philosopher, or anybody, written anything that could in any way be taken as a remotely plausible physical account of mental disorder [7]. Given psychiatry's biological aspirations, that step would seem fairly elementary, but it appears to have been overlooked. Without it, Insel's twenty-billion-and-counting positivist research program was built on expectations, hopes and - dare we say it? - unproven metaphysical assumptions.

Fortunately, these assumptions have been analysed at depth by philosopher, Daniel Stoljar, who sounded a serious warning:

> The first thing to say when considering the truth of physicalism is that we live in an overwhelmingly physicalist or materialist intellectual culture ... the standards of argumentation required to persuade someone of the truth of physicalism are much lower than the standards required to persuade someone of its negation. (The point here is a perfectly general one: if you already believe or want something to be true, you are likely to accept fairly low standards of argumentation for its truth) [22].

In a meticulous analysis of physicalism, Stoljar [22] concluded that there is no possible version of the physicalist thesis which is both true and worthy of the name. The claim that the ultimate nature of the universe is physical is either true but boring and of no explanatory value, or an interesting idea that seems helpful but turns out to be wrong. We can therefore take it as read: mental disorder will never be explained by reducing it to the physical substance of the brain.

My case is that the reductionist program is inherently contradictory. Mental function depends on the brain's manipulation of symbols, but symbols cannot be reduced to or explained by their physical substrate just because they cease being symbols [23]. It's like the coins in my pocket: they have a value, but if I try to explain that value by melting them down to the raw metal, they cease being coins. In the absence of any evidence to the contrary, it appears reductionist biological psychiatrists are operating without warrant. *The burden of proof rests upon them.*

The state of theorising in psychiatry: the Biopsychosocial Model

Of the remaining options listed above...

b) It is all a matter of individual psychology
c) It is all a matter of social pathology
d) All of the above in various forms

...only (d) the mixture has any current standing. Those psychiatrists who have not converted to the positivist faith accept that it is important to look at the patient's biology, individual psychology, and social standing. This is known as the biopsychosocial model, attributed to the gastroenterologist George Engel (1913-99) of Rochester, NY.

Engel believed that the prevailing, reductionist "biomedical model" (the one that has never been written) missed important features of illness. Medicine needed a new, holistic model, he believed—one able to incorporate the relevant biological, psychological, and social factors to arrive at a full understanding of the patient's condition. This he named the biopsychosocial (BPS) model and although it was originally intended to replace the biomedical approach, it has largely been adopted by psychiatrists.

I have published extensively on this topic [24, 25, 26] so there is no need to repeat that material. Suffice it to say that large numbers of influential psychiatrists around the world, supported by some equally influential philosophers, believe that the model exists—and is not just helpful to practice, but defines psychiatry as a unique specialty. Without it, psychiatry would struggle to justify itself.

My case is that there is no BPS model, just because Engel didn't write one and nobody else has, either. I have outlined the reasons I think he made such an egregious mistake [25] and it is now up to psychiatry to consider those reasons. Failing to do so leaves psychiatry open to the charge of deception of the profession, of our patients, of the wider public, and of the funding agencies [26]. That should be enough to frighten the profession into a careful examination of the matter but, as the following example shows, it has had no effect.

In an opinion piece, *Looking forward to a decade of the biopsychosocial model*, published in the *British Journal of Psychiatry Bulletin*, philosopher and psychologist Derek Bolton reiterated his previous, very strong support for Engel's BPS model:

> The topic of this article is the biopsychosocial model. My main
> contention is that – notwithstanding doubts as to what exactly it is,

or indeed whether it is anything – there is a coherent account of it, in terms of both applications to particular health conditions and mechanisms with wide application ... The problem that we don't know exactly what the model is naturally gives rise to the worry that it isn't anything, and a decade or so ago this worry was being voiced loudly and clearly by experts in medicine generally and psychiatry in particular ... the biopsychosocial model has to do with many or all types of health conditions, professions and specialties, and so we should hardly expect it to be *simple* [27, p 228; his emphasis].

Because we have "...major new explanatory theories that integrate biopsychosocial factors across very wide ranges of health conditions..." [27, p 229], and lacking any indicators of biological causes of mental disorder, Bolton argued that we should devote the coming decade to studying the role of psychosocial factors, not just in causing and prolonging mental disorder but also their role throughout general medicine. Concerning the absence of formal models in the entire field, he asked: "But ... what exactly is the biomedical model (that Engel had criticised)?" This is important as there is no such model. But, crucially, that's also true of the BPS model. In the matter of psychiatrists misleading themselves due to unstated metaphysical assumptions, one need not go further than this paper (as Bolton is a philosopher, this is actually a case of psychiatrists eagerly publishing misleading material because it suits them).

To begin with, and coming in the same sentence as his admission that it may not exist, Bolton's claim that there is a "coherent account" of the BPS model is not just false but is absurd. Over the years, Bolton has put a great deal of effort into the BPS model. Rather than confronting the longstanding criticism that Engel never wrote his model—because that would ruin the narrative of a caring, empathic psychiatry—Bolton mentions *en passant* there were some minor objections to it ten years previously. The clear implication is that there were no others, and even they didn't amount to much. Instead of dealing with the killer objection (it doesn't exist, and Bolton himself has quoted the 1998 paper that said it doesn't), he switches the focus to all the interesting research that could be done on psychosocial contributors to mental and physical illness.

That's always a good debating move as psychiatrists would much rather hear how their profession is on the verge of a major scientific breakthrough (and, unstated, their social acceptance as real doctors). He, thereby, airbrushes out of the narrative the uncomfortable fact that psychiatry doesn't actually have an articulated model of its subject matter. This raises the very real possibility that psychiatrists do not have the education to distinguish between a scientific model and a wish-fulfilling fantasy — or they are wilfully deceptive [26]. Or both.

Conclusion: Toward a post-positivist psychiatry

Psychiatry is in a bind. Lured into a rigid and dehumanizing positivist worldview, it has hurled itself into basic biological research in the hope of finding something in the brain — a chemical switch, as it were — that can be flipped and — hey, presto! — all will be well. In the process, it has converted itself from what may once have been a caring profession into a sterile production line where "patients" are first classified and then drugged and/or shocked until they stop complaining or stop causing complaints.

This is done entirely without the benefit of a formal model that says, "This is the nature of mind, this is the process by which minds go astray and this is how to correct them." There is no biomedical model, it doesn't exist [7]. Yet billions are spent every year in searching for the "biological causes" of mental disorder, and tens of billions are spent on chemicals to "treat" the disorders. Driven by human desperation, the money keeps rolling into an industry that regards empathy and compassion as silly hangovers from the distant, unscientific past.

Electroconvulsive treatment (ECT) is widely used in the US and in Australia, far more so than in most other countries in the world; the single most important factor in its overuse is the enormous and effortless financial returns it generates [28]. Now, in transcranial magnetic or direct current stimulation, psychiatrists have new avenues of generating similar profits. However, for those relatively few psychiatrists who aren't wedded to the reductionist biological approach, there is the fig leaf of the "biopsychosocial model." Once again, there is no model but this time, psychiatry seems to be taking active steps to conceal that fact. How this will turn out depends on how the general public will react when they learn they've been led astray.

Leaving aside these theoretical considerations, it is true that all this is costing us a lot of money—so where is the benefit? How is society better off because of modern psychiatry? In fact, there is no evidence to suggest the mental health of the country is improving. For a profession that claims to be "evidence-based," this is shocking.

What we are seeing is not a "science of mental disorder"—akin to the science of immunology that gave us Covid vaccines in record times—but an ideology of mental disorder. Instead of open discussion of the theoretical shortcomings of the specialty, we have propaganda pieces such as that by Bolton, published in prestigious journals by a fully complicit editorial staff appointed and actively supported by the most senior figures in the profession. It is exceedingly rare for mainstream journals to publish material critical of their stance; critics can expect to be marginalised, or worse.

That, however, is the reality of psychiatry today: as Buckminster Fuller said, "You never change something by fighting the existing reality. To change something, build a new model that makes the existing model obsolete." A post-positivist psychiatry is long-overdue.

References

1. Hahn H, Neurath O, Carnap R (1929). *The Scientific Conception of the World: The Vienna Circle.* Ernst Mach Society, University of Vienna.

2. Schlick M (1930). Die Wende der Philosophie. *Erkenntnis* 1: 4-11. Translated as *The Turning Point in Philosophy*. Available online.

3. Ryle G (1949). *The Concept of Mind.* London: Hutchinson. Reprinted (1973) Penguin University Books.

4. Holman HR (1976). The 'Excellence' Deception in Medicine. *Hospital Practice*, 11:4, 11-21.

5. Scull A (2022). *Desperate Remedies: Psychiatry and the mysteries of mental illness.* London: Penguin.

6. Guze SB (1992). *Why psychiatry is a branch of medicine.* New York: Oxford University Press.

7. McLaren N (2013). Psychiatry as Ideology. *Ethical Human Psychology and Psychiatry* 15: 7-18.

8. McLaren N (2012). Chapters 12, 13 in *The Mind-Body Problem Explained: The Biocognitive Model for Psychiatry.* Ann Arbor, MI: Future Psychiatry Press.

9. Carrier, R (2005). *Sense and Goodness Without a God: a defence of metaphysical naturalism.* Bloomington, IN: AuthorHouse.

10. Guze SB (1989). Biological psychiatry: is there any other kind? *Psychological Medicine,* 19: 315-323.

11. Kupfer DJ, Kuhl EA, Wuisin L (2013). Psychiatry's integration with medicine: the role of DSM5. *Annual Review of Medicine* 64: 385-92.

12. Insel TR, Cuthbert BN, Garvey M, et al (2010). Research Domain Criteria (RDoC): toward a new classification framework for research on mental disorders. Commentary. *American Journal of Psychiatry,* 167: 748-751.

13. Insel TR (2009). Disruptive insights in psychiatry: transforming a clinical discipline. *Journal of Clinical Investigations* 119: 700–705.

14. Insel TR (2010). Faulty Circuits. *Scientific American* April 2010, p. 45.

15. Andreasen NC (1984). *The Broken Brain: The biological revolution in psychiatry.* New York: Harper and Row.

16. Kendler K (2016). The nature of psychiatric disorders. *World Psychiatry.* 15(1): 5–12.

17. Kandel ER (2005). *Psychiatry, psychoanalysis and the new biology of mind.* Washington, DC: American Psychiatric Publishing.

18. Kandel ER (2006). *In search of memory: the emergence of a new science of mind.* New York: Norton.

19. Thagard P (2008). Mental Illness from the Perspective of Theoretical Neuroscience. *Perspectives in Biology and Medicine,* 51(3): 335-52.

20. Rogers A (2017). Star Neuroscientist Tom Insel Leaves the Google-Spawned Verily for ... a Startup? *Wired Science* May 11 2017.

21. Stoljar D (2021). Physicalism. *Stanford Encyclopedia of Philosophy*. At: https://plato.stanford.edu/entries/physicalism/.

22. Stoljar D (2010). *Physicalism*. Oxford: Routledge.

23. McLaren N (2021). *Natural Dualism and Mental Disorder: The biocognitive model for psychiatry*. London, Routledge.

24. McLaren N (1998). A critical review of the biopsychosocial model. *Australian and New Zealand Journal of Psychiatry*. 32; 86-92.

25. McLaren N (2020). The Biopsychosocial Model: the end of a reign of error. *Ethical Human Psychology and Psychiatry*. 22:71-82.

26. McLaren N (in press). The Biopsychosocial Model and Scientific Deception. *Ethical Human Psychology and Psychiatry*, TBA.

27. Bolton D (2022). Looking forward to a decade of the biopsychosocial model. *British Journal of Psychiatry Bulletin*, 46: 228–232.

28. McLaren N (2017). Electroconvulsive Therapy: A Critical Perspective. *Ethical Human Psychology and Psychiatry* 19: 91-104.

Toward a Post-Positivist Psychiatry: The Biocognitive Model of Mental Disorder

Niall McLaren

Abstract: *In the absence of a formal account of mental disorder, psychiatry lacks the most basic element in any field wishing to be seen as scientific: a model of its subject matter. The problem lies in psychiatry's unthinking embrace of the principles of positivism, which eschew any talk of mental life as "metaphysical." A new model of mental disorder has been proposed, the biocognitive model for psychiatry, which gives a formal account of mind as a rational, emergent phenomenon which can be understood in informational terms. This leads directly to a model of mental disorder, and to an understanding of personality and thence to personality disorder. Mental disorder, in this model, is almost entirely a psychological phenomenon occurring in the setting of a healthy brain. This has profound consequences for our apprehension and treatment of the mentally-troubled in our midst.*

Introduction: Who has the model of mental disorder?

There is growing awareness that the institution of psychiatry serves itself better than it serves the community [e.g. 1, 2]. There are many reasons why this is the case but, as outlined in my prior chapter in this volume, they all devolve to a single point: under the influence of an uncompromising positivism, psychiatrists have never articulated a scientific model of mental disorder.

The point of a model is that it tells you what you should and shouldn't do; without it, you can't claim to know what you are doing. History is full of examples of bad models leading to bad or dangerous practice [3, 4] and not just in psychiatry. General Washington didn't die of malaria; he was bled to death by his physicians who believed that fevers were caused by an excess of hot blood. Given that model of disease, venesection made perfect sense. Its fatal consequences were invariably excused because (a) the doctors did everything they could but (b) obviously the patient had a very bad attack of whatever it was. That is, the patient let the doctors down.

Driven by the ideological belief that the patient's biological state tells us all we need to know, psychiatry dismisses problems of mental life as irrelevant [5]. Why does this happen? Because a model doesn't only tell you what you should and shouldn't do—it also tells you what observations are "solid evidence" and what must be discarded as meaningless. Convinced that mind can be reduced to brain, psychiatry threw itself on the biological bus, thereafter refusing to consider that "mere mental stuff" could cause mental disorder.

That this vastly expensive project is going nowhere is dismissed by the "true believers" who run psychiatry today. Their response to suggestions of failure is always "More of the same: more researchers, more laboratories, more and bigger machines." Their efforts would be better directed at trying to develop a reductionist model of "mental disorder as biology" because the effort would tell them it can't be done. That does not, however, mean adopting an eclectic or "biopsychosocial" model, because that just licences "anything goes" [6] and we're back to where we started.

Because the positivist approach has failed, I have proposed a novel alternative: the biocognitive model [7]. Unlike the existing *approaches* (not models)—loosely, "biomedical" and "biopsychosocial," which start with preconceptions as to the nature of mental disorder—the biocognitive model starts with first principles. It asks: What is the nature of the human animal such that we can experience mental disorder? This leads to a dualist concept, but a natural dualism—not the classic or Cartesian substance dualism which is so widely derided by positivists (e.g. throughout [8]).

The new dualism says that the universe consists of two realms: the familiar realm of matter and energy interacting in a time-space matrix, and another, so familiar that we don't see it, of information. Unlike any previous theories in psychiatry, the biocognitive model relies on a theory of information, the lack of which propelled the early positivists into their doctrinaire position that if we can't measure it, it doesn't exist. By these means, they dismissed the critical informational element in human life (experienced as mentality) and tried to turn us into "biological critters."

Since it is causally efficacious, information is real but also insubstantial and unlocalised. From this, we have to construct an integrative theory of body and mind to provide a formal basis for a model of mental disorder. However, in order to avoid the hand-waving so common among positivists [8], every step on the way has to be spelled out in detail. That this has never been done in psychiatry is established fact: the "biopsychosocial model" consists of just three words with no further development while the "biomedical model" has never been written. By contrast, the biocognitive model consists (so far) of 80,000 words. What follows is a very brief summary of that work.

The biocognitive model: constructing an integrative psychiatry

We start with the irrefutable evidence of our senses: I look outside and see green trees against a blue sky, yet there is nothing green or blue inside my head. I taste chilli, and it is something that chocolate is not; I am amused, but pain is not a joke. These things must be explained, not dismissed as "unscientific" or explained away, as Dennett tries to do [8, p 220].

For dualism, the problem has always been how to get sensory experience from the body to the mind and, then, behavioral instructions back from mind to body. The clue is to rephrase the problem to read: How does information get from sensory receptors to brain, thence to mind, and back again to the effector organs? In principle, the resolution is simple: If the mind is itself an informational state, then there is no discontinuity between the information coursing through the body and a mental state.

The information carried in an afferent nerve doesn't leave the physical world and jump into a supernatural world, as naive positivists believe [8], but it transits the data processing systems of the brain as information, and is then despatched to the effector systems, still as information. In order to make sense of this, we need a theory of information.

There are two problems in talking of a theory of information. The first is that, as Luciano Floridi glumly concludes, we don't have one:

> The concept of information has become central in most contemporary philosophy. However, recent surveys have shown no consensus on a single, unified definition of semantic information. This is hardly surprising. Information is such a powerful and elusive concept... [9, p 351]

His more recent primer on information offers descriptions of information at work but does not define it. Even his major work, entitled *The Philosophy of Information*, says only: "Information is still an elusive concept" [10, p 30].

The second problem stems from what appears to be an historical error. Most people believe that, yes, we do have a theory of information—it comes from The Father of Information Theory, Claude Shannon. This is incorrect. As the title of his book makes perfectly clear, Shannon wrote a *mathematical theory of communication*. He was very careful to say what can be *done* with information but not what it *is*:

> The fundamental problem of communication is that of reproducing at one point either exactly or approximately a message selected at another point. Frequently the messages have meaning; that is, they refer to or are correlated according to some system with certain physical or conceptual entities. These semantic aspects of communication are *irrelevant* to the engineering problem [11, emphasis added].

Shannon's concern was how to shove data down a tube while ensuring that what emerged at the other end accurately recreated what had gone in. As an engineer, he wasn't concerned with what went into the tube, be it philosophy or pornography (engineers are like that)—only its accuracy. The entire IT revolution is based on what you can *do* with information (and how much money you can make from it), not on the idea of what information *is*. A theory of mind based in information, however, needs a non-circular account of what information actually *is*, for which we turn to history.

In 1847, a largely self-taught and unknown English mathematician working in the remote town of Cork, in the far south of Ireland, published a small pamphlet titled *A Mathematical Analysis of Logic*. At the age of just 32 years,

George Boole (1815-64) outlined the revolutionary notion of translating logic into a mathematical form. Boole wanted to show that reasoning (the process of using logical methods to reach valid conclusions) is non-metaphysical in nature and, as an independent and universal science, could therefore be reframed in a mathematical notation that anybody could learn and apply. Over the next seven years, he developed his project, publishing it in 1854 as *An Investigation of the Laws of Thought* [12].

Boole's "science of logic" was based on the notion of a *dual-valued calculus*, originally developed by Gottfried Leibniz (1646-1716). A calculus (Latin for stone) is defined as *any formal system in which symbolic expressions are manipulated according to fixed rules*. His "Laws of Thought" are the laws governing a dual-valued calculus, most of which he derived and proved himself. Insofar as human thought can undertake any process of reasoning, he said, it must rely *in some sense* on the fundamental logical rules that he described. That is, the laws of logic are also the laws of reasoning or thought.

Early in the twentieth century, logicians formalised the concept of truth tables, a means of setting out the logical relationships between two or more propositions as they are subjected to different logical operations (all according to Boole's laws, generally known as Boolean algebra). Truth tables are important for two reasons. Firstly, they again show that the processes of logic are essentially very ordinary mechanical steps with no room for imagination. Schoolboys can learn them, so logic is no longer the exclusive domain of Olympian intellects—and the egos that often go with them. Second, the laws governing truth functors are not *physical* laws. Logic exists in a semantic world, or world of meaning (the bit that *didn't* interest Shannon), entirely separate from the material realm of physics and thermodynamics, etc. Most importantly, semantic laws cannot be reduced to physical laws, a point which is fatal to attempts to reduce mind (including mental disorder) to brain. These concepts are critically important in arriving at a natural dualist theory of mind.

Moving ahead, in 1936 a young British mathematician published a forbiddingly complex paper in which he outlined the essential principles of machine-based intelligence. Alan Turing worked on the Enigma project during World War II but continued his research post-war, asking in 1950 whether machines can think [13]. His answer was that it doesn't matter—it's good enough if they can fool us. In this paper, he showed that any question can be reduced to such simple steps that a machine could answer just by choosing between two options. Intelligence, he argued, is not magic, a point which has long eluded positivists. Shannon had already shown that simple electrical relays could mimic the input-output states of truth tables, producing what we now know as logic gates [14]. This meant that a proven physical basis for intelligent operations existed and could be built in any factory.

The biocognitive model [7] proposes that logic gates encoded in the cell walls of neurons convert each neuron into a microprocessor, able to implement the logical processes outlined by Boole 175 years ago. Information coded into afferent neurons as spike impulses enters the computational systems of the brain to be manipulated by coded instructions. A decision is reached and is despatched, still coded in the form of neuronal spike impulses, to the effector organs, whatever they are. There is no disjunction between informational input, computation, and output; they are in the same form, but the significance changes, depending on where they are and, above all, by the different forms of connector neurons.

During the process of computation, a range of sensory experiences emerges, each unique to the part of the brain subserving it. This is postulated as a matter of coding, but it is highly unlikely that we will ever know the nature of the codes as there is no conceivable input-output "port" through which they can be read. This says that mind is an emergent process of brain computation, which satisfies the criteria of Descartes' "thinking substance" but, critically, gives an internal structure to its actions so they no longer come across as magic. They are simply Boole's Laws of Thought in action. This is central to the model.

Philosopher David Chalmers has long championed the idea of a natural dualism [15]. He proposed that the mind supervenes upon the brain structure and functions by psychophysical laws that we can potentially understand. Chalmers has not elaborated on his proposed laws of supervenience but, at this stage, it appears Boole's laws of binary algebra (logic) meet the conditions he has proposed [7, Chapters 4-6]. From this formulation, we see an essential point which eluded the early positivists: the difference between the informational "machinery" which constitutes the mind, common to all humans (and certainly many other animals), and the informational content unique to each individual which cannot be gainsaid.

Positivism conflated all brain-based information. Instead of distinguishing clearly between the informational mechanism of mind, and the information it was acting on, they dumped the lot as "meaningless metaphysics." I cannot emphasise this point enough. It is legitimate to talk of the mental mechanisms just as it is legitimate to discuss theorems, or plans or design specifications, or systems of laws, etc, as these are closed systems and, thus, amenable to "logical analysis," whereas the *products* of mind (fiction, fantasy, paranoid political beliefs etc) as open (unlimited) systems are not.

Thus emerges an integrative model of the mind as a causally-efficacious and wholly mental entity that *cannot be reduced* to the brain. This has profound significance for psychiatry, as a model of this nature leads directly to models of personality (and thence of personality disorder), and to a concept of mental disorder as a primary disturbance of psychological function in a perfectly healthy brain. In the absence of any remotely plausible account of mental disorder as a disorder of the physical brain, the concept of a "chemical imbalance of the brain" is exposed as a pseudo-explanation, a misleading trope in the same dangerous class as the idea of "hot blood" causing the fevers of malaria.

The biocognitive model of personality

It must not be forgotten that mainstream psychiatry does not have a model of personality or personality disorder. It has a categorical classification (the DSM and ICD systems), but a classification is not a model.

The notion that we can distinguish between an informational mechanism and the content it processes is now basic to our way of life: there is an informational *mechanism* called Facebook (usually called software) which operates on a physical mechanism, called hardware. Finally, there is all the *content* that people load. In the brain, we have the physical cerebral mechanism ("wetware"), the informational (mental) mechanism called the mind, and, finally, the content of each person's mind. Biological reductionists, including psychiatrists, want to conflate the two entirely different forms of mechanism—the neuronal and the informational—to say they are one and the same thing. Most emphatically, they are not.

We have innate cognitive processes, common to all humans and, therefore, innate cognitive biases, which are a separate subject. But we are individuals, otherwise known as personalities. A very large part of the processing system consists of rules acquired by life experience. Many of these form common systems, such as the rules of language, but the rest are the product of the individual's unique experiences. These amount to the personality, defined as:

> Personality is the *total set* of explicit and implicit mental rules (including attitudes, beliefs, etc) that, in the stable adult mode of behavior, *generates* the uniquely distinguishing habitual patterns of interaction between healthy, sober individuals and their environments [7, Chap. 8].

Because rules and their outcome vary dimensionally, the idea that we can build a categorical classification of personality disorder is shown to be false. If an individual's rules are internally consistent and work harmoniously with the rules of the larger society, we say that person has a normal personality. If the rules are internally inconsistent or contradictory, thereby generating erratic behavior and/or persistent emotional distress and/or repeatedly bring the individual into conflict with the larger society, then that is personality disorder.

As the product of the individual's total life experiences, mainly early but also later, personality is entirely a matter of psychology. This is also true of the post-traumatic conditions in which an experience of massive psychological stressors during adolescence or adulthood can change the individual's fundamental belief system for the worse. That is to say, what is now called "PTSD" is not a "mental disease caused by brain damage"; it is a personality change which leads to damaging emotional and behavioral outcomes. For example, from seeing the world as a pleasant, helpful sort of place, the victim now sees the world and its occupants as dangerous and destructive, and reacts accordingly. That is not an illness in any convincing sense of the word, and drugs and other physical treatments can be no more than briefly helpful in acute cases.

While acute distress can respond to certain classes of drugs, personality disorder itself cannot be treated by drugs. Any directed treatment will have to be a form of cooperative psychotherapy, just because nothing else can work. However, due to its inability to treat a major factor in mental disturbance, mainstream psychiatry is engaged in a huge program of re-diagnosing people with a primary personality disorder as mentally ill and, therefore, able to be drugged [16, Chapters 14-16]. While failing to deal with the primary problem, drugs produce an iatrogenic disturbance which leads to further treatment, and so the process becomes self-sustaining—and immensely profitable to drug companies and psychiatrists.

Mental disorder in the biocognitive model

How many times do people have to search for the Loch Ness Monster before they finally admit it doesn't exist? In any information-processing system, errors are highly likely. The first and most obvious type is at the level of the physical system that implements the data processing—in this case, the brain. After nearly a century of diligent search costing untold billions, biological psychiatry has produced not a single interesting cause or biomarker of mental disorder [17]. The biocognitive model says that mental disorder, including the most damaging forms, can and does arise in a perfectly healthy brain entirely as the result of psychological causes. However, biological psychiatrists can't admit defeat because theirs is an ideological crusade, not science [18].

The next level is the informational processing mechanism itself, the settings of the logic gates, as it were. The logic gates are fine. There is nothing wrong with them—they just aren't set for optimal benefit. That is the result of learning, of early childhood experiences producing a distorted perception of the world and the self. In particular, the biocognitive model sees anxiety as the basis of practically all mental disturbance [19].

If, as a result of early life experiences, a person has a poor self-perception ("I'm ugly and stupid and nobody could possibly like me"), then this will necessarily lead to repeated hurts and rejections, even if they weren't intended that way. That will lead to anxiety, withdrawal, loss of social supports, failure and then to recurrent depression and/or drug and alcohol abuse and/or everything else and, finally, even to suicide. All mental events have a mental cause, not a physical cause; it is the job of the psychiatrist or therapist to find them and deal with them, not bury them under a flood of psychoactive chemicals.

Finally, there is the level of disordered informational input. The person gets the wrong idea and reacts accordingly, but this causes trouble with the surroundings. However, people believe what they want to believe: out of the range of possibilities, they choose the interpretation that fits with their prior belief system [5, Chap. 11], so this level of error very often devolves to an error at the level of the coded rules that comprise the personality.

For example, a person may believe that his hero was cheated of the election; that goes back to a deep-seated mistrust of authority and a firm conviction that there is always more going on behind the scenes than is being released (in other words, a conspiracy). In turn, this goes back to being brought up by parents who lied and cheated and were always concealing things. With a proper explanatory model, mental disorder makes sense.

The notion of levels of disturbance is complicated by feedback systems, the chief of which is physiological arousal; that is, the difference between being drowsy or alert. The biocognitive model places great emphasis on this concept. Because of their belief systems, people can quickly become over-aroused, which produces cognitive distortions, errors in its own right, and leads to loss of sleep. Lack of sleep can cause sensory malfunctions, perceived as hallucinations, which further intensify the arousal.

This is the basis of the biocognitive concept of mental disorder as a self-reinforcing loop of agitation producing more and more disturbance until the individual loses contact with reality. Highly agitated people are not amenable to psychological intervention until the agitation is settled and they can explain what has happened and begin to understand it themselves. However, psychotherapy is the mainstay of management. Psychosis requires a modification of the model, but the principle remains the same: the specific disturbances seen in a psychotic state can be adequately explained as the predictable outcome of a range of psychological factors affecting a dualist interactional (mind-body) system.

Civil detention

In his final report to the UN Human Rights Commission, Special Rapporteur Prof. Dainius Puras pointed to the excessive reliance of mental health services worldwide on involuntary custodial management of the mentally disturbed using physical and chemical means [20]. Without ever having broken a law, the mentally troubled are subjected to measures that would not be tolerated in any other section of the community. Just on the basis of mental disturbance of whatever cause, a person can be forcibly detained; taken to a mental hospital; stripped of all possessions, civil rights and dignity; injected with unknown chemicals by unknown people; locked in a single room indefinitely; denied visitors; forcibly subjected to involuntary ECT; and generally treated far worse than any convicted murderer.

Most citizens in most countries have only a vague idea that this still goes on. What they don't know is that this practice is devoid of any form of medical, legal, social, or ethical justification, yet it persists in our midst [21]. Periodically, a detained person dies by suicide or by neglect; these cases attract very little publicity but if a mentally disturbed person commits a crime, the media have a field day. What this says is that, despite repeated government assurances that the mentally troubled will be "treated with the respect and consideration they need and deserve," underneath, nothing really changes.

The biocognitive model does not offer any support for these practices. Governments who wish to justify them must look elsewhere than science.

Conclusion

Newton's first law of motion states: "A body remains at rest, or in motion at a constant speed in a straight line, unless acted upon by a force." This is true not just of physical bodies, but also of human social systems. This is especially the case when influential people are benefiting from the existing social system, such as making lots of money or gaining power they wouldn't otherwise have.

In the case of mental disorder, the present system will continue to roll along because the people making money from it are making a very great deal of money; the people who enjoy power because of it have essentially unlimited power; and the people who lose from it are denied their civil right to protest by the very people who are profiting from their deprived status. This will not change until the world becomes aware of the fact that psychiatry is operating without a theoretical warrant, and a new model of mental disorder takes its place. The biocognitive model of mind for psychiatry is the first entirely novel model since Freud, and the first articulated integrationist model of mind and body in medicine.

References

1. Whitaker R, Cosgrove L (2015). *Psychiatry Under the Influence: Institutional Corruption, Social Injury, and Prescriptions for Reform.* New York: Palgrave MacMillan.

2. McLaren N (2017). Electroconvulsive Therapy: A Critical Perspective. *Ethical Human Psychology and Psychiatry* 19: 91-104.

3. Scull A (2022). *Desperate Remedies: Psychiatry and the mysteries of mental illness.* London: Penguin.

4. Harrington A (2020). *Mind Fixers: Psychiatry's Troubled Search for the Biology of Mental Illness.* New York: Norton.

5. McLaren N (In press). *Charting the Labyrinth: Theories in Psychiatry.* Ann Arbor, MI: Future Psychiatry Press.

6. McLaren N (1996). The myth of eclecticism. *Australasian Psychiatry*; 4: 260-61.

7. McLaren N (2021). *Natural Dualism and Mental Disorder: The biocognitive model for psychiatry.* London, Routledge.

8. Dennett DC (1991). *Consciousness Explained.* Boston: Little Brown. Page numbers refer to the Penguin edition (1993).

9. Floridi L (2005). Is Semantic Information Meaningful Data? *Philosophy and Phenomenological Research* 70:(2): 351-71

10. Floridi, L (2011). *The Philosophy of Information*. Oxford: University Press.

11. Shannon CE (1948). A Mathematical Theory of Communication. *Bell System Technical Journal* 27: 379–423, 623–656 (July, October).

12. Boole G (1854). *An Investigation of the Laws of Thought, on which are Founded the Mathematical Theories of Logic and Probabilities.* Dover Classics of Science and Mathematics. New York: Dover. Also available through Google Books.

13. Turing AM (1950). Computing machinery and intelligence. *Mind*; 59: 433-60.

14. Shannon CE. "A Symbolic Analysis of Relay and Switching Circuits," unpublished MS Thesis, Massachusetts Institute of Technology, Aug. 10, 1937.

15. Chalmers DJ (1996). *The Conscious Mind: in search of a fundamental theory.* Oxford: University Press.

16. McLaren N (2012). *The Mind-Body Problem Explained: The Biocognitive Model for Psychiatry.* Ann Arbor, MI: Future Psychiatry Press.

17. Kingdon D (2020). Why hasn't neuroscience delivered for psychiatry? *BJPsych Bulletin,* 44:107–109.

18. McLaren N (2013). Psychiatry as Ideology. *Ethical Human Psychology and Psychiatry* 15: 7-19.

19. McLaren N (2018). *Anxiety: The Inside Story.* Ann Arbor, MI: Future Psychiatry Press.

20. Puras D (2020). UN Human Rights Council. Report of the Special Rapporteur on the right of everyone to the enjoyment of the highest attainable standard of physical and mental health. UNHRC Document A /HRC/44/48. Final report: July 16th 2020, UN Doc. A/75/163.

21. Wipond R (2023). *Your Consent is Not Required: the rise in psychiatric detentions, forced treatment, and abusive guardianships.* Dallas, TX: BenBella Books.

There's Nothing as Practical as a Good Theory: Trouble is, it's Hard to Find a Good Theory

Timothy A. Carey and Robert Griffiths

Abstract: *People who like to help others might think spending time understanding theories of behaviour and helping is not a good use of their time. We disagree. Our position is that everyone has a theory about things like why they do what they do. Even the most strident non-theorists can provide some explanation about why they used this technique at that time with that particular individual. We think, however, that, by and large, the theories that relate to behaviour, mental health, contentment, and well-being aren't very good theories. And that's a problem. We are in complete agreement that people should not spend time acquainting themselves with poor theories. In fact, we would advocate avoiding poor practices as well as substandard theories. A good theory, however, enables you to be more targeted in the helping practices you adopt and more effective and efficient in the help you provide. In this chapter, we will explain a theory which we think is a better-than-good theory. This is a robust, scientific explanation of life as it is being lived. We will explain why that is important and provide some indications of what it means for our helping practices. When people's practices are informed by the principles of an accurate explanation that is consistent with other facts we have established about our physical and social world, the help that is offered might become much more helpful so that people experience less torment and anguish for shorter periods of time leading to contentment and social harmony on a much grander scale.*

Introduction

To many people, theories are boring. Mention the word "theory" and people can quickly find some other urgent tasks that needs their attention. It's common for people to claim that they don't need to understand how something works in order to use it effectively. Lots of people drive cars, for example, without in-depth knowledge of how an internal combustion engine works. People use computers and the internet without understanding all the intricacies involved.

For the most part, we agree with the general consensus about theories. Many theories are boring or incomprehensible or impossibly detailed and complex or all of these things at once. And lots and lots of theories about people and the complexities of social living are completely nonfunctional. What we mean is, they don't work. And not only do they not work, but they also can't be made to work without fundamentally changing them.

What does it mean to say a theory "works"? Well, we think of a theory as a kind of a story about why something occurs the way it does. The theory of plate tectonics, for example, explains the way the landscape is shaped into the forms it takes based on the result of movements below the Earth's surface. The "working" aspects of the theory are the mechanisms it suggests as responsible for propelling bits of the earth in various directions. The theory integrates different pieces of evidence and builds models that simulate the way the theory suggests landforms arise.

When we discuss this kind of subject matter, we use the terms "theory" and "model" to refer to slightly different things. We think a theory is a succinct statement that explains how and why something occurs the way it does. And we think of a model as an expression of that statement that puts the ideas conveyed in the statement into action. Essentially, a theory states how something might occur, and a model shows how something does occur according to the specifications of the theory.

With regard to psychological distress, we think a good and useful theory should provide a plausible account of how it arises and how it is resolved. Our standard of plausibility means we think the narrative about psychological distress should be consistent with other generally accepted explanations about the world we live in. We would regard attributing the manifestation of psychological distress to misdemeanours from a past life as implausible because the topic of past lives is not consistent with other generally accepted explanations of human functioning. A theory of past lives would not fit snugly into the network of facts and ideas that are already well established with regard to human form and function.

To use this theory would mean having to ignore or dismiss a large body of well-regarded information. That doesn't mean we shouldn't do it, but it does mean there would need to be very compelling reasons for taking this approach and there must not be a better alternative available. From our perspective, there is a much better alternative that is readily available.

The Importance of Theories

So why might it be important to understand how something works? Well, for the most part, as we suggested with the car example, it isn't important to understand how something works. It only becomes important to understand how something works when that something isn't working the way it's supposed to. When your car isn't motoring as you would like it to, if you want to rectify this it is essential to find someone who knows about the mechanical goings on of your auto.

Similarly, our ability to organise large amounts of plastic, metal, fabric, and other material into a form that flies through the air like a bird only came about when some very clever people figured out how gravity, aerodynamics, and other important aspects of physics worked. Working out how things work is an absolute must if you want to be able to fix things or improve things systematically.

The word "systematically" is important here. If your car broke down and you had lots of time and money, you could perhaps invite people from your community to suggest various activities to fix it. Sooner or later, it might be the case that someone happened to turn the right bit or change the broken part so that your vehicle started humming again. Generally, people don't have lots of time and money. When something is not working in the way that people would like, they would usually prefer to have it fixed sooner rather than later.

If you're as good at helping others as you like to be, then what we discuss here probably won't have any benefit for you or be of interest to you. We like to continually reflect on our practice and identify areas in which we could improve. To that end, we have found a sturdy, scientific theory to be invaluable in helping our work get better and better. For people who would like to reflect on their helping practices with a view to making adjustments as and when they are required, the information we provide here might be of some benefit.

So, we think a good theory is expressed in such a way that models can be built that simulate the thing the theory is explaining. Unfortunately, current theories of behaviour are not that kind of a theory. Most behaviour theories, or any other theory of human activity, are guesses about the way something might arise, but no models based on these hunches are ever built to simulate the thing that is being explained and to test the theoriser's theorising.

Some of these theories even refer to "mechanisms" but the mechanisms that are described are not mechanistic in the sense of making any tangible or physical thing happen. In a recent systematic review, for example, we tried to identify whether any functional mechanisms have been proposed that seek to explain how psychotherapy works (Carey et al., 2020). Such a theory would explain the mechanisms through which psychotherapy helps people feel less distressed by their problems. Unfortunately, we were unable to find any mechanisms that were described in functional terms.

Even when there is good evidence that theories are wrong, many people still subscribe to them. For decades, people have tried and failed to find credible evidence for the chemical imbalance theory of psychological distress, yet it continues to be an explanation that people use. Almost as soon as it was first proposed, the idea that problems we might call "depression" or "schizophrenia" were caused by an imbalance of brain chemicals was considered to be highly implausible. The lack of evidence for this idea has not acted as an impediment to its widespread dissemination (Ang et al., 2022; Moncrieff, 2009; Moncrieff et al., 2022).

The explanations that give rise to labels such as depression and schizophrenia are also highly dubious (Timimi, 2014), but regardless of their shortcomings, these explanations have been tremendously influential. Unfortunately, in many ways, these less than adequate explanations have created problems in addition to any they may have solved. In fact, the main problem they may have solved is how pharmaceutical companies can steeply increase their profits (Healy, 2012).

To reiterate, many theories of human life are not scientific explanations in the sense of being expressed in such a way that models can be built to simulate the phenomena being explained. We think this is a problem because it means that when there are difficulties with human life—when day-to-day-living is not proceeding in the way that is desired—we can only correct it serendipitously. Without a systematic approach, it is likely that many difficulties persist for much longer than they otherwise might. A different kind of theory would allow us to tackle problems systematically rather than serendipitously.

We know a theory that we think is different in the way we have been describing. The theory is Perceptual Control Theory (PCT), and, for us, it is a theory worth paying attention to.

Perceptual Control Theory

Perceptual Control Theory, or PCT, was developed by the renowned American medical physicist and control systems engineer, William (Bill) T. Powers (Powers, 2005). Perhaps Bill's approach to testing theories by building models was shaped by his background in physics. For Bill, a model was something that simulates or mimics the thing it is a model of. A model of behaviour, for example, should be able to produce the behaviour it is supposed to be explaining.

The standard activity for testing PCT is a tracking task in which a person sits in front of a computer screen and uses the computer mouse to keep a little vertical line matched up to another little vertical line. At the same time that the person is controlling the position of the line, a computer program is also affecting the position of the line so that if the person did not move the mouse at all, the line would just wander horizontally backwards and forwards across the screen according to the specifications of the computer program.

When the person uses the mouse to control the line on the computer screen, a record of the person's actions is collected and then the PCT model simulates those actions. PCT is such an accurate theory that the model simulates the behaviour very, very closely. There is typically an extremely high correlation between the behaviour and the model. When we say "extremely high," we mean correlations like 0.99! You can try out these PCT activities for yourself at the website www.mindreadings.com/demos.htm

Such an accurate explanation of behaviour has some lessons which we have found extremely useful in our work helping people achieve greater contentment and well-being—and living a life they value. For now, we will focus on one of the lessons we think is most valuable. The references we provide will be good sources to find out about more of these ideas.

Behaviour à la PCT

PCT explains that there is a "relativity" to life. Knowing about this relativity can be useful when thinking about the causes of behaviour and understanding why problems happen when they do. In fact, PCT upends the way we generally think about causality. Before we explain and explore the relativity dimension and what it means for how we understand causality, however, it first might be helpful to outline the PCT idea of behaviour.

Although the word "behaviour" is used freely in both the scientific and non-scientific literature, it has been devilishly difficult to define accurately and precisely. We won't spend time discussing all the difficulties and complexities there are in clarifying exactly what is meant by the term, but we think PCT offers a helpful perspective. PCT suggests there are three elements to all behaviour: perception, comparison, and action (Powers, 1998). These elements are processes that are all happening simultaneously all the time. We could just have easily written them as: comparison, action, perception or action, perception, comparison. The general idea is that, for any behaviour to occur, we have to be able to: *perceive* certain things, *compare* what we perceive to what we want to perceive, and *act* to make what we perceive match and keep matching what we want to perceive.

Some examples might help to illustrate. Think about the behaviour of driving. To drive your car along the road, you have to be able to *perceive* where your car is, how close it is to other cars, how fast it's going, and so on. You have to be able to *compare* where your car is right now (and every other right now that follows) with where you want it to be. And you have to be able to *act* in order to keep where your car is right now matching what you have in mind for where it should be. If we stopped one of these—let's say, you shut your eyes or took your hands off the steering wheel—your driving behaviour would quickly halt!

We could also think of something mundane like baking a cake. To bake a cake, you have to be able to *perceive* the ingredients, *compare* the state of the ingredients at the moment with the state you want them to be in, and *act* to make the state they are in and the state they should be in be the same state.

The Big Deal About Behaviour

Spending time understanding behaviour from the PCT perspective can provide some very helpful insights for how we go about living our lives. For example, the PCT account of behaviour suggests that our familiar ideas about cause and effect don't really apply in a straightforward way. Suppose a car in front of you suddenly brakes. Does that event, sudden braking, *make* you take action? We suspect if we asked a lot of people that question, just about everyone would say something like, "Of course it does! They braked, so I had to brake!".

We would say "not so fast!" If we use the *perceive-compare-act* lens, we would explain that when the car in front braked, you perceived the brake lights coming on and the car getting much closer to you than you wanted it to, so you acted to keep the distance between you and the car ahead how you wanted it to be. From this point of view, your action arose from what was happening in the environment (the car in front braking suddenly) *and also* your goal of maintaining a certain distance between you and the car in front. Both the event and your goal *are jointly and equally responsible* for your action.

If you had a different goal—let's say, for some reason you want to create a car crash—then you would take different action. Every action, all the time, is just one part of the process of people making their worlds be the way they want them to be and keeping them that way. Our actions are always connected to a goal from inside a person *and* events from outside the person. The point of any action is to keep perceptions of what is going on outside matching what your inside goals and plans say *should* be going on. It is this joint effect that makes it very difficult to ever pinpoint specific causes of behaviour. What we think might have caused a behaviour for one person will have a different impact on another person in a different environment with different goals.

The PCT explanation allows us to understand why the same apparent "cause," such as the car in front braking suddenly, doesn't have exactly the same effect for different people. This is not really the way the physical world is supposed to work. If you push on a rock, or some other inanimate object, the rock moves in direct proportion to the force you apply to it given its mass. If you push on a person, however, the response is not so straightforward. The person might push back, run away, double the force that you applied to them in return, or snuggle in closer for a bit more contact. How the person responds depends on the impact the push has on the goal states the person cares about. Rocks don't care if they're pushed. People do.

A Little Bit About Causality

In society at the moment, we are brought up to think that some things cause other things. Often, the language isn't as straightforward as A causes B, but the general pattern is still there. For example, we're told that red meat leads to cancer or high cholesterol results in heart disease or food additives produce hyperactivity. The list goes on. We can also find statements that suggest that reading to your child means they will do well at school or delaying gratification means you'll end up being more successful.

The idea of a neat path from cause to effect is even reflected in popular cultural mythologies and other beliefs. If you're a good boy or girl, for example, Santa Claus will bring you gifts at Christmas time. And if you live a good life, then you'll go to heaven when you die. Although it's nice and simple to think in this way, as we indicated at the end of the previous section, PCT informs us that when it comes to the behaviour of living things, this particular way of thinking isn't right. At best, it's incomplete.

For people, causality is a circle not a straight line. Whenever an event happens, there is always something going on before that event and there is always something occurring after the event. When a child is bullied in the school playground, there were circumstances occurring before the bullying event. The child didn't just magically happen to be in that specific place in the playground at that particular time. And there are always things going on after the event. The reason this is important is because bullying will be experienced differently by different children.

From a PCT perspective, the problem with bullying is that it upends certain aspects of a person's world. If you're a child, bullying might disrupt your sense of safety or confidence or even your worth as a person. If you're an adult being bullied at work, it might be your career aspirations that are being shattered. On the other hand, being bullied could be a student's way of getting other students into trouble or getting to spend more time with a teacher they admire. This is not at all to imply that victims of bullying contrive to be bullied. Our only suggestion here is that being bullied is not the same experience for all those who are bullied.

In order to help someone who is being bullied in a way that they find helpful, we have to know what aspects of their world are being trampled on. In what way is bullying a problem? What does being bullied mean to them? It depends. It depends what aspect of the bullied person's life is being disturbed. There is a relativity to living that is fundamentally important but easily overlooked. Does money cause happiness? It depends. Do adverse childhood experiences cause mental health problems? It depends.

It Depends: Some Implications of the Relativity of Life

Keeping in mind the relativity of living through the "it depends" slogan helps us remember the importance of perspective when we are helping others. The question of "when is helping, helping?" really comes down to perspective. If we interact with others in a way that they don't find helpful, then what we are doing is not helping regardless of what our intentions are. PCT is a theory of living from a first-person perspective rather than from an observer perspective. From a PCT point of view, it makes sense to adopt a framework of "patient-perspective care" rather than the more familiar "patient-centred care" (Carey, 2017).

Anamorphosis is a technique used in the visual arts whereby an image will appear distorted or abstract unless it is viewed from a specific perspective.

One of the most famous examples of anamorphic art was produced by the Swiss painter, Hans Holbein the Younger (c. 1497-1543). His painting "The Ambassadors" is a double portrait that features an apparently distorted image placed between the two subjects. Viewed from a certain angle, however, the distorted image reveals itself to be a depiction of a skull.

We think that there are parallels here with the ways that mental health services approach their work with people experiencing psychological distress. Within these services, there is often a question of whose perspective is prioritised, particularly when there is disagreement about the best course of action to be taken. What service should the patient be referred to? When should someone be discharged from acute mental health inpatient services? What medications should someone be prescribed and in what form should they be administered? How many sessions of psychological therapy should someone receive? And who should make that decision?

Frequently, it appears to be the case that decisions about what support is offered and how that support should be delivered are made by practitioners working within mental health services, and the views and preferences of patients are deprioritised or entirely overlooked. We think it would be useful to give some examples to illustrate what we mean when we say that patients' perspectives are often deprioritised.

This is by no means an exhaustive list. There are many other examples we could have highlighted. One example is that within mental health services, practitioners frequently discuss their perception of a patient's level of "insight." What appears to be meant by the term insight is the extent to which the patient recognises and accepts that they have a "mental illness" (Osatuke et al., 2008; Thirouioux et al., 2019). In practical terms, decisions about a patient's level of insight really have to do with the extent to which they agree and comply with the practitioner.

The argument seems to follow that rejecting the label of "mental illness" is an indication of a lack of insight, which is itself further evidence that the patient does, indeed, have a mental illness. Rejecting the "mental illness" label, therefore, is both evidence of and a product of a lack of insight. This is the kind of logic that readers of Lewis Carroll's Alice in Wonderland might find eerily familiar. What this approach to conceptualising insight does not take into account is the plethora of views that exist regarding how we understand the nature of mental health and psychological distress. It instead places a great deal of emphasis on the perspective of the practitioner and seems to give very little regard to the patient's views on the matter.

Another example would be the use of outcome measures that are completed from the practitioner's perspective. The Global Assessment of Functioning (GAF) Scale is a widely used assessment of the severity of patients' difficulties in the domains of social, psychological, and occupational functioning (Pedersen et al., 2018). It asks the practitioner to make judgments about whether the patient's symptoms are mild, moderate, or severe—or whether "life's problems never seem to get out of hand" for the person. This approach, again, seems to prioritise the perspective of the practitioner over the patient's view of their own difficulties.

Even with self-report instruments, the routine use of the term "measure" seems to equate these questionnaires with blood pressure monitors, scales, or thermometers. From the perspective of PCT, it would be more accurate to refer to these resources as reporting devices. Sometimes the practitioner uses them to report their perspective and sometimes the patient is able to use them to report their perspective. It's all perspective. Our view is that, as with anamorphic artworks, psychological distress only makes sense when viewed from a particular perspective. The perspective that really counts, in this context, is the patient's.

The PCT principle of relativity stipulates that any single "symptom" of a mental health problem is unlikely to be distressing when taken in isolation. Feeling anxious, low in mood, or hearing voices are not problematic per se. These things become problematic when they create a conflict for a person. This helps us to understand why it is the case that so many people report having experiences like hearing voices but are apparently not sufficiently troubled by these experiences to seek help from mental health services (e.g., van Os et al., 2009). Some people might even be inspired by the voices they hear. If hearing voices makes you feel anxious in social situations, however, and this prevents you from meeting your goal of socialising with friends, you might begin to view this experience as more problematic. Only the person experiencing the problem is in a position to understand exactly which goals are in conflict, and how that conflict might be resolved.

Referring again to the PCT perceive-compare-act explanation of behaviour helps explain why perspective is so critical. No one else can do your perceiving for you. No one else knows what is inside your mind that is being compared to what is currently perceived and no one else can act to make your perceptions match your internal comparison standard. Understanding behaviour as a perceive-compare-act process can help explain why advice and suggestions are unhelpful.

Nobody can advise another person what to perceive or how to move their body to make their perceptions be right. Distress is individually owned and experienced and must be individually solved. If something is distressing for someone, then it is distressing regardless of how someone else considers the distressing event or information. On the other hand, if some particular occurrence is *not* distressing to a certain individual, then it is not distressing to them regardless of how much someone else insists that it is.

There is currently a great deal of discussion about the personalisation of care in healthcare (e.g., NHS England, 2019). One recent policy statement, for example, sets out an ambition that people should expect to have "...the same choice and control over their mental and physical health that they have come to expect in every other aspect of their life" (NHS England, n.d.). We think the move towards personalised care is a laudable development. Our reservation, however, is that while there are moves to give patients greater control over the support they receive, it is questionable whether this is being implemented in a meaningful way.

It often appears that patients are only given control over minor or superficial aspects of care delivery while the substantial decisions continue to be made by practitioners. For example, practice guidelines still recommend how many sessions of psychological therapy patients should receive (e.g., National Institute for Health and Care Excellence [NICE],

2014; NICE 2022). Such practices make little sense when considered in relation to the PCT principle of relativity. The appropriate number of sessions of therapy someone requires to adequately resolve their difficulties is something that only the individual themselves can determine. In important ways, the question of how many sessions of therapy someone should have is much like the question, "How long is a piece of string?" It depends.

Perhaps an even more important consideration is who gets to answer the question of how many sessions are required. We think that should be the patient. Current approaches to "personalisation" often remind us of the famous quote from Henry Ford that "a customer can have a car painted any colour he wants as long as it's black." Healthcare systems are creating an illusion of patient choice and control without actually relinquishing meaningful control over those aspects of care that really matter. We also find it a little disconcerting that a nationwide health service would be introducing something called a "personalisation agenda" as a service innovation in the 21st century. We wonder what has been delivered up to this point if it hasn't been personalised healthcare.

Concluding Comments

Not all theories are created equal. While many theories might sound reasonable, our standard for a theory we are willing to pay attention to is one that can simulate to a high degree of accuracy the thing that it is supposed to be an explanation of. For us, PCT is one of those theories. We have barely scratched the surface of all that PCT has to offer but, in terms of increasing our helpfulness to those who experience psychological turmoil, we have found the characterisation of the phenomenon of control as the ongoing interplay of perceiving, comparing, and acting to be enormously helpful. Understanding the primary importance of a first-person perspective as well as the relativity of what we experience has also been invaluable.

PCT offers the opportunity to fundamentally reimagine the way we consider how it is that people go about their day-to-day business and the things that can interfere with that. Not everyone needs to understand the mechanics of control but, if you are in the business of helping people live the life they wish for, having an accurate sense of what it means to live is a huge advantage. We enjoy imagining a time when control is taken for granted as much as stimulus and response are now.

It was Powers who said, "The childhood of the human race is far from over. We have a long way to go before most people will understand that what they do for others is just as important to their wellbeing as what they do for themselves" (as quoted in Carey et al., 2021, p. 155). When the global community recognises themselves and others as controllers, along with all that that implies, we will achieve contentment, wellbeing, and social cohesion on a scale that is currently unimaginable. We hope this chapter helps, even a little bit, to move us in that direction.

References

Ang, B., Horowitz, M., & Moncrieff, J. (2022). Is the chemical imbalance an 'urban legend'? An exploration of the status of the serotonin theory of depression in the scientific literature. *SSM - Mental Health, 2*, 100098. https:/doi.org/10.1016/j.ssmmh.2022.100098

Carey, T. A. (2017). *Patient-perspective care: A new paradigm for health systems and services.* London: Routledge.

Carey, T. A., Griffiths, R., Dixon, J. E., & Hines, S. (2020). Identifying functional mechanisms in psychotherapy: A scoping systematic review. *Frontiers in Psychiatry, 11.* https://doi.org/10.3389/fpsyt.2020.00291

Carey, T. A., Tai, S. J., & Griffiths, R. (2021). *Deconstructing Health Inequity: A Perceptual Control Theory Perspective.* Cham, Switzerland: Palgrave Macmillan.

Healy, D. (2012). *Pharmageddon.* Berkeley, CA: University of California Press.

Moncrieff, J. (2009). A critique of the dopamine hypothesis of schizophrenia and psychosis. *Harvard Review of Psychiatry, 17*(3), 214–225. https://doi.org/10.1080/10673220902979896

Moncrieff, J., Cooper, R. E., Stockmann, T., Amendola, S., Hengartner, M. P., & Horowitz, M. A. (2022). The serotonin theory of depression: a systematic umbrella review of the evidence. *Molecular Psychiatry, June 2021*, 1–14. https://doi.org/10.1038/s41380-022-01661-0

National Institute for Health and Care Excellence (NICE). (2014). Psychosis and schizophrenia in adults: Prevention and management. In Nice. https://doi.org/10.1002/14651858.CD010823.pub2.Copyright

National Institute for Health and Clinical Excellence. (2022). Depression in adults: Treatment and management NICE guideline. NICE Guideline, June. www.nice.org.uk/guidance/ng222NHS

NHS England. (2019). *The NHS Long Term Plan.* https://www.longtermplan.nhs.uk/online-version/

NHS England. (n.d.). *Personalised Care.* Retrieved October 31, 2023, from https://www.england.nhs.uk/personalisedcare/

Osatuke, K., Ciesla, J., Kasckow, J. W., Zisook, S., & Mohamed, S. (2008). Insight in schizophrenia: A review of etiological models and supporting research. *Comprehensive Psychiatry*, 49(1), 70–77. https://doi.org/10.1016/j.comppsych.2007.08.001

Pedersen, G., Urnes, Ø, Hummelen, B., Wilberg, T., & Kvarstein, E. (2018). Revised manual for the Global Assessment of Functioning scale. *European Psychiatry*, 51, 16-19. doi:10.1016/j.eurpsy.2017.12.028

Powers, W. T. (2005). *Behavior: The control of perception* (2nd ed.). New Canaan, CT: Benchmark.

Powers, W. T. (1998). *Making sense of behavior: The meaning of control.* New Canaan, CT: Benchmark.

Thirioux, B., Harika-Germaneau, G., Langbour, N., & Jaafari, N. (2019). The relation between empathy and insight in psychiatric disorders: Phenomenological, etiological, and neuro-functional mechanisms. *Frontiers in Psychiatry*, 10, 966. https://doi.org/10.3389/fpsyt.2019.00966

van Os, J., Linscott, R. J., Myin-Germeys, I., Delespaul, P., & Krabbendam, L. (2009). A systematic review and meta-analysis of the psychosis continuum: Evidence for a psychosis proneness–persistence–impairment model of psychotic disorder. *Psycho-logical Medicine*, 39(2), 179–195. https://doi.org/10.1017/S0033291708003814

Varieties of Suffering in the Clinical Setting: Re-envisioning Mental Health Beyond the Medical Model

Paul T. P. Wong and Don Laird

Abstract: *We argue for the need to rethink mental health. Given the universality of human suffering, people often wrestle with existential questions such as "Why struggle when all life ends in death?" Existential positive psychology (EPP or PP2.0) was developed to address existential concerns. We provide clinical case studies to demonstrate the advantages of this broader existential framework. According to EPP, mental illness is reconceptualized as both deficiency in knowledge and skills in coping and the neglect of the Soul's yearnings for faith, hope, and love. We propose meaning therapy to equip people with the needed skills to achieve healing and wholeness.*

Acknowledgement: This book chapter was originally published as Wong, P. T. P., & Laird, D. (2023). Varieties of suffering in clinical setting: Re-envisioning mental health beyond the medical model. *Frontiers in Psychology,* 14. https://doi.org/10.3389/fpsyg.2023.1155845. The authors have obtained permission from Frontiers in Psychology to have their article republished.

Introduction

The era of coronavirus disease 2019 (COVID-19) has ushered in a global mental health crisis (De Kock et al., 2022; de la Rosa et al., 2022; Wong et al., 2022a). We need to rethink mental health beyond the medical model and the Diagnostic and Statistical Manual of Mental Disorders (DSM-5; American Psychiatric Association, 2013) because most human suffering cannot be diagnosed by the DSM-5. For example, many people suffer from the frequent mass killings (Metzl et al., 2021) and overloading of bad news (Huff, 2022), but this type of social suffering is not covered by the DSM-5.

After the pandemic, people have generally learned to accept the fact that no human being is immune from suffering. This creates an opening for a broader conversation regarding the various effects of suffering on mental health. Most people do not realize that suffering is not always bad for us, because suffering and wellbeing are intertwined in a complex way (Anderson, 2014). That is why a science of suffering is needed to develop a taxonomy of suffering and the different outcomes of suffering depending on how individuals react to it.

A preliminary taxonomy of suffering encompasses at least four kinds of suffering: physical suffering (physical injury or pain in one's body), psychological suffering (the ego, painful emotions and inherent human limitations), social and interpersonal suffering (injustice, interpersonal conflicts and crimes; Kleinman et al., 1997; Moghaddam, 2022), and existential suffering (struggling with the ultimate concerns and unmet spiritual needs for meaning; Bates, 2016; Wong and Yu, 2021).

Given the universality and complexity of suffering, it is only natural for people to wonder "How could we find happiness when suffering is an inescapable part of life?" and "What is the point of striving when all life ends in death?" Neither existential philosophy nor positive psychology can by itself provide a complete answer to the human quest for meaning and happiness. We need a broader, integrative, and interdisciplinary framework to address the existential angst of common people regarding the ultimate concerns (Yalom, 1980), the meaning of life and suffering (Frankl, 1985), and the meaning of love in a multicultural society (Wong and Mayer, 2023). We also need an inviolable narrative of human beings' role in the world and beyond (Feder, 2020). Existential positive psychology (EPP or PP2.0) was developed to provide a such holistic and interdisciplinary framework for mental health beyond medical model (Wong, 2020a).

In this chapter we first explain the inherent limitations of the medical model in today's complex and fragmented society and why EPP is both necessary and beneficial for both mental health. We then provide illustrative case studies to demonstrate the advantages of this broader alternative framework for case conceptualization and interventions.

According to EPP, mental illness can be reconceptualized as both deficiency in knowledge and skills in coping with the demands and suffering of life and deficiency in meeting the basic needs for livelihood and mental health. Finally, we introduce integrative meaning therapy as a therapeutic framework to achieve healing, wholeness, and sustainable flourishing even in times of suffering.

The medical model and the Diagnostic and Statistical Manual of Mental Disorders

The medical model is essentially a biomedical model which "posits that mental disorders are brain diseases and emphasizes pharmacological treatment to target presumed biological abnormalities" (Deacon, 2013). Accordingly, by design, the Diagnostic and Statistical Manual of Mental Disorders (DSM) inherently implies that something is wrong with a person and that they are ill.

The stigmatizing effects of the DSM have been documented for a long time (Piner and Kahle, 1984; Corrigan and Penn, 1999). Diagnostic labels derived from the DSM can also lead clinicians to "implicitly adopt a disease model which may have negative consequences for the process of psychotherapy, such as less empathy for the client as a fellow human being." (Honos-Webb and Leitner, 2001, p. 38) Recently, Raskin et al. (2022) found that nearly 90% of psychologists used the DSM despite being dissatisfied with it. For many people, their psychological problems can be attributed to the circumstances of their lives. Focusing only on the individual misses the complex relational context and malfunctioning social structures (Robbins et al., 2017). Therefore, the first goal of any therapist should be to recognize the source, nature and context of the client's presenting problems.

Unfortunately, the DSM cannot assess the complex human experiences that are central to the human condition, such as existential loneliness or existential anxiety. Pathologizing these fundamental human experiences actually prevent the psychotherapist from offering the needed help. The cartesian approach is insufficient for realizing the complexities and nuances of the lived human experiences (Bradford, 2009).

Any manual bold enough to monopolize an entire profession inevitably lacks the necessary scope to include all the causes of psychological suffering, as we have alluded to in the introduction. It would be more helpful for the psychotherapist to understand clients' struggles for reasons of living in an absurd world or their need for guidance and wisdom to resolve common problems such as how to relate better with their spouses and their bosses.

Likewise, cognitive-behavioral therapy (CBT) handbooks are promoted to explain away any kind of psychic pain in terms of irrational thinking—thus, either blaming or clinically gaslighting clients. In a post-pandemic world, this approach often ignores clients' existential struggles for meaning and happiness and the macro problems such as climate change, internet scams, abuse of AI for personal gains, and the potential for international wars in Europe and Asia.

Mental health is more than an individual issue. It is also interpersonal, societal, cultural, and transcendental. Furthermore, it is not helpful to pathologize normal human reactions to complex and difficult life situations. Therefore, a new narrative of mental illness is needed to reduce the stigma by recognizing that other factors such as nature, society, and fate are often beyond individual control and can negatively impact one's mental health.

What is EPP? Why is it a necessary and beneficial framework for mental health?

EPP is based on Wong's five decades of research on suffering, clinical practice on suffering, and the integration of the East and West such as ancient Chinese wisdom of the dialectical principles of Yin and Yang (Wong and Cowden, 2022; Wong, n.d.-a).

Culture plays an important role in shaping our attitude toward suffering. Traditionally, children in China were taught by their parents and schools that the most important lesson in life is the ability of "eat bitterness" [不吃苦, 不成人]. This simple Chinese proverb means that if you do not learn how to endure hardships, you will never amount to anything in life. An analogy is that if you do not develop deep roots, you cannot grow into a tall tree. To me (Wong), this is a truism, but this worldview is not widely accepted in the West.

In Western culture, the dominant worldview is to enjoy life; that is, if we focus on the positives, the negatives simply go away. In some way, it is desirable to be happy-go-lucky people who have both the temperament and economic resources to enjoy life without much worry. The downside of this approach is that they are ill prepared when their comfortable life is disrupted by the inescapable storms of life such as a pandemic, death of a loved one, bitter divorce, or terminal cancer.

Human nature does not change. At the deepest level, what is personal is also universal. The existential universals are the same for all cultures. These existential givens are our ultimate concerns such as personal mortality, existential loneliness, the meaning of human existence, and the meaning of suffering. Repressed existential anxiety may manifest itself in other forms (Yalom, 1980).

Another existential universal is that we all have experienced the civil war between good and evil (Challa, 2020). Yet, it is painful to confront our dark side; as a result, we do not know how to relate to our Shadow, which is part of our true self (Perry, 2015). The lack of deep self-knowledge often leads to bad decisions. Denial or covering up our mistakes only make things worse.

Perhaps, the biggest existential challenge for anyone is going through the pain, isolation, and fears of the unknown during the last stage of life. As an 86-year-old man, I (Wong) have gone through a near death experience more than once. More than 10 years ago, I was rushed to the hospital by an ambulance after collapsing in a pool of blood. I gave a blow-by-blow account of the horrors of being "to hell and back" (Wong, 2008). This experience led my discovery of mature happiness (Wong and Bowers, 2018).

Recently, I had another close encounter with death and went through all the painful procedures and aftermaths of surgery (Wong, 2023a). Strong belief in self-efficacy and all my research on successful aging was not enough to cope with the existential crisis of the end-of-life stage. One needs all the existential competences, and spiritual and social support in order to go through the crisis with inner peace and equanimity (Wong and Yu, 2021; Wong, 2023b).

In view of the above, we need to recognize that suffering remains a missing link in wellbeing research (Anderson, 2014; Fowers et al., 2017; Soper, 2020; Clifton, 2022; Wong et al., 2022) and a promising direction of future research on human flourishing. According to EPP, the new science of flourishing through suffering involves not only research on different types of suffering, but also the processes and the outcomes of sustainable wellbeing.

The following represents some of the advantages of the EPP framework integrating East and West and intertwining suffering and happiness, which expands wellbeing research beyond the binary approach:

1. The process of navigating the dialectical interactions between Yin-Yang in order to discover the adaptive balance or the middle way between positives and negatives (Wong, 2012a; Wong, 2016a; Wong and Cowden, 2022).
2. The process of transcending suffering, inherent limitations, and duality through self-transcendence (Kaufman, 2020; Wong, 2020a; Wong et al., 2021a,b).
3. The outcome of true positivity of seeing the light in the darkness such as tragic optimism (Leung et al., 2021), existential gratitude (Jans-Beken and Wong, 2019), chaironic happiness (Wong, 2011), and mature happiness (Carreno et al., 2023). This type of happiness is characterized by achieving some kind of inner peace, balance, and harmony through the difficult process of adapting to suffering or difficulty (Lomas, 2021).

There are hopeful signs of a paradigm shift (Harvard Human Flourishing Program, 2022; Wong et al., 2022a). Various recent publications (Bloom, 2021; Cain, 2022; Ho et al., 2022; Rashid and Brooks, 2022) also emphasize the need to integrate suffering for happiness and flourishing. Buddhist psychology has been the strongest advocate of ending suffering as the precondition for happiness. Its first noble truth is that life is suffering because our desires for carnal happiness and our ignorance of the impermanence of life (Thera, 2004; Targ and Hurtak, 2006; Cowden et al., 2021).

The need to embrace suffering and transform it into something meaningful is a recurrent theme in philosophy, literature, and religion (Heller, 2015). EPP is simply an extension of existential psychology (May, 1969; Yalom, 1980; Frankl, 1985) into a new science of suffering by developing a comprehensive account of the effects of suffering and its complex interactions with wellbeing (Wong, 2019; Wong et al., 2021b, 2022b). The following examples serve to illustrate the advantages of the broader EPP framework for mental health and psychotherapy.

Illustrative examples of suffering in clinical settings[1]

Many of my (Wong) clients came to me because they were attracted to my meaning-centered therapy and counseling.

Case one

Jackie suffered from depression. She was a 39-year-old attractive woman with a five-year-old son. Her husband was a very successful developer who worked seven days a week and seldom came home for dinner. She used to work as a real estate agent together with her husband; they used to struggle together in the early years of their marriage. Those were the happiest times of her life. After the birth of their first son, she became a stay-at-home housewife. Even though she was able to hire two helpers and had lots of time to do whatever she liked, she could not get rid of her sense of loneliness and emptiness. Her marriage no longer gave her happiness. That was why she wanted a divorce, hoping that this would solve her problems.

During joint sessions, it became clear that her husband was a good, responsible man who really loved and adored his wife. He thought that by working hard, he could provide more financial security and a better future.

---

[1] The case illustrations provided here are fictional characters based on similar cases. Their personal characteristics and identities are disguised so that no one can identify a real person from these case adaptations.

As a result of meaning therapy, he decided family was more important than money, and that he needed to better manage work-family balance; as a result, he drastically cut down his projects so that he could spend more time at home. Jackie discovered that her depression was because she was bored with life and did not have an outlet for her love for creative work. She decided to return to college to pursue her interests in internal design. As a result of the above changes, she no longer needs antidepressive medication or desires a divorce.

Case two

Oscar suffers from anxiety. He is a very successful medical professor teaching in an Ivy League university. His main problem is that his 10-year-old son has Type One diabetes, and he feels guilty for his inability to help his son medically in spite of all the honors and awards he has received in his medical field. In addition, he also suffers from his inability to see his son as much as he wants since his estranged wife (now living in separation) manipulates his visiting time in order to squeeze out more money from him. His previous psychologist advised him to divorce his wife and win the child custody case, but he is reluctant to go to court because of his concern for his son's wellbeing. These problems caused him immense pain and anxiety.

Existential answers for Oscar's problems revolved around the following themes: (a) the Stoic wisdom of changing ourselves rather than changing others (e.g., Aurelius, 2016); (b) cultivating the wisdom of loving his son, but with some emotional detachment so that he would not suffer so intensely; (c) treating his wife with kindness and forgiveness even though she remains a manipulative and deceitful woman (he wants to believe that love will eventually prevail over evil); and (d) learning to endure the pain with joy and gratitude since his suffering has brought him closer to God and made him a very successful surgeon due to his extraordinary skills and compassion toward patients. Oscar finds Stoic philosophy most helpful in its emphasis on doing what is within his control and what matters most to him. In addition, he finds some inner peace from the principle of acceptance, enduring and praying to God for what is beyond his control.

Space would not allow me to provide more cases. My clients over the last 30 years include successful movie stars, lawyers, physicians, scientists, professors, bankers, and CEOs. These individuals possess everything people can only dream of, yet they still suffer in their private hell including marital problems, work stress, inner emptiness, and disillusion with life. Therefore, there is the need for a more holistic and meaning-centered narrative for mental health.

Varieties of suffering in the clinical setting: a new conceptualization

As illustrated by Wong's examples, many clinical cases are simply normal human reactions to the inescapable sufferings from one or any combination of the four sources of suffering. We propose that most psychological disorders can be contributed to different types of deficiencies, such as:

1. Deficiency in meeting one's basic physical needs such as sleep, food, or exercise (Columbia University Department of Psychiatry, 2022).
2. Deficiency in caring for the soul's yearning or spiritual meaning for hope (for a meaningful future), love (loving relationships with others), and faith in protection and help from God or a higher power (Wong, 2023b).
3. Deficiency in emotional regulations (temper tantrum, frequent mood swing, or lack of emotional intelligence), self-control, and discipline (indulgence in pleasure, addiction, or bad habits such as laziness and gluttony).
4. Deficiency in meaning attribution (exaggerated common attribution biases such as claiming credit for success and blaming others for failure).
5. Deficiency in responsibility for one's wellbeing and future in addition to failing to take responsibility for one's words and deeds (Arslan and Wong, 2022).
6. Deficiency in relational skills such as listening and speaking truthfully and clearly.
7. Deficiency in basic human decency or virtues such as honesty, integrity, and kindness.

8. Deficiency in coping resources and skills (Wong et al., 2006).
9. Deficiency in endurance and tolerance of suffering and people one does not like (Wong, 2004).
10. Deficiency in life intelligence (LQ; Wong, 2017) or existential intelligence (Gardner, 2020).

Integrative meaning therapy (IMT)

The above examples illustrate that most inorganic psychological difficulties can be re-conceptualized as existential concerns and difficulties in coping with various suffering in life. Therefore, integrative meaning therapy (IMT; Wong, 2010, 2016b, 2020b) seems most appropriate because it focuses on the fundamental human needs for meaning, relationship, and spiritual faith in addition to the human quest for meaning as its central organizing construct and inner peace as its desirable outcome. IMT reduces the stigma of mental illness because it focuses on unleashing people's natural power of meaning for healing and flourishing.

Meaning is one of the core experiences of human existence. The important role of meaning and purpose for our wellbeing is supported by a mountain of empirical research (e.g., Wong, 2012b; Hicks and Routledge, 2013). At present, many people are wrestling with finding meaning and purpose in their work, marriage, or life in general.

As illustrated by the first case study, one's primary need for meaning is replaced or suppressed by one's blind pursuit of happiness and success. Ironically, research has shown that such pursuit is a main source of suffering (Schumaker, 2006; Wong, 2007; Zerwas and Ford, 2021). In addition, toxic positivity has attracted increasing public attention (Scully, 2020; Kaufman, 2021; Princing, 2021; Villines, 2021; Cain, 2022).

The advantages of cultivating a meaning-mindset (Wong, 2011) includes: (1) allowing one to facilitate the discovery of meaning in situations and in one's life overall; (2) adding a spiritual perspective to everyday activities; (3) allowing an individual to orient themselves to the values of eudemonia and self-transcendence; (4) contributing to personal growth and becoming a fully functioning person; and (5) increasing one's likelihood of success in having a meaningful purpose.

The good news is that research has shown meaning to be an antidote to the perils in the pursuit of happiness and success when meaning is defined as a self-transcendence reorientation (Frankl, 1988; Wong, 2014; Wong et al., 2021a). Self-transcendence can be illustrated by the following widely cited saying from Dalai Lama: "Our prime purpose in this life is to help others. And if you cannot help them, at least do not hurt them."

IMT focuses on meaning-centered coping which includes (a) finding benefits or lessons from suffering, (b) leaning to accept and transcend inescapable suffering, (c) praying to God or a Higher Power for help, (d) reframing suffering into something more manageable and positive, (e) linking suffering to some meta narrative or mythology, and (f) integrating suffering with something positive or meaningful (Wong et al., 2006; Eisenbeck et al., 2022). Meaning is a common factor in all kinds of therapies (Vos, 2018). Here are 10 characteristics of a meaning-centered psychotherapist:

1. Holds a hopeful view of every client and treats them with respect and dignity.
2. Makes effective use of the self—the therapist is the therapy.
3. Helps clients move toward both healing and wellbeing simultaneously.
4. Sees both the big picture and situational problems.
5. Integrates different modalities around the central construct of meaning.
6. Integrates the art and science of meaningful living.
7. Considers meaning as both personally and socially constructed.
8. Empowers clients to take personal responsibility to develop their own potentials.
9. Equips clients with skills of making the right decision and effective coping.
10. Takes a holistic view of wellbeing, including spiritual wellbeing.

In sum, IMT involves how to manage the three broad themes of human existence: (1) how to live a fulfilling and meaningful life, (2) how to become better and stronger though overcoming and transforming suffering into something meaningful, and (3) how to love and relate well to others in a multicultural society (Wong, n.d.-b).

Total wellbeing and why the best possible life is a deep life

From the perspective of EPP, we can enjoy total wellbeing when we are able to transcend our limitations, suffering, and cultural differences. In doing so, we can enjoy living a meaningful life involving all four dimensions of our personhood – bio, psycho, social, and spiritual.

According to the American Psychological Association (2023), wellbeing is defined as "a state of happiness and contentment, with low levels of distress, overall good physical and mental health and outlook, or good quality of life." The World Health Organization (2021) has a broader conception of wellbeing beyond physical and mental health as follows:

> Well-being is a positive state experienced by individuals and societies. Similar to health, it is a resource for daily life and is determined by social, economic and environmental conditions. Well-being encompasses quality of life and the ability of people and societies to contribute to the world with a sense of meaning and purpose. Focusing on well-being supports the tracking of the equitable distribution of resources, overall thriving and sustainability. A society's well-being can be determined by the extent to which they are resilient, build capacity for action, and are prepared to transcend challenges (World Health Organization, 2021).

Thus, it calls for total mobilization of all sections and all citizens to be involved in actions of promoting wellbeing in societies in which all people can enjoy some good quality of life. Toward this goal, we have developed a tripartite meaning management model of focusing on managing three existential universals for sustainable wellbeing: meaningful living, meaningful suffering, and meaningful relationships in a multicultural society.

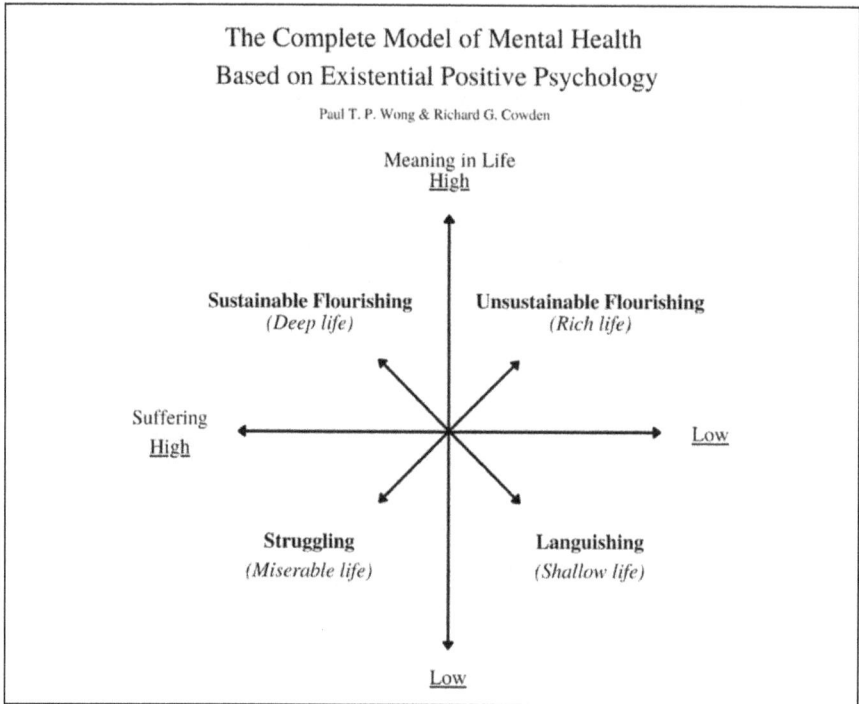

Figure 1: *The complete model of mental health based on existential positive psychology*

Research has also shown that illness can be viewed as a spiritual phenomenon according to Dame Cicely Saunders' ground-breaking concept of total suffering as comprising physical, emotional, social, and spiritual sources of pain (Balboni and Balboni, 2018). By the same token, we can also have total wellbeing which includes the spiritual-existential source of wellbeing (Wong, 2023b).

A complete model of mental health depends on how well we manage suffering and to what extent we embrace meaning. Figure 1 explains both the importance of suffering and meaning as well as the need for balance.

Regarding the four quadrants, in times like this when life is full of suffering and stress, the best possible life is a deep life or sustainable flourishing. It may sound counter-intuitive because we instinctively avoid suffering. Figure 2 provides the reasons why suffering is necessary for a deep life.

The second-best life is where the privileged can avoid most of the pain common folks suffer from and engage in all kinds of desirable experiences. This kind of life has been described as the rich life. According to Oishi and Westgate (2022), "Unlike happy or meaningful lives, psychologically rich lives are best characterized by a variety of interesting and perspective-changing experiences." (p. 790).

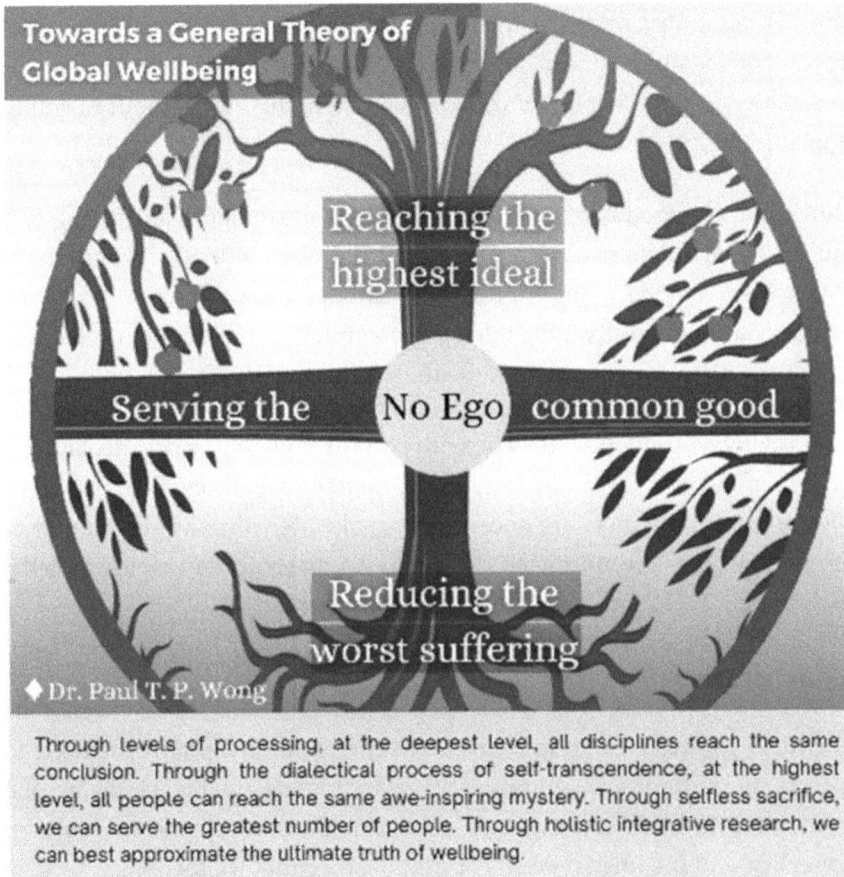

Towards a General Theory of Global Wellbeing

Reaching the highest ideal

Serving the   No Ego   common good

Reducing the worst suffering

♦ Dr. Paul T. P. Wong

Through levels of processing, at the deepest level, all disciplines reach the same conclusion. Through the dialectical process of self-transcendence, at the highest level, all people can reach the same awe-inspiring mystery. Through selfless sacrifice, we can serve the greatest number of people. Through holistic integrative research, we can best approximate the ultimate truth of wellbeing.

Figure 2: *Towards a general theory of wellbeing*

But a rich life is unsustainable in the long run because when one encounters a tough patch of life, struck by unexpected tragedy or trauma, one does not have the solid foundation or resilience to maintain their rich lifestyle.

The quadrant of languishing refers to the ordinary shallow life of the eat-work-sleep cycle. A boring, meaningless existence can be described as a shallow life. "Happiness without meaning characterizes a relatively shallow, self-absorbed or even selfish life, in which things go well, needs and desire are easily satisfied, and difficult or taxing entanglements are avoided" (Baumeister et al., 2013).

The last quadrant refers to the worst possible life full of suffering and devoid of meaning. It can be called a wasted life or miserable life. A miserable life may be a better description of a living hell without meaning transformation.

Our tripartite model of meaningful living, meaningful suffering, and multicultural relationship can also be translated into the evolutionary psychology of the pain-brain-culture model of wellbeing. From an evolutionary perspective, the main thing animals or human beings have to contend with is danger, pain, or death in order to stay alive.

That is why learning how to cope with painful experiences or suffering is a matter of survival and striving, not a matter of pathology or sickness. Meaning and happiness are necessary to make life worth living in order to prevent us from committing suicide or giving up (quiet suicide). This is the logic Soper (2020) and Wong (2022) have argued for.

Conclusion

The main contribution of this chapter is threefold: it explains the need to incorporate suffering as an important factor for sustainable wellbeing, the need for IMT and learning how to live a meaningful life in times of adversity, and the importance of spiritual-existential wellbeing.

We have made the case that suffering is necessary for sustainable wellbeing and flourishing. If we focus only on the negative events in our life, we will be swallowed up by the black hole of depression and anger. However, if we focus on the meaning of suffering and learn to see light or be the light in the darkest hours though practicing hope, love, and faith, we will be strengthened and blessed.

As a new narrative beyond the medical model, our EPP framework encourages the following new trends which may help resolve the current mental health crisis.

1. From a symptom-based approach to a holistic approach to total wellbeing.
2. From clinical treatment to practical guidelines for living fully and vitally.
3. From adhering to a particular school of thought to integrating multiple modalities.
4. From Western-ethnocentric psychology to multicultural and indigenous psychology.
5. From depending only on the medical profession to including educational and other social institutions.

References

American Psychiatric Association (2013). *Diagnostic and statistical manual of mental disorders.* 5th Edition. Washington, DC: American Psychiatric Assoc Pub.

American Psychological Association (2023). Well-being. APA Dictionary of Psychology. Available at: https://dictionary.apa.org/well-being

Anderson, R. E. (2014). *World suffering and quality of life.* New York: Springer.

Arslan, G., and Wong, P. T. P. (2022). Measuring personal and social responsibility: an existential positive psychology approach. *J Happiness Health* 2, 1–11. doi: 10.47602/johah.v2i1.5

Aurelius, M. (2016). Meditations. (Hanselman, S., Trans.). London, UK: Profile Books. Balboni, T. A., and

Balboni, M. J. (2018). The spiritual event of serious illness. *J. Pain Symptom Manage.* 56, 816–822. doi: 10.1016/j.jpainsymman.2018.05.018

Bates, A. T. (2016). Addressing existential suffering. *BCMJ* 58, 268–273.

Baumeister, R. F., Vohs, K. D., Aaker, J. L., and Garbinsky, E. N. (2013). Some key differences between a happy life and a meaningful life. *J. Posit. Psychol.* 8, 505–516. doi: 10.1080/17439760.2013.830764

Bloom, P. (2021). *The sweet spot: The pleasures of suffering and the search for meaning.* New York: Ecco.

Bradford, G. K. (2009). Revisioning diagnosis: A contemplative phenomenological approach. *J. Transpers. Psychol.* 41, 121–138. Available at: https://www.atpweb.org/ jtparchive/trps-41-02-121.pdf

Cain, S. (2022). *Bittersweet: How sorrow and longing make us whole.* New York: Crown.

Carreno, D. F., Eisenbeck, N., Greville, J., and Wong, P. T. P. (2023). Cross-cultural psychometric analysis of the mature happiness scale-revised: mature happiness, psychological inflexibility, and the PERMA model. *J. Happiness Stud.* 24, 1075–1099. doi: 10.1007/s10902-023-00633-7

Challa, B. (2020). *The war within – Between good and evil: Reconstructing morality, money, and mortality.* New Delhi: Gyan Publishing House.

Clifton, J. (2022). *Blind spot: The global rise of unhappiness and how leaders missed it.* Washington DC: Gallup Press.

Columbia University Department of Psychiatry. (2022). How sleep deprivation impacts mental health. Available at: https://www.columbiapsychiatry.org/news/how-sleep-deprivation-affects-your-mental-health

Corrigan, P. W., and Penn, D. L. (1999). Lessons from social psychology on discrediting psychiatric stigma. *Am. Psychol.* 54, 765–776. doi: 10.1037/0003-066X.54.9.765

Cowden, R. G., Counted, V., and Ramkissoon, H. (2021). "Place attachment and suffering during a pandemic" in *Place and post-pandemic flourishing: Disruption, adjustment, and healthy behaviors.* eds. V. Counted, R. G. Cowden and H. Ramkissoon (New York: Springer), 45–54.

De Kock, J. H., Latham, H. A., and Cowden, R. G. (2022). The mental health of healthcare workers during the COVID-19 pandemic: a narrative review. *Curr. Opin. Psychiatry* 35, 311–316. doi: 10.1097/YCO.0000000000000805

de la Rosa, P. A., Cowden, R. G., de Filippis, R., Jerotic, S., Nahidi, M., Ori, D., et al. (2022). Associations of lockdown stringency and duration with

Google searches for mental health terms during the COVID-19 pandemic: a nine-country study. *J. Psychiatr. Res.* 150, 237–245. doi: 10.1016/j.jpsychires.2022.03.026

Deacon, B. J. (2013). The biomedical model of mental disorder: a critical analysis of its validity, utility, and effects on psychotherapy research. *Clin. Psychol. Rev.* 33, 846–861. doi: 10.1016/j.cpr.2012.09.007

Eisenbeck, N., Carreno, D. F., Wong, P. T. P., Hicks, J. A., María, R. G., Puga, J. L., et al. (2022). An international study on psychological coping during COVID-19: towards a meaning-centered coping style. *Int. J. Clin. Health Psychol.* 22:100256. doi: 10.1016/j.ijchp.2021.100256

Feder, S. (2020). Religious faith can lead to positive mental benefits, writes Stanford anthropologist. Stanford News. Available at: https://news.stanford.edu/2020/11/13/deep-faith-beneficial-health/#

Fowers, B. J., Richardson, F. C., and Slife, B. D. (2017). *Frailty, suffering, and vice: Flourishing in the face of human limitations.* Washington DC: American Psychological Association.

Frankl, V. E. (1985). *Man's search for meaning.* New York: Washington Square Press.

Frankl, V. E. (1988). *The will to meaning.* London, UK: Penguin Group.

Gardner, H. (2020). A resurgence of interest in existential intelligence: Why now? Available at: https://www.howardgardner.com/howards-blog/a-resurgence-of-interest-in-existential-intelligence-why-now

Harvard Human Flourishing Program. (2022). *Lighting the darkness of suffering.* Cambridge, Massachusetts: Harvard University.

Heller, S. (2015). Finding meaning in suffering. Psych Central. Available at: https://psychcentral.com/pro/finding-meaning-in-suffering#1

Hicks, J. A., and Routledge, C. (2013). *The experience of meaning in life: Classical perspectives, emerging themes, and controversies.* New York: Springer.

Ho, S., Cook, K. V., Chen, Z. J., Kurniati, N. M. T., Suwartono, C., Widyarini, N., et al. (2022). Suffering, psychological distress, and well-being in Indonesia: a prospective cohort study. *Stress. Health* 38, 879–890. doi: 10.1002/smi.3139

Honos-Webb, L., and Leitner, L. M. (2001). How using the DSM causes damage: a client's report. *J. Humanist. Psychol.* 41, 36–56. doi: 10.1177/0022167801414003

Huff, C. (2022). Media overload is hurting our mental health. Here are ways to manage headline stress. *Monit. Psychol.* 53:20.

Jans-Beken, L. G. P. J., and Wong, P. T. P. (2019). Development and preliminary validation of the existential gratitude scale (EGS). *Couns. Psychol. Q.* 34, 72–86. doi: 10.1080/09515070.2019.1656054

Kaufman, S. B. (2020). *Transcend: The new science of self-actualization.* New York: Tarcher Perigee.

Kaufman, S. B. (2021). The opposite of toxic positivity: tragic optimism. The Atlantic. Available at: https://www.theatlantic.com/family/archive/2021/08/tragic-optimism-opposite-toxic-positivity/619786/

Kleinman, A., Das, V., and Lock, M. M. (Eds.) (1997). *Social suffering. 1st* Edn Berkeley: University of California Press.

Leung, M. M., Arslan, G., and Wong, P. T. P. (2021). Tragic optimism as a buffer against COVID-19 suffering and the psychometric properties of a brief version of the life attitudes scale (LAS-B). *Front. Psychol.* 12:646843. doi: 10.3389/fpsyg.2021.646843

Lomas, T. (2021). Life balance and harmony: Wellbeing's golden thread. *Int J Wellbeing* 11, 50–68. doi: 10.5502/ijw.v11i1.1477

May, R. (Ed.) (1969). *Existential psychology. 2nd* Edn. New York: Random House.

Metzl, J. M., Piemonte, J., and McKay, T. (2021). Mental illness, mass shootings, and the future of psychiatric research into American gun violence. *Harv. Rev.* Psychiatry 29, 81–89. doi: 10.1097/HRP.0000000000000280

Moghaddam, F. M. (2022). *How psychologists failed: We neglected the poor and minorities, favored the rich and privileged, and got science wrong.* Cambridge, MA: Cambridge University Press.

Oishi, S., and Westgate, E. C. (2022). A psychologically rich life: beyond happiness and meaning. *Psychol. Rev.* 129, 790–811. doi: 10.1037/rev0000317

Perry, C. (2015). The Jungian shadow. The Society of Analytical Psychology. Available at: https://www.thesap.org.uk/articles-on-jungian-psychology-2/about-analysis-and-therapy/the-shadow/

Piner, K. E., and Kahle, L. R. (1984). Adapting to the stigmatizing label of mental illness: foregone but not forgotten. *J. Pers. Soc. Psychol.* 47, 805–811. doi: 10.1037/0022-3514.47.4.805

Princing, M. (2021). What you need to know about toxic positivity. Right as Rain. Available at: https://rightasrain.uwmedicine.org/mind/well-being/toxic-positivity

Rashid, R., and Brooks, A. C. (2022). A new formula for happiness. The Atlantic. Available at: https://www.theatlantic.com/podcasts/archive/2022/11/happiness-formula-howto-age/672109/

Raskin, J. D., Maynard, D., and Gayle, M. C. (2022). Psychologist attitudes toward DSM-5 and its alternatives. *Prof. Psychol. Res.* Pract. 53, 553–563. doi: 10.1037/pro0000480

Robbins, B. D., Kamens, S. R., and Elkins, D. N. (2017). DSM-5 reform efforts by the society for humanistic psychology. *J. Humanist. Psychol.* 57, 602–624. doi: 10.1177/0022167817698617

Schumaker, J. F. (2006). The happiness conspiracy. New Internationalist, 391. Available at: http://www.newint.org/columns/essays/2006/07/01/happiness-conspiracy/

Scully, S. M. (2020). 'Toxic positive' is real – and it's a big problem during the pandemic. Healthline. Available at: https://www.healthline.com/health/mental-health/toxic-positivity-during-the-pandemic

Soper, C. A. (2020). *The evolution of life worth living: Why we choose to live.*

Targ, R., and Hurtak, J. J. (2006). The end of suffering: Fearless living in troubled times… or, how to get out of hell free. Newbuyport, MA: Hampton Roads Publishing.

Thera, N. (2004). Why end suffering? Access to Insight. Available at: https://www.accesstoinsight.org/lib/authors/nyanaponika/whyend.html

Villines, Z. (2021). What to know about toxic positivity. Medical News Today. Available at: https://www.medicalnewstoday.com/articles/toxic-positivity/

Vos, J. (2018). *Meaning in life: An evidence-based handbook for practitioners.* London, UK: Palgrave Macmillan.

Wong, P. T. P. (2004). The power of endurance [President's column]. Positive Living Newsletter. Available at: https://www.meaning.ca/article/the-power-of-endurance/

Wong, P. T. P. (2007). Perils and promises in the pursuit of happiness review of the book. In: *Search of happiness: Understanding an endangered state of mind,* by J. F. Schumaker]. PsycCRITIQUES, 52. doi: 10.1037/a0010040

Wong, P. T. P. (2008). To hell and back and what I have learned about happiness. International Network on Personal Meaning. Available at: http://www.meaning.ca/archives/archive/art_hell_and_back_P_Wong.html

Wong, P. T. P. (2010). Meaning therapy: an integrative and positive existential psychotherapy. *J. Contemp.* Psychother. 40, 85–93. doi: 10.1007/s10879-009-9132-6

Wong, P. T. P. (2011). Positive psychology 2.0: towards a balanced interactive model of the good life. *Can. Psychol.* 52, 69–81. doi: 10.1037/a0022511

Wong, P. T. P. (2012a). "Toward a dual-systems model of what makes life worth living" in *The human quest for meaning: Theories, research, and applications.* ed. P. T. P. Wong. 2nd ed (Oxfordshire, UK: Routledge), 3–22.

Wong, P. T. P. (Ed.) (2012b). *The human quest for meaning: Theories, research, and applications.* 2nd Edition. Oxfordshire, UK: Routledge.

Wong, P. T. P. (2014). "Viktor Frankl's meaning seeking model and positive psychology" in *Meaning in existential and positive psychology.* eds. A. Batthyany and P. Russo-Netzer (New York: Springer), 149–184.

Wong, P. T. P. (2016a). Acceptance, transcendence, and yin-yang dialectics: the three basic tenets of second wave positive psychology. Positive Living Newsletter. Available at: www.drpaulwong.com/inpm-presidents-report-november-2016

Wong, P. T. P. (2016b). "Integrative meaning therapy: from logotherapy to existential positive interventions" in *Clinical perspectives on meaning: Positive and existential psychotherapy.* eds. P. Russo-Netzer, S. E. Schulenberg and A. Batthyány (New York: Springer), 323–342.

Wong, P. T. P. (2017). *Lessons of life intelligence through life education [presentation].* Tzu Chi University, Hualien, Taiwan.

Wong, P. T. P. (2019). Second wave positive psychology's (PP 2.0) contribution to counselling psychology. *Couns. Psychol. Q.* [Special Issue] 32, 275–284. doi: 10.1080/09515070.2019.1671320

Wong, P. T. P. (2020a). *Made for resilience and happiness: Effective coping with covid-19 according to Viktor E. Frankl, E and Paul T. P. Wong* Toronto, Canada: INPM Press.

Wong, P. T. P. (2020b). Existential positive psychology and integrative meaning therapy. *Int. Rev. Psychiatry* 32, 565–578. doi: 10.1080/09540261.2020.1814703

Wong, P. T. P., Cowden, R. G., Mayer, C.-H., and Bowers, V. L. (2022). "Shifting the paradigm of positive psychology: Toward an existential positive psychology of wellbeing" in *Broadening the scope of wellbeing science: Multidisciplinary and interdisciplinary perspectives on human flourishing and wellbeing.* Ed. A. H. Kemp. (Palgrave Macmillan), 13–27.

Wong, P. T. P. (2023a). Hope keeps us moving forward [President's column]. Positive Living Newsletter. https://mailchi.mp/meaning.ca/pldt-mar-11967588

Wong, P. T. P. (2023b). Spiritual-existential wellbeing (SEW): the faith-hope-love model of mental health and total wellbeing. *Int J Existential Posit Psychol*, 12.

Wong, P. T. P. (n.d.-a). Pioneer in research in existential positive psychology of suffering and global flourishing: Paul T. P. Wong. *Appl. Res. Qual. Life*

Wong, P. T. P. (n.d.-b). "An existential perspective on positive psychology: towards a general theory of global flourishing" in *APA handbook of humanistic and existential psychology.* ed. L. Hoffman

Wong, P. T. P., Arslan, G., Bowers, V. L., Peacock, E. J., Kjell, O. N. E., Ivtzan, I., et al. (2021a). Self-transcendence as a buffer against COVID-19 suffering: the development and validation of the self-transcendence measure-B. *Front. Psychol.* 12:4229. doi: 10.3389/fpsyg.2021.648549

Wong, P. T. P., and Bowers, V. (2018). "Mature happiness and global wellbeing in difficult times" in *Scientific concepts behind happiness, kindness, and empathy in contemporary society.* ed. N. R. Silton (Hershey, Pennsylvania: IGI Global), 112–134.

Wong, P. T. P., and Cowden, R. G. (2022). Accelerating the science and practice of psychology beyond WEIRD biases: enriching the landscape through Asian psychology. *Front. Psychol.* 13:1054519. doi: 10.3389/fpsyg.2022.1054519

Wong, P. T. P., Cowden, R. G., Mayer, C.-H., and Bowers, V. L. (2022a). "Shifting the paradigm of positive psychology: toward an existential positive psychology of wellbeing" in *Broadening the scope of wellbeing science: Multidisciplinary and interdisciplinary perspectives on human flourishing and wellbeing.* ed. A. H. Kemp (London, UK: Palgrave Macmillan), 13–27.

Wong, P. T. P., Ho, L. S., Cowden, R. G., Mayer, C.-H., and Yang, F. (2022b). A new science of suffering, the wisdom of the soul, and the new behavioral economics of happiness: towards a general theory of wellbeing. *Front. Psychol.*

Wong, P. T. P., and Mayer, C.-H. (2023). The meaning of love and its bittersweet nature. *Int. Rev. Psychiatry* 35, 33–41. doi: 10.1080/09540261.2023.2173001

Wong, P. T. P., Mayer, C.-H., and Arslan, G. (Eds.). (2021b). COVID-19 and existential positive psychology (PP 2.0): the new science of self-transcendence. Available at: https:// www.frontiersin.org/research-topics/14988/covid-19-and-existential-positive-psychology-pp20-the-new-science-of-self-transcendence

Wong, P. T. P., Reker, G. T., and Peacock, E. (2006). "The resource-congruence model of coping and the development of the coping schemas inventory" in *Handbook of multicultural perspectives on stress and coping.* eds. P. T. P. Wong and L. C. J. Wong (New York: Springer), 223–283.

Wong, P. T. P., and Yu, T. T. F. (2021). Existential suffering in palliative care: an existential positive psychology perspective. *Medicina* 57:924. doi: 10.3390/medicina57090924

World Health Organization. (2021). Glossary of terms. Available at: https://www.who.int/publications/i/item/9789240038349

Yalom, I. D. (1980). *Existential psychotherapy.* New York: Basic Books.

Zerwas, F. K., and Ford, B. Q. (2021). The paradox of pursuing happiness. *Curr. Opin. Behav. Sci.* 39, 106–112. doi: 10.1016/j.cobeha.2021.03.006

Languaging the Other:
Diagnosis and Ways of Seeing

Craig Newnes

Abstract: *This chapter critiques the psy agenda of diagnosis and suggests alternative ways of labelling conduct.*

Modernist professionals, including psychologists and psychiatrists, tend to act as if their present knowledge results from the accumulation of many years of trial and error, history inevitably leading us to a new enlightenment.[1] It is difficult to remember, as do some post-modernists, that any knowledge is little more than a way of emphasizing (privileging) certain ways of seeing – ways that serve interest rather than describing immutable truths.[2]

A technocracy such as psychology will emphasize ways of seeing the world, and those within it, which can be measured. Such measurement may take the form of quantifying assumed internal characteristics (intelligence, introversion, depression) of individuals. Hence the popularizing of computerized Cognitive Behaviour Therapy (CBT) for those whose conduct can be conveniently divided into discrete, de-contextualised elements of thought, emotion and behaviour; each element to be then separately modified with the aid of a computer programme. In such a scheme morality disappears as, without context, there is no way of discovering what is right, only what the person wants – what is to stop a person asking to convert their behaviour and mindset into that of a serial killer?[3]

Many people that psychologists see have already been branded via psychiatric diagnoses, itself a curious parody of the scientific method.[4] Arbitrary and unrelated behaviours have been observed or reported before being clustered into seemingly random concepts – depression, schizophrenia, etc.[5] This sleight of hand obscures the fact there is no reason that, say, visual hallucinations or voice hearing should be investigated as part of the same syndrome, yet psychiatric researchers set about looking for a single cause (genetic or bio-chemical) or various interacting causes (environment, up-bringing, genetic predisposition, etc.) underlying the diagnosed malady.

Since its inception in 1952 the *Diagnostic and Statistical Manual* (DSM) of the American Psychiatric Association (APA) has increased the defined diagnoses from a mere 162 to 365 in the current DSM-V. For several years an APA committee, heavily influence by pharmaceutical company subsidies, has been working on which new diagnoses to *vote* into the sixth edition. If any person's behaviour isn't covered, that person is going to feel lonely indeed. It is remuneration for research and psychological services that drives the increase in diagnoses, something first noted by Spitzer and his colleagues when revising *DSM-III*: *TIME* magazine reported from the first of their meetings that the most important thing, "… is that *DSM-III* is of crucial importance to the profession [because] … its diagnoses are generally recognized by the courts, hospitals and insurance companies."[6]

University researchers in the United Kingdom are similarly constrained as research funding is based on successful publication in American Psychological Association (APA) approved journals that insist on the use of diagnosis. A publication from the Division of Clinical Psychology (DCP) of the British Psychological Society (BPS) decrying the use of psychiatric diagnosis was produced by a much-respected group of clinical and critically inclined psychologists, the majority of whom had used diagnoses unapologetically when previously publishing in APA approved journals.[7]

Alternatives

Jose Luis Borges (quoted in Foucault[8]) suggests an intriguing typology (of animals) rather different from our own: those which have just knocked over the water pitcher and those which from a distance look like flies, beasts owned by the Emperor, and so on. It is possible to imagine a similarly challenging typology of persons, less reductionist and more visible, than that currently embraced by psychiatry, psychology, and related professions.

A walk along a crowded beach in summer can give us a starting point. We might categorize people in the following, less technical, ways: those that play with children, those that show off their bellies (tanned or otherwise), those that can balance a football on the back of the neck, those that scream as they run into the sea, and more, ad infinitum. Such ways of seeing people can be developed in more subtle and equally easily verifiable ways.

Let us continue: those that regard history as a biased account of the past, those that see God in everything, those that understand planting rhythms, those that smoke to change their consciousness (albeit briefly) and those that do so out of habit, those that prefer touch (healing) to talk (mouthfuls of air[9]), those that prefer giving to receiving oral sex. The list is endless.

Ways of Seeing

Historiography here is key. It is all too easy to forget that belief systems come and go. Ways of seeing change too. Historians can write as if history systematically uncoils to the present, entire systems of thought being replaced along the way. But systems of thought move in cycles, privileging certain principles (the importance of theism or rationality, for example) for centuries before moving again to a previously discarded doctrine. We are, for example, inclined to see various schools of therapy or psychological theories as ineluctable and logical truths destined to last many lifetimes. But Freudian concepts are just a hundred and twenty years old, Beck's theory is not yet seventy. Compare such theories with Catharism, a credo surviving over two hundred years or the views of Anselm, a determined theistic rationalist who was influential for centuries.[10]

Systems of thought are maps. And as any cartographer will tell you, maps constantly change. Indeed, cartography is a more revealing instance of the way interest shapes practise – the Indian sub-continent shrank at the hands of Mercator, keen to give the impression that the countries around the Mediterranean were more important.[11] Maps are, of course, *never* the territory. A brain scan tells you nothing of love, pacifism, or gloominess. Even memory is almost entirely contextual, being triggered by events or actions. A map of the temporal lobe will tell you little of how concert pianists play nocturnes – recall is through their fingers, not their brains.

To return to the temporary and cyclical nature of conceptual systems: in the world of academic psychology, the extraversion-introversion split was popularized by Eysenk but simply didn't exist as a way of seeing until the mid-twentieth century. Even depression, so beloved of drug companies and psychiatry, was not in common parlance in the 1960s; even in the late 1970s when working as a probationer clinical psychologist, this author received many referrals of people labelled agoraphobic, but none for depression.

Jackson[12] explores theories of the construction and treatment of depression and its forebear, melancholia, charting the history of the diagnosis from humoral postulants of the 5th century BCE to the publication of *DSM-III* in 1980. He notes numerous attempts by, amongst others, Samuel Johnson, Tuke, Pinel, Esquirol, Morel, Krafft-Ebing, Kraepelin, Meyer, Henry Maudsley and Freud to categorise and delineate forms of distress variously described as melancholia, involutional melancholia, insanity and psychoneurosis; "depression," he notes as, "a relative latecomer to the terminology for dejected states."[13] In 1725, Blakemore writes of "being depressed into deep Sadness and Melancholy" while in 1801, David Daniel Davis's translation of Pinel's *Treatise on Insanity* rendered *l'abbattement* as "depression of spirits."

To summarize. History moves in cycles, its recording determined by vested interests. Professional theory and practice are at a point on the cycle, not some glorious endpoint. Rationality is only a system of thought, not *the* system. Persons can be categorized according to any system (the very *existence* of persons can only be inferred, not logically proven[14]). That system could be based on visible conduct rather than invisible, wholly imagined, attributes. Psychology itself is simply a system, with no way of discerning either truth or the order of things. What might be the implications of all this?

A Nod Towards Utility

We could begin by asking what the most useful system might be for selecting therapists, politicians, friends, etc. Would you rather if your therapist could play with children, or had an IQ of 135 and a low score on the Beck Depression Inventory? Would you vote for a politician who was an extravert with an average rating on the *Hamilton Anxiety and Depression Scale* or smiled in a way that warmed your heart and played card games for pebbles? Do you want friends who help you out or see a bat perfectly clearly on card V of the Rorschach? Of course, such descriptors are not mutually exclusive. It is perfectly possible that your therapist has a high IQ and helps people off buses. For all I know, many psychotherapists can decipher Derrida *and* tell you the best time to plant onion sets.

For those presently at the receiving end, there may be some surprising results at its crudest a version of "What are you complaining about?" For example, under the present system you might approach a therapist saying that you feel miserable and occasionally hear distressing voices. Under the new system, hearing voices and being miserable have no diagnostic utility. The therapist will only have been trained to help people develop, say, kindness and a certain sensuousness in the way they walk. A previous diagnosis of "schizophrenia" here is irrelevant (unless medication is playing havoc with motor skills or attempts to withdraw have resulted in potentially lethal reactions[15]).

The advantage of a new typology is that it has immediate, non-technical meaning to the majority. Barely literate people understand real kindness, calm and intimacy. If such constructs were to be emphasized in the professional worlds of psychology and psychiatry, we might, just, develop a useful way of being with others. In the order of things, both professions might struggle. To outlast the Cathars would be achievement enough.

References

1. Calder, J. (2005). Histories of abuse. In: C Newnes & N Radcliffe (eds) *The Making and Breaking of Children's Lives*. Ross-on-Wye: PCCS Books.

2. Smail, D. (2005). *Power, Interest and Psychology*. Ross-on-Wye: PCCS Books.

3. Murdoch, I. (1992). *Metaphysics as a Guide to Morals*. London: Chatto & Windus.

4. Parodic because the psy professions are scientistic rather than scientific – it is impossible to remove subjective interpretations the assessor/observer from interviews with patients.

5. Boyle, M. (1999). Diagnosis. In: C Newnes, G Holmes & C Dunn (eds) *This is Madness: A critical look at psychiatry and the future of mental health services.* Ross-on-Wye: PCCS Books.

6. Leo, J. (1985). Battling over masochism. TIME, Dec. 2, 764.

7. Cooke, A. (2014). *Understanding Psychosis and Schizophrenia* Leicester: BPS Publications

8. Foucault, M. (1971). *The Order of Things.* (Trans. A Sheridan). New York: Random House.

9. Burgess, A. (1992). *A Mouthful of Air: Language and languages, especially English.* London: QPD.

10. Stenfert Kroese, W. (2005). The way ahead. St Anselm, rationality and the modern world. *Journal of Critical Psychology Counselling and Psychotherapy, 5* (2), 79–84.

11. Crane, N. (2002). *Mercator: The man who mapped the planet.* London: Weidenfeld & Nicholson

12. Jackson S. W. (1986). *Melancholia and Depression.* New Haven, CT: Yale University Press.

13. Ibid., p. 5

14. Russell, B. (1912/1991). *The Problems of Philosophy.* Oxford: OUP.

15. Lehmann, P. and Newnes, C. (eds) (2023). *Withdrawal from Prescribed Psychotropic Drugs.* Lancaster, UK: Egalitarian Publishing Ltd.

DSM: Formist Roots and Contextualist Alternatives

Jay S. Efran and Jonah N. Cohen

Abstract: *Formism, an explanatory model that seeks to classify phenomena based on similarities, underpins the architecture of the Diagnostic and Statistical Manual of Mental Disorders (DSM). This approach toward understanding mental disorders is problematic—linguistically, theoretically, and practically. This article reviews common linguistic confusions that are inherent to formist constructions, including the DSM. Contextualism is suggested as a more promising explanatory framework.*

In 1942, Stephen C. Pepper described six ways to understand the world. One of these—formism—emphasizes classification and list-making. It is the strategy on which the *Diagnostic and statistical manual for mental disorders* (DSM; American Psychiatric Association, 2022) is based. In this paper, we discuss the limitations of the formist approach and argue that contextualism—another of Pepper's strategies—would be more useful to clinicians. Unlike formism, contextualism (i.e., the telling of stories about unfolding life events) focuses on narratives rather than groupings.

Formism classifies phenomena by identifying similarities between objects and/or events. In other words, it is the "if it looks like a duck, it must be a duck" approach. This works reasonably well in some fields of study, such as botany: Plants can be grouped and understood in terms of their structural similarities. For instance, do they have similar leaf patterns, the same number of petals, and so on?

However, this strategy breaks down when dealing with the complexities of human behavior. Its use as the basis for the DSM is particularly problematic because that system combines a mishmash of different classificatory principles, many of which hinge on highly subjective, unreliable, culture-bound judgements.

Moreover, the exact mix of principles shifts from one disorder to another. Thus, it is possible for two individuals to carry the same diagnosis without having any characteristics in common. For instance, the diagnosis of Persistent Depressive Disorder requires exhibiting at least two symptoms out of a possible list of six. Thus, one person could qualify by complaining of poor appetite and insomnia (criteria 1 and 2) whereas another might manifest low self-esteem and decision-making difficulties (criteria 4 and 5).

Because of these foundational flaws, attempts to clean up the DSM have had little success, and it seems unlikely that future efforts will be any more successful. Thus, the DSM will remain an unwieldy concoction that lacks desirable levels of reliability, validity, and utility. At best, it provides limited assistance in establishing causes, selecting treatments, or predicting outcomes. Practitioners often rely on it to justify insurance payments. Even in that realm, however, it is a clunky system that invites deception. Unable to accurately portray their patients' conditions, clinicians choose labels that maximize the possibility of receiving reimbursement while minimizing the risk of stigmatizing patients.

These weaknesses are thoroughly discussed elsewhere (e.g., Cantú, 2023). Rather than rehash them here, we want to highlight two linguistic hazards that derive from the DSM's formist roots.

The Nominal Fallacy

In *The Imaginary Invalid*, Moliére's 1673 farce, a physician is asked to explain why opium puts people to sleep. He replies with great self-assurance that it is because opium has "dormitive properties." This is the classic, literary example of the nominal fallacy—a fancy name that masquerades as a sophisticated explanation.

Years ago, one of the authors informed his internist that he was experiencing digestive distress. Without a moment's hesitation, the internist diagnosed the problem as "gastritis." The author was impressed with the internist's diagnostic ability. He was able to identify the problem even before conducting a physical examination or administering any diagnostic tests. Later, the author realized that "gastritis" is simply the medical term (from Ancient Greek roots) for "stomach inflammation." By itself, the word conveyed very little information about the cause, treatment, or prognosis of the author's condition. However, it sounded good. Note that it was only the author who, in his naiveté, was impressed by the use of the term. The internist knew full well that the details of the author's illness were yet to be determined.

The danger of the nominal fallacy is that it prematurely halts investigation, creating the illusion that the phenomenon in question has already been adequately explained. Unfortunately, the mental health field contains a goldmine of potential nominal fallacies. For example, calling sadness "depression" sounds informative but explains very little. Similarly, fear is neither nullified nor explained by calling it a symptom of an anxiety disorder. We are reminded that maverick psychiatrist Thomas Szasz (1973) often called psychiatric jargon a "language of defamation" and worked to call attention to some of the field's more grievous nominal fallacies.

Map-Territory Confusion

The DSM is usually considered a "biopsychosocial approach" because it cites biological, psychological, and social determinants. Similarly, mental health workers often describe mental disorders as "psychosocial," "biopsychosocial," and "neuropsychological." These co-joined (or hyphenated) terms are well-intended attempts to capture the complexity of mental illness. However, all such formulations represent unrecognized map-territory confusions (Korzybski, 1995).

The specialized languages human beings invent, such as those of biology, sociology, chemistry, neurology, electronics, and psychology, are navigational tools—maps to aid in the exploration of particular experiential terrains. However, it is easy to forget that none of these maps *owns* any of the territories to which it is applied. In other words, just because the biological map has been successful in deciphering important aspects of our lives, that does not make humans biological creatures. Humans are no more biological than they are chemical, psychological, sociological, spiritual, cosmic, electronic, or neurological.

Each of those terms identifies an explanatory language and privileges a particular level of analysis. However, no linguistic analysis is synonymous with the object, event, or phenomenon being studied. Moreover, new languages—yet unimagined—will undoubtedly be called upon to explain aspects of our experience that are now puzzling. Also, certain descriptions that once seemed relevant will fall by the wayside as no longer effective. For instance, the "possession" theory of illness has now been largely abandoned in Western cultures, and exorcisms are now rare events. Similarly, the versions we call cathartic rituals have also lost popularity.

Because describing the symptoms of, for example, diabetes in chemical terms works well for many purposes, the illusion is that diabetes really is chemical rather than spiritual or socioeconomic. In other words, accomplishments using the language of chemistry seduce us into thinking of diabetes as a chemical event and nothing but a chemical event. Equating the *experience* of diabetes with chemistry is an illegitimate transformation. The disadvantage of that sort of equation is that we become less likely to analyze the phenomenon—in this case, diabetes—from other potentially profitable perspectives. Diabetes, for instance, can be usefully understood in terms of economics, dietary practices, and systemic oppression. As it turns out, America is among the five largest producers of sugar, Americans consume about 100 pounds of it per capita per year, and structural racism plays a significant role in the progression of the disease (Egede, et al., 2023).

Of course, we are always permitted to apply more than one language map to any aspect of our lives. However, there is a danger in combining such vocabularies in a helter-skelter fashion. This is the problem of conjoined mental illness maps of the "biopsychosocial" variety. How is one to decide how much of a particular condition is "bio," how much "psycho," and how much "social." What are the combinatorial rules? Should we assign percentages? Will the percentages be different in different cases? In the absence of clear guidelines that determine how and when to apply which sub-language, expressions such as biopsychosocial disintegrate into theoretical incoherence; they become mere slogans.

A far better approach is for specialists—psychologists, sociologists, economists, biologists, geneticists, and so on—to each try their hands at solving current problems using the vocabulary (and methods) of their respective disciplines. This comes close to what personality theorist George

Kelly (1991a, 1991b) had in mind when he created the theory of "constructive alternativism."

From Kelly's perspective, if a physician thought that he could make some sense of a panic attack using a stethoscope, he was welcome to try. On the other hand, Kelly objected to that same physician claiming that panic attacks were medical events and that non-medical explanations or interventions were illegitimate. He also considered it foolhardy for professionals, including psychologists, to suddenly speak the language of a different profession—one for which they had not been trained. Thus, when he designed his theory, he was careful to provide fully psychological definitions of terms such as "anxiety" and "guilt" so that psychologists would not be tempted to periodically lapse into biology-speak. He would certainly have gotten a chuckle out of those therapists who are now showing clients before and after brain scans to prove that psychotherapy works, as if only neurophysiological evidence matters.

Contextualism in the Clinic—A Better Alternative

Because formism deals in labels and classifications, it is particularly susceptible to the linguistic muddles we have described. On the other hand, contextualism—another of Pepper's six models—avoids such confusions and may be a more appropriate explanatory strategy for clinicians. It highlights narrative description rather than classification.

In *Mind and Nature* (1979), Gregory Bateson recounts a tale in which an advanced computer is tasked with determining the essence of being human. After many days of computation, the device spits out a tape that reads: "That reminds me of a story." Bateson's point is that we live in our stories—they are the glue that holds the self together. In our stories, we reveal who we are, both to ourselves and to others. Stories describe where we have been, where we are, and where we are going. It is the ideal medium for understanding a client's experiences in context.

Contextualism encourages great flexibility. One can choose how much of a person's existence to explore, and with what level of granularity. In fact, the freedom to determine a story's starting and end points can be one of the most useful tools in a therapist's arsenal (Hussong & Efran, 2023). The therapist can expand the problem focus to include the person's childhood or narrow it to the current week's events. George Kelly, who worked within the contextualist paradigm, wrote that "whatever exists can be reconstrued," adding that some constructions "open fresh channels for a rich and productive life" whereas others "offer . . . no alternative save suicide" (1969, p. 227-228).

In other words, our stories are consequential. In fact, an entire psychotherapy can be built around assisting clients to reorganize their stories, shorten or lengthen time perspectives, and revise the list of featured players. Kelly's (1991a) fixed-role therapy went a step further, encouraging clients to step out of their own narrative and spend a few weeks in another person's shoes. They could then make use of what they had learned about the world having peered at it through a different set of glasses.

Contextualism is a pragmatic approach. Constructions are valued in terms of their usefulness for the project at hand—not in terms of some metaphysical certainty. For instance, there is no requirement to construct a detailed family genogram if a simple series of exposures will eliminate the person's snake or spider phobia. Similarly, although there are multiple theories about hallucinations, including Julian Jaynes's (1976) fascinating thesis that hallucinating used to be a commonplace occurrence, one need not choose among these theories if a low dose of a psychotropic medication will eliminate the images that the individual finds disturbing.

Summary

It is unlikely that insurance companies will abandon the DSM anytime soon, nor will mental health diagnosis spring free of its formist roots and the related linguistic muddles. As George Albee (2000), former president of the American Psychological Association, notes, mental health workers long ago sold their souls to the devil when we agreed to accept the classification of mental illness as a branch of medicine and were bribed to define psychotherapy as a form of treatment. These "category mistakes" (Ryle, 1949) have haunted us ever since. However, it is foolish to keep struggling to convert the DSM into something it is not. At least in the psychology clinic, it seems more promising to explicitly shift to a contextualist model.

References

Albee, G. (2000). The Boulder model's fatal flaw. *American Psychologist, 55*(2), 247-248. https://doi.org/10.1037//0003-066X.55.2.247

American Psychiatric Association. (2022). *Diagnostic and statistical manual of mental disorders* (5th ed., text rev.). American Psychiatric Publishing. https://doi.org/10.1176/appi.books.9780890425787

Bateson, G. (1979). *Mind and nature: A necessary unity*. E.P. Dutton.

Cantú, A. (2023). It is time to replace the DSM: a critical review of social work and the biomedical model of practice. *Ethical Human Psychology and Psychiatry, 25*(1), 38-56. https://doi.org/10.1891/EHPP-2022-0002

Egede, L. E., Campbell, J. A., Walker, R. J., & Linde, S. (2023). Structural racism as an upstream social determinant of diabetes outcomes: A scoping review. *Diabetes Care, 46*, 667–677. https://doi.org/10.2337/dci22-0044

Hussong, D., & Efran, J. S. (2023). Rediscovering interpersonal punctuation. *American Journal of Psychotherapy, 77*, 1-4. https://doi.org/10.1176/appi.psychotherapy.20230009

Jaynes, J. (1976). *The origin of consciousness in the breakdown of the bicameral mind*. Houghton Mifflin.

Kelly, G. A. (1969). *Clinical psychology and personality: The selected papers of George Kelly* (Brendan Maher, Ed.). John Wiley & Sons.

Kelly, G. A. (1991a). *The psychology of personal constructs: Vol. 1. A theory of personality*. Routledge. (Original work published 1955)

Kelly, G. A. (1991b). *The psychology of personal constructs: Vol. 2. Clinical diagnosis and psychotherapy*. Routledge. (Original work published 1955)

Korzybski, A. (1995). *Science and sanity: An introduction to non-Aristotelian systems and general semantics* (5th ed). International Non-Aristotelian Library Publishing Company, Institute of General Semantics.

Pepper, S. C. (1942). *World hypotheses: A study in evidence*. University of California Press.

Ryle, G. (1949). *The concept of mind*. Hutchinson University Library.

Szasz, T. S. (1973). *The second sin*. Doubleday.

Medical Model of Treatment vs. the Psychosocial Model: How the Choice Impacts Lives Starting in Childhood

Elizabeth E. Root

Abstract: *The author proposes to demonstrate the imperative for choosing the appropriate treatment for emotional distress in the early stages of life. The author's examples from experience treating children in the public sector contrast divergent trajectories of emotional development between the two models. Her examples demonstrate the process of downward spiral in youngsters being treated by the psychiatric (medical) model. On the contrary, those treated without psychotropic medications (psychosocial model) experience happier outcomes and less time in treatment. The author details the risks associated with psychiatric treatment. Some discussion is given to the reasons for the reported increase of emotional distress among children and youth as well as to suggestions to remediate the stresses they face.*

Introduction

I know adults who struggle with chronic emotional and, sometimes, physical distress caused by their reliance on multiple psychotropic medications since childhood or adolescence. Indeed, the reliance is now real since the brain is by now seriously compromised. Even when one desires to get free of the medications, it is unlikely a psychiatrist or any doctor is available to titrate a large combination of drugs.

This comprises my case for early healthy choices when parents or caregivers face a need for help with a distressed child. The informed mental health provider can often perceive causes that lie in the family rather than in the individual child who might just be the one expressing the pain—and this statement sets the stage for all that follows.

I intend to demonstrate the superiority of the psychosocial model over the medical through discussions of related topics that include informed consent, comparison of methods used in the two treatment models, and the common pitfalls associated with the medical model. These include diagnosis using the *Diagnostic and Statistical Manual of Mental Disorders (DSM)*, psychotropic medications, and identification with the disorder.

Examples from my 19 years of clinical practice in the public sector illustrate my points. A related and final topic presents the work of specialists who address the ever-increasing phenomenon of distressed American children. These professionals cite educational changes and insufficient time in play as contributing causes.

Informed Consent

High-spirited Alice Compton[1] has entered first grade with gusto. Her teacher, Ms. Smith, begins complaining to Mrs. Compton about Alice's rambunctiousness. One day she calls to suggest maybe Alice should be "tested" for attention-deficit/hyperactivity disorder (ADHD) because Alice cannot sit still and focus on her seatwork, and she sometimes disrupts the rest of the class by speaking out of turn. She suggests medication might help Alice to stay focused. Since Alice is Mrs. Compton's oldest child, she hasn't had much experience with teachers. Alice's mother takes Ms. Smith's complaint to heart because Ms. Smith is the authority and Mrs. Compton wants Alice to succeed at school. She and Alice are referred to the local mental health clinic and Alice is evaluated by a clinical social worker. Mrs. Compton asks about this medication the teacher mentioned and the evaluator tells her Alice has to meet with the clinic psychiatrist for that.

The two present to Dr. Hamilton and they repeat basically the same procedure as with the social worker in a forty-five-minute session. Mrs. Compton tells Dr. Hamilton how Alice has always been strong-willed, high spirited, and energetic. She admits that Alice can be a challenging child who doesn't easily take orders and often argues and connives to get her way. She tells him Ms. Smith suggested medication. Dr. Hamilton responds with the various brand-name stimulants of the day. Mrs. Compton asks if there are side effects. He replies that some children have diminished appetite and that sometimes they have trouble sleeping. However, he states that he can prescribe another pill to help with the sleep. Mrs. Compton asks if he has any literature about ADHD and the medication. He readily hands her a booklet about the Attention Deficit Disorders and standard treatment. He also refers her to the CHADD[2] website.

At home, Mrs. Compton reads the pamphlet and gleans information from the CHADD website. Both tell her that a stimulant drug sometimes combined with counseling is the treatment of choice. They state unequivocally that medication is the crucial element in treatment. They also claim ADHD is a biological or neurological disorder and that stimulant medication corrects a chemical imbalance or anomaly in the brain. It seems to make sense. What is Mrs. Compton to do?

This scenario is played out every day in mental health clinics that serve children. Most parents believe in the validity of the information provided by the doctor. Mrs. Compton may have friends who report that their child's behavior and school performance improved with medication. Often the adults in the child's life make such claims based on their objective opinion. But if the child were asked, his or her subjective experience might be quite different. Many children complain that they do not like the feeling induced by the drug despite the praise of adults who find them more manageable.

In fact, the consent by Mrs. Compton to medicate Alice based on the information provided at the clinic is not an informed one. Dr. Hamilton failed to explain that the stimulant medications are all versions of either amphetamine or methylphenidate, which is a synthetic derivative of amphetamine and nearly identical in chemical structure and function—and that their effect on the brain is virtually identical to that of cocaine. Had Mrs. Compton thought to ask about that "test" for ADHD mentioned by the teacher, Dr. Hamilton would have had to admit that his diagnosis is only based on his judgment of Alice's behavior in his office and the little information Mrs. Compton gave him.

She didn't notice the tiny print on the back of the ADHD information booklet signifying that it is published by one of the drug companies that makes stimulant medication. Additionally, the CHADD website didn't mention its close alliance with drug companies and the American Psychiatric Association (APA). Every day doctors prescribe psychiatric medications without telling the parents the whole story. Often, doctors don't know the whole story because they are selective in their reading material and often base their recommendations on information (or misinformation) provided them by drug company salespeople who frequent their offices.

It is critically important for parents to be armed with the information they need to make informed choices in the treatment of their children for perceived problem behavior. Among clinicians in typical community mental health clinics, it is rare to identify one willing or even able to fill the vacuum of non-information or to correct misinformation. This author can attest that doing so is usually a swift path to unemployment.

I was fired from three of five positions for questioning the diagnoses of the staff psychiatrist or for going against the grain of the majority staff views. However, the clinical director of my fifth position respected my knowledge and requested I present in-service training to my peers. He had me invite Peter Breggin,[3] with whom I had made an acquaintance, to speak to our staff. Breggin presented his views in a friendly, even-handed manner and was well received. The clinic psychiatrist did not attend. During meetings I challenged this psychiatrist's actions as well as the drug salespeople's claims as they fed us their pitch along with gourmet food. I observed that one salesman met regularly with our psychiatrist to illegally push drugs not approved for children.

Attending educational planning meetings in schools was part of my job. Teachers and school administrators colluded with the mental health system in pursuit of diagnoses that allowed eligibility for special educational services. Ultimately, the goal was to get children on medication. Educators were so keen on getting students "tested" for labels that New York State changed the rules during my tenure, making it illegal to suggest diagnoses. They got around the rule by recommending "medical assessments."

Two Treatment Models

The Medical Model

The late George Albee, past president of the American Psychological Association (APA) and sage in the discipline of psychology, spoke at the 2004 Conference of the International Center for the Study of Psychiatry and Psychology.[4] Throughout his long career, he advocated for a preventive approach to emotional distress to replace the medical model of treatment. He pressed his conviction that psychologists made a tragic error when they borrowed the medical model from psychiatry at the dawn of their profession. Clinical social workers, the largest component of psychotherapists in our country, followed suit along with most other mental health professionals.

It is unfortunate that medical doctors laid the groundwork for mental health treatment because undoing their paradigm of diagnosing a disease and prescribing a medical solution has proved challenging. For purposes here, I'll refer to mental health practitioners who apply the medical model as "neurobiologists." They maintain that emotional distress is "mental illness" caused by a defect in brain chemistry and often with a genetic component. This remains the standard of diagnosis and treatment in most public and non-profit community mental health clinics.

The Psychosocial Model

I and many other clinicians embrace the psychosocial perspective, a view that diverges from the neurobiological in many respects. We believe that emotional distress stems from adverse life events to which people vary in response. Some people are more resilient and experience a mild upset; others become so overwhelmed by catastrophic events that they become irrational and temporarily flee from reality as a defense mechanism. Our opposition to the chemical imbalance theory is supported by the fact that decades of experimentation have produced no proof that emotional dysfunction is caused by faulty brain chemistry.

In working with children, it is relatively easy to identify the causes for temper tantrums, rages, or misbehavior. All the social, environmental, and familial influences that have impacted the child comprise the psychosocial history. When the primary caregivers disclose this history, the causes of misbehavior are usually evident to the impartial professional and sometimes to others close to the child who are often interviewed as part of the evaluation process. The causes are often not as obvious to parents who are too close and immersed in their child's life to be objective.

The psychosocially oriented therapist believes misbehaviors are normal child-like responses to extraordinary stress. Common stressors on children include divorce (especially when there is acrimony between parents), troubles associated with school, loss of significant friends or caregivers, multiple relocations, verbal or physical violence, and disability in a family member. The absence of such stressors means seeking elsewhere for explanation of the perceived problem. Sometimes the components of misbehavior like high energy, intensity, irritability, and temperament can only be explained by a child's innate personality, inherited character traits, or by some congenital anomaly.

A specialist who can diagnose or rule out a medical condition should evaluate unusually troubling behavior that may contribute to the problem. If a cognitive impairment such as a learning disability or mental retardation is suspected, psychological testing may be part of the evaluation. Cognitive impairments can also be difficult to diagnose, but knowledge of disability enables caregivers and teachers to obtain appropriate accommodations and form realistic expectations.

The Risks of Typical Mental Health Care

The fortunate child comes to the clinic with a problem that is solved relatively easily, and the family gets back on track in a timely fashion. Too often, though, the child enters a downward spiral that can lead to iatrogenic chronic illness due to being labeled, medicated long-term, possibly hospitalized repeatedly, and/or placed in a mental health day care program. The following are risks that can precipitate unfortunate outcomes.

Diagnosis with the DSM[5]

The first risk is posed when the clinician assigns a diagnosis to the child. Commensurate with the medical model, the clinician decides which, among the mental disorders listed in the *DSM*, matches the child's presenting condition. Most practitioners are bound by the rules of medical insurance companies that require diagnostic codes and precise prescriptions for treatment in order to receive payment. To this extent, the clinician is hijacked into the medical model regardless of any objection to the process. Moreover, often the parent requests or the referring source mandates further evaluation by the clinic psychiatrist. The great majority of children who visit this doctor leave with a prescription for psychotropic medication.

The *DSM-5* was unveiled in 2013 with changes that affect the diagnoses of children. The four diagnoses along the autism spectrum were subsumed under the title Autism Spectrum Disorder. According to Zur and Nordmarken,[6] a benefit is that it should result in less labeling because the criteria are more accurate and specific. However, many families with children carrying the dropped diagnoses (notably, Asperger's) feared losing educational services that were contingent on the diagnosis. These authors counter that educational services might more appropriately be delegated by educational professionals rather than by a manual designed to diagnose mental disorders.

A new diagnosis, Disruptive Mood Dysregulation Disorder (DMDD), was introduced, affecting children aged 6 and above and youth to age 18, and typified by frequent severe temper tantrums and all-around irritability or anger between them. The National Institutes of Mental Health (NIMH)[7] reports that research is ongoing to determine the best treatment for DMDD. In the meantime, treatment with medications used for other disorders that share symptoms of irritability, temper tantrums, ADHD, anxiety disorders, Oppositional Defiant Disorder (ODD), and Major Depression are recommended. This would include stimulants, antidepressants, and atypical antipsychotics.

For the psychosocial-minded clinician, it does not bode well that medication is the first recommendation. After medication, NIMH lists psychological treatments that include psychotherapy, parent training, and, for affected youth, computer-based training.

Pediatric Bipolar Disorder (PBD) was dropped from *DSM-5* because research indicated that youngsters with that label did not mature to adults with typical Bipolar. A study by Parry et.al.[8] concluded that Bipolar Disorder is very rare in childhood as well as adolescence, and when applied it fails to correlate with adult Bipolar Disorder. These authors state that even though early diagnosis is important, over-diagnosis risks adverse iatrogenic consequences.

Unfortunately, the risk proved real in many cases—some tragically so as in the well-publicized death of 4-year-old Rebecca Riley in 2006. Beginning at age 2 ½, she endured a regimen of 10 strong medications daily (many not approved for children) such as Seroquel (atypical antipsychotic), Depakote (anti-seizure medicine used as mood stabilizer) and clonidine (blood pressure medicine used as sedative). She died of an overdose of clonidine. Other child and adolescent deaths and injuries have been documented, many attributed to antidepressants as well.

To psychosocial clinicians, the elimination of PBD seems like a good thing. However, its loss together with the addition of DMDD can cause confusion. DMDD applies to children ages 6 and up, but younger children can still be labeled bipolar without clear diagnostic criteria for very young children. Furthermore, all pose characteristics similar to Oppositional Defiant Disorder.

Allen J. Frances, M.D.,[9] who was lead author of the *DSM-IV*, has been a most outspoken critic of the *DSM-5*. Frances cogently articulates long-held views of psychosocial-oriented therapists. His title, "*DSM-5* Diagnoses in Kids Should Always Be Written in Pencil," with the subtitle "Mislabelling children and adolescents is frequent and can haunt them for life" succinctly says so much and validates my own convictions formed over years working with children.

Frances reports that in the past 20 years, rates of the ADHD diagnosis tripled and rates of Autism and kiddie (his word) Bipolar have multiplied an incredible 40 times. He attributes these to powerful external factors. For example, drug companies provide very generous "research grants" to psychiatrists who invent new diagnoses such as pediatric bipolar to sell more and stronger drugs to children, the motive being to establish life-long customers.

My clinic experience substantiates the explosion of bipolar diagnoses in very young children just around the year 2002 following publication of many articles citing the work of a team of psychiatrists at Massachusetts General Hospital. The team claimed that bipolar could be caught early and treated with atypical antipsychotics, anticonvulsants, and other drugs that were previously prescribed only for adults. The consequences were devastating as the team wielded great influence. In some areas, evaluators were sent into pre-schools and homes overseen by department of social service workers to "test" for bipolar! All children with behavior issues were in peril of this regimen. Hopefully, this is alleviated with the *DSM-5* changes. However, I've no doubt that psychiatrists and drug companies continue their collaboration as Frances describes to exploit any revisions.

Frances blames the explosion of Autism diagnoses on the addition of Asperger's in the *DSM-IV* in addition to the fact that the diagnosis allowed eligibility for enhanced school services (just as the explosion of ADHD followed its inclusion in school special services in the early 1990s). Frances asserts that *DSM* diagnoses are inappropriate criteria for entrance to special educational services, that these decisions should be assessed by educators using educational tools, and they should be based on the child's educational needs.

Medication

Medication is the next risk factor following diagnosis. Years of observing children deteriorate following the introduction of chemicals into their brains via medication convinced me that doing so worsens the original problem. A worst-case scenario is when a second diagnosis is driven by a child's reaction to medication prescribed for the original diagnosis. If it seems to not "work," the psychiatrist may decide the first diagnosis was wrong or a second medication is prescribed to address a side effect of the first.

Absurd as it sounds, doctors sometimes claim the medication revealed a more serious underlying condition. They then assign or add a more serious diagnosis in which case the prescribed drugs will get stronger and multiply. Hence, the child's likelihood of developing lifelong iatrogenic illness rises significantly. I, sadly, observed this unfold many times during my tenure.

I worked with many children in the foster care system. The mandates of child protective services often rendered me impotent to provide the help I deemed appropriate. Virtually all the children were required to meet with the psychiatrist and were medicated with the usual downward spiral, often because it often took many months for the case to be settled. Sometimes the parents, likewise, rendered impotent, disparaged the process. Many times, I testified in family court on behalf of children and family.

> Jake was placed in foster care at age 9. I'd known the family for some years and believed the placement was unfounded. Caseworkers cited his ongoing conflict with school authorities as cause. Jake had been heavily medicated since age 6 with a changing regimen of drugs that included stimulants, atypical antipsychotics, and adjunctive drugs. In his first foster home, out of ignorance or carelessness, he overdosed on Depakote. Jake had continuous vomiting for days. This exacerbated his usual ridicule and denigration by teachers and caseworkers.
>
> When the psychiatrist documented his dangerously high blood level of Depakote, I used this information in family court in one of my attempts to bring Jake home. The dubious judge and social services lawyer were not moved despite the proof I provided with the doctor's document. Jake and his family suffered physically and emotionally for over another year before we succeeded in reuniting them.

Children are severely wounded by separation from their loved ones and medication is not the answer. I love what a presenter said years ago at a Point Park University symposium, "A broken heart is not a mental illness."

Identification with the Diagnosis

Especially devastating is the final risk factor that logically follows from a diagnosis and a chemical remedy. The child and parents are led to believe that the problem lies within the child. Getting a diagnosis and taking medicine support this erroneous belief that something is wrong with the child.

> Twelve-year-old Mary returned with her mother to our clinic after a time away. Her mother introduced the problem: "Mary's acting up. Sometimes I don't know if it's her bipolar or her ADHD that is coming out. I don't think the medicine is working, it probably needs to be increased." I turned to Mary then and asked how she felt things were going. Her response: "I got in trouble last week at school for fighting with a girl. And my grades went down this marking period." I asked if she could identify a reason for her difficulties, such as trouble with friends or a teacher she wasn't getting along with. She responded: "My friends don't understand about me being bipolar. The pills were helping me with my schoolwork before."

> Mary was revealing how she identified with a perceived disorder and felt something wrong with her negatively affected her friendships. Her diagnosis became a self-fulfilling prophecy. She attributed her success or deterioration to her medicine rather than taking credit or responsibility for the ups and downs typical for her age. I had known Mary since she was nine and felt she was a pretty typical youngster. She was vivacious and prone to outbursts that I deemed normal for the person she was. But her mother insisted on seeing the clinic psychiatrist because she, herself, and others in the family were bipolar and on medication—and Mary was just like her. The psychiatrist predictably agreed with mother and started the drug regimen at that time. She had been on and off various pills ever since and discontinued counseling except when prompted by a concern between doctor's visits. Scheduling an extra visit with the psychiatrist mollified this concern. But I knew Mary's future was jeopardized by an illness unwittingly created through the collusion of her mother and the psychiatrist.

Sadly, this is a common scenario where parents believe the problem resides in their child. They seem unwilling to look for other possible causes of unwanted behavior such as negative family interactions or other factors. They want the "quick fix" they have been led to believe lies in a pill. In Mary's case, her mother had believed for years that bipolar or some other disorder was inevitable because of family history—not necessarily of mental illness—but a history of dependence on medication to solve emotional distress.

It is very hard to convince parents like Mary's to try a psychosocial approach that reaches to the source of the distress and ameliorates emotional pain that cycles through generations. I could not help children like Mary who are destined to believe they have a mental illness that requires a lifetime of powerful medication. We can hope for a favorable turn of events before their brains or their lives are irrevocably damaged. Otherwise, these children face poor prognoses.

Steve Balt[10] offers an interesting viewpoint that would help people like Mary. Balt's blog has more to do with the often quite rancorous criticism of the *DSM-5*, but his insight and discussion applies to all *DSM* diagnoses. He points out that the label arrived at says little to nothing about the presenting complaint and nothing about how it should be treated. It's merely a means of satisfying an insurance requirement. Symptoms presented by the patient are subjective descriptions of the problem and what might be at its roots. That may be the information the clinician uses for diagnosis.

As for treatment, consideration of socio-cultural roots and all information gathered in a comprehensive evaluation comprise a basis for addressing the unique needs of the individual. Balt cites the new DMDD diagnosis, saying it may suggest something about the child's behavior or experience. However, given the heterogeneity of the population of kids getting the diagnosis, probing deeper is a must in order to decide on a potential remedy. Balt would say the good practitioner doesn't treat the DMDD, but he or she treats *the person with* (italics his) the DMDD. If only the psychiatrist treating Mary had adopted this view, Mary would have been less likely to identify herself with her diagnosis.

Balt stops short of what I perceive as a logical consequence of his directive; that the medical model is insufficient beyond applying a *DSM* diagnosis. It requires the psychosocial model to fairly treat the person with the presenting condition.

Childhood Distress

Much discussion has focused on the treatment of children. Missing are explanations for the eruption of distress among American children. Peter Gray cites research[11] that shows the steepest rise in children's mental health distress occurred in the 1980s when school standardized testing took precedence to the detriment of recess and other self-directed creative activities, which were cut. First priority became better performance on one-right-answer multiple-choice tests.

Gray[12] calls it fallacious that schools are addressing the crisis by hiring more school psychologists and developing socio-emotional learning (SEL) courses intended to teach students how to be sensitive toward others and reduce negativism; and yet, it's the schools themselves causing the distress. Not only do long periods of sedentary and boring micromanaged tasks and stiff competition for grades stress students out. He fails to mention the pressure teachers feel due to mandated testing; their stress also affects students. Gray nails a key cause of mental health distress in children, but it does not tell the whole story.

The 1980s was a transition time in our culture for families. Many went from one working parent to two, which necessitated childcare (both pre- and after-school). This meant loss of neighborhood play for the majority of children. Families vary in their capacity to make up for the expansive freedom of play that older generations enjoyed. Some have the ability to provide a close proximity.

But for most, the norm has become supervised activity all day long for children. Child development experts have written volumes emphasizing the importance of free imaginary play[13] and its requirement for healthy development. Space does not allow for elaboration on this very important topic. I refer the reader to Chapter 8 in my book[14] for a summary of some of these authors' revelations.

Given the changes discussed above, one might ask how our kids are doing in school and what is America's educational success rate. According to the Pew Research Center,[15] the United States' standing among developed nations is mediocre. Academic achievement among 15-year-olds in 2017 yielded the following: seventeen countries outranked the U.S. in Science; thirty-five in Math; and fourteen in Reading. Yet, Dominic Rushe[16] reports that the U.S. funds more per pupil than any other country. These statistics beg for remediation.

Summary

The model chosen, psychosocial or medical, influences the therapist's attitude toward clients. Psychosocial-oriented therapists focus on the strengths of their child clients believing, for example, that super-abundant energy rightly directed can be an asset. They collaborate with family members, believing that a suffering child does not stand alone, but rather is one member of a system of caring individuals, each willing to make adjustments. Psychosocial proponents believe our model enriches the quality of life for children and all family members.

The medical model devotee treats the child client as ill and applies a chemical remedy to that individual, denying the family the opportunity to get to the source of emotional distress and make system changes. Problems are likely to emerge on a continuous basis for years. Treatment gone terribly wrong was evidenced in client records at our clinic. Charts inches thick and sometimes divided into multiple volumes contained the stories of children made chronically ill by the treatment to which they were subjected.

One cause for the epidemic of distressed children lies within our schools where recess and opportunities for creative expression have been drastically reduced due to the introduction of competitive achievement testing. These exams stress both teachers and students due to achievement expectations on these tests. School stress is a macro-system phenomenon, burdensome to resolve.

Family life too has changed, diminishing the time available for children to have free, unsupervised play, which is a healthy deterrent of distress.

Childcare centers vary in their allotment of free time for kids in their care. Where this is lacking, some families are able to arrange alternatives for their children that allow for free play. Ideal is when extended family members are available to provide homecare, or when the primary caregivers can juggle schedules to allow more time together at home with their children.

References

1. All names are pseudonyms.

2. CHADD is an acronym for Children and Adults with Attention Deficit Disorder. It is a nationwide organization of lay people diagnosed with ADHD. It endorses neurobiological theory and stimulant medication.

3. Peter Breggin, M.D. is a long-time, well-known critic of the medical model and has published volumes on its myriad pitfalls as well as on positive alternative models.

4. Albee, George. "A Radical View of the Causes, Prevention, and Treatment of Mental Disorders." Plenary presentation at the 2004 Conference of the International Center for the Study of Psychiatry and Psychology, Flushing, NY October 8-10, 2004.

5. The *Diagnostic and Statistical Manual of Mental Disorders* is a publication of the American Psychiatric Association (APA) and is used nationwide by mental health professionals to assign diagnoses to their patients or clients.

6. Zur, Ofer PhD and Nordmarken, Nola MFT. "DSM-5 Diagnosing for Status and Money." Web page https://dzur.com/dsm-critic/

7. https://www.nimh.nih.gov/health/topics/disruptive-mood-dysregulation-disorder-dmdd/disruptive-mood-dysregulation-disorder

8. Parry, P., Allison, S. & Bastiampillai, T. "Pediatric Bipolar Disorder rates are still lower than claimed: a re-examination of eight epidemiological surveys used by an updated meta-analysis." *International Journal of Bipolar Disorders* 9, 21 (2021). https://doi.org/10.1186/s40345-021-00225-5

9. Frances, Allen J. M.D. "DSM-5 Diagnoses in Kids Should Always Be Written in Pencil; Mislabelling children and adolescents is frequent and can haunt them for life." *Psychology Today*. October 31, 2016

https://www.psychologytoday.com/intl/blog/saving-normal/201610/
dsm-5-diagnoses-in-kids-should-always-be-written-in-pencil

10. Balt, Steve, MD, MS. "Is the Criticism of DSM-5 Misguided?" Taken from
    Dr. Balt's blog at *http//thoughtbroadcast.com/2011/12/15/is-the-critism-of-the-
    dsm-misguided/*

11. Gray, P. (2013). "The decline of play and rise of psychopathology in
    children and adolescents." *American Journal of Play*, 3, 443-463.

12. Gray, Peter PhD. "More Play and Less Therapy for Students: Schools
    produce anxiety and depression and then hire therapists to reduce them."
    *Psychology Today. https://www.psychologytoday.com/us/blog/freedom-
    learn/202207/more-play-and-less-therapy-students*

13. Olfman, Sharna. "Where Do the Children Play?" in *Childhood Lost*, ed.
    Sharna Olfman (Westport, CT: Praeger Publishers, 2005), pp. 203-215.

14. Root, Elizabeth. *Kids Caught in the Psychiatric Maelstrom.* (Santa Barbara,
    CA: Praeger Publishers, 2009).

15. "U.S. students' academic achievement still lags that of their peers in many
    other countries." DeSilver, Drew. https://www.pewresearch.org/fact-
    tank/2017/02/15/u-s-students-internationally-math-science/

16. Rushe, Dominic. "The U.S. spends more on education than other
    countries. Why is it falling behind?" https://www.theguardian.com/us-
    news/2018/sep/07/us-education-spending-finland-south-korea

25 Alternative Models to the Psychiatric Model

Eric Maisel

Abstract: *In this chapter, the author provides a conceptual overview of alternative models to the psychiatric model of mental health treatment, arguing that the psychiatric model, while entrenched, is only one way of thinking about what can help sufferers. Because it is a flawed, pseudo-medical model whose legitimacy has recently been widely questioned, the psychiatric model is ready to be replaced by more helpful models, and in this chapter, the author describes and discusses twenty-five such alternative models.*

What are some real alternatives to the psychiatric model? What are some theoretical alternatives? Which of these alternative models currently exist and function? Who are they intended for? Which ones are the better ones and which are the worse ones and which are the more practical ones and which are the more impractical? How are they similar and how do they differ? And so on!

These questions vex us for four main reasons. First, they encompass everything about our species. To try to create models that take into account a French lad acting out in school, a farmer in Topeka who hates his wife, an executive in Damascus who is afraid of his government, an African tribeswoman hearing voices and having visions, a gay woman in a fundamentalist town, a child born with very high intelligence and a child born more anxious than average—to try to create models that take *all of this* into account, and everything else human, boggles the mind and feels like folly.

Second, our models butt up against our ignorance. When it comes to anything on our radar—let's say, "depression"—we will never know what is causing it in a given individual because cause-and-effect is human affairs is both complicated and opaque. We understand why the seven ball is rolling toward the pocket—because we hit it with the cue ball. That is the epitome of simple cause-and-effect. But the second we ask the next order questions: why did I strike the cue ball, and why did I happen to wander into this pool hall, and what was I looking for on this seedy side of town, and so on ... the second we ask about that infinite regress of causes and effects, we fall down the rabbit hole. That problem plagues our models, as we are simply too ignorant to know "what really" is causing that "depression" .... or anything.

Third, people do not mean the same thing by things which may be named in the same way. And they do not hold the same intentions for similarly named things. A shaman, a priest, a Buddhist monk, a spiritually-oriented psychotherapist, a spiritually curious sufferer, and even an atheist who believes in mystery may all say that what helps is "in the realm of the spiritual"—but is there any chance that they are speaking about the same things or holding the same intentions? If and when we posit a "spiritual model," who do we have in mind as the practitioner and what do we suppose that he or she might be proposing? An exorcism? A shamanic journey? An acid trip? Accepting God? Letting go of gods? Or what?

Fourth, we do not know what we mean by "mental wellness" or "mental illness." Is it more "well" to hate killing strangers during a war and return home with PTSD or more "well" to come home indifferent to your experiences because killing doesn't bother you at all? The first soldier is "mentally ill" and the second soldier is "well-balanced"? Is someone who believes that his phone is tapped "mentally ill" and someone who believes in made-up gods and heaven and hell "well-balanced"? Is someone who follows orders, when those orders harm others, just fine, mentally speaking? Is that the sort of person we want to anoint as mentally well: the one who is undisturbed by killing, who follows orders, who believes in made-up gods, and who plays a good round of golf?

So, let us accept that the task is impossible. We are not like the blind men in the famous Sufi tale of the elephant: their only problem was not knowing that they were feeling an elephant. What a simple problem, compared to ours! Our problem is much graver. We know we are dealing with an elephant. But we are asking impossible questions like "What is that elephant thinking?" and "Will that elephant turn on us one day?" That we are entertaining such impossible-to-answer questions should make us shake our head, chuckle a little, and settle for a hot chocolate. But we are indeed entertaining them.

In this chapter, let me describe twenty-five alternative models to the psychiatric model, chat about each one briefly, give a sense of its premises, and maybe open the door to some thinking. Each model is slippery and can easily change its shape and become more like some other model. Let us be easy with that reality and that shapeshifting, relax, and proceed.

The psychiatric model

On the one hand, it is very hard to say what the psychiatric model is, which is one of the reasons it holds such sway. On the other hand, it is easy to describe. It takes the position that there is something called mental illness, that we can easily identify those mental illnesses by virtue of their symptom pictures, that they are clearly caused by biopsychosocial causes, and that medicine is readily available for most of them. It is interesting how easily that sentence flows off the tongue and how much it looks like a reasonable vision of "what's going on." That it is completely false is startling and shows how amazing language is to lure and to falsify.

To say that something is "biopsychosocial" is to say absolutely nothing. To make believe that medicine diagnoses on the basis of symptom picture alone is nonsense. To make believe that these *are* "symptom pictures" when it comes to "mental illness" is to lie. But that, in a nutshell, is the model: human distress is a medical issue to be treated with chemicals fancifully called medication.

The logic of the model: mental distress is a broken brain sort of thing and requires the "medical treatment" afforded by psychiatrists.

Alternative 1: The medical model

The medical model is different from the psychiatric model. The medical model involves real medicine. It doesn't say that your child is suffering from a biopsychosocial problem. It says that your child has a tumor on the brain, which explains his explosive behavior. It then goes on to say what it can or can't do for the tumor—that is, it tackles talking about intervening at the causal level and not at the symptom level. If it can't intervene at the causal level—if, say, the tumor is inoperable—then it moves on to palliative care, symptom reduction, and other ideas having to do with "making it easier" on the child. But there is a clear distinction made between trying to tackle the cause and shifting to symptom remediation.

There are of course many, many instances where it is hard to know if the medical model is the appropriate model: think autism, for example. It is crazy-making that we often do not know and can't know if what we are seeing aligns with a medical intervention or doesn't. In theory, this "helping practice" is straightforward to understand; in practice, it can get profoundly murky.

The logic of the model: Some emotional and behavioral problems, and some forms of distress, are caused by genuine medical issues requiring medical intervention.

Alternative 2: The psychological model

Put simply, the psychological model announces that human beings have personalities (whatever that means precisely), that they have minds (whatever that means precisely), that they are some (unknown) combination of roiling forces, that their experiences matter, that the causes of their distress are rooted in their "psychology," and that with awareness of "their psychology" comes the possibility of "growth, healing, and change." Unlike the textbook definition of psychology as "the science of behavior," psychologically-minded practitioners do not typically believe that enough is known about the inner workings of human beings to call what they do "science."

But by the same token they often do want to act as if they do know: that, for instance, to presumptuously announce that Vincent van Gogh's troubles were caused by his "latent homosexual feelings." Of course, there are a hundred variations on a theme here: Freudian psychology, Jungian psychology, gestalt psychology, cognitive-behavioral psychology, positive psychology, etc. All, however, share the following core belief: that human beings are dynamic creatures with minds, that human beings think and feel, that human beings are relatively unaware of their motivations and conflicts, that human beings relatively often make their own misery, and that *more insight and greater awareness matter*.

The logic of the model: Unseen, deep in that roiling, messy place called the mind, are the forces that cause human anguish. Get those forces out into the bright light of daylight and exposed, and the person will feel better and do better.

Alternative 3: The talking model

The talking model is ubiquitous. But where did we get the rather odd idea that just "talking about it" could help so very much as to be all that a person might need to feel better and do better? Your father is beating you—let's talk about it. Your company makes a product that is poisoning millions. Let's talk about it. Your husband is sleeping with your best friend. Let's talk about it. Mixed up together in this model are two contradictory-feeling realities: that "just talking about it" does often help and that "just talking about it" can't possibly be enough in many instances.

The logic of the model: talking to another person often does a lot of good, whether that is talking to a friend, talking to a stranger, talking to a paid professional, or, who knows, talking to an AI robot (designed to be warm and supportive). All of psychotherapy, counseling, coaching, etc. is not only based on this model but relies on it.

Alternative 4: The talking-plus-action model

One version of the talking model is built on the idea that talking is enough: that, for example, airing a problem provides both relief and insight—and those are good things, whether or not they lead to change. Another version has it that "insight must be followed by work": that insight alone is insufficient for a sufferer to get the real relief he needs, and that real relief only comes by turning insight into action.

Life coaches, to take one group, want their clients to talk about things but then to actually do things. In everyday life, one friend might "just listen" to your woes and another, "pushier" friend might press you to take certain actions: for instance, leave your bullying spouse, ask for that raise at work, etc.

The logic of the model: dealing with distress is essentially a two-step process, where the sufferer gains insight and can name what he or she needs to do next in life, and then attempts to do that. The model does not suppose that the doing will be easy or successful—only that such doing is essential.

Alternative 5: The self-help model

Side-by-side with the idea that sufferers need "professional help" or need "outside help" in the form of social services or economic relief is the idea that sufferers can take good care of their emotional well-being all by themselves if they "do the work" that self-help implies: if, for instance, they grow in awareness, make cognitive changes, rid their life of toxic people, become less co-dependent, etc.

This model, which is not a stoic, grin-and-bear-it model but rather an optimistic, you-can-do-much-better model, plays on the following core ideas: that human beings can think and can come to understand themselves and their situation; and that they are free, or free enough, to build on that self-knowledge, make necessary changes, and radically improve their lives exclusively by their own efforts.

The logic of the model: human beings have all the inner resources they need to deal with any emotional or "mental health" problem that might arise. Yes, the actions they decide to take may require them to deal with the outside world—dealing with their critical boss, their bullying father, etc.— but, at the end of the day, they can arrive at a place of "wellness" through their own efforts.

Alternative 6: The custodial model

This model makes the following simple, clear assertion: society has rights. If you are a "danger to yourself or others," society has the right to intervene. If you are "incapable of taking care of yourself," society has the right to intervene. If you commit a crime while "not in your right mind," society has the right to remove you from society.

If, in certain countries, you are a dissident and you do not agree with those in power, those in power have the right to call you "insane" and lock you away. In these and in similar instances, the model takes no particular interest in your concerns, inner workings, or desires: it boldly announces that society's needs come first. The particular custodial situation may be more or less humane, but even if it is "humane," it is still a coerced situation where the individual's rights have been abrogated.

The logic of the model: If you are "mentally ill" — or, more precisely, when a so-called expert or panel of experts say that you are "mentally ill" — society has the right to segregate you from the rest of society, for their good and also "for your own good." You have been identified as a problem and society has no better way of rectifying "you as problem" than by separating you from "normal people" and taking complete control of your life.

Alternative 7: The village model

The village model is an idea, an ideal, or an idealized version of what is possible or could be possible: the idea that everyone in a community looks out for everyone else and, when it comes to a little Johnny who is different in some way or difficult in some way, the whole community accepts little Johnny as "different" or "special," does not stigmatize little Jonny, actively helps little Johnny when he's lost or runs afoul of some rule, and continues helping him and accepting him when he becomes Big Johnny. This model presumes that members of a community know one another, care about one another, and accept community interventions.

The logic of the model: Built into this model is the idea that people "are who they are" and "can't really change" and therefore need to be supported without criticism or judgment and without any hope that they "will improve." This model takes personality as relatively or absolutely immutable and, in that sense, it is a pessimistic model; but at the same time, it is a humane and supportive model, announcing that, "with everyone's help," even "the least equipped and the most troubled" community members can live a decent life.

Alternative 8: The therapeutic community model

Sometimes actual, real-world therapeutic communities are created that are typically residential in nature—that is, "guests" live there. In these "intentional communities," the intentions are to refrain from psychiatric medication (though sometimes they are employed); to refrain from constraint and the custodial model; to treat the folks served as human beings and as equals; to provide them with simple real-world duties, like gardening or tending to livestock, duties that support the community and provide a stress-free daily routine; and to "think as a team" with respect to each "guest." Many of these therapeutic communities have actually existed and some handful continue to exist.

The logic of the model: the model is rooted in a set of philosophical principles; that human beings, no matter how distressed or disturbed, can be significantly helped simply by treating them with respect and by having their situation simplified and "normalized"; and that these troubled or "disorganized" individuals do not need and will not benefit from psychiatric labeling or psychiatric interventions like chemicals and electroshock. This is a sophisticated, intentional, spelled-out version of the village model.

Alternative 9: The activities model

The activities model is a modest model. It holds as a core conviction that a troubled, anxious, or otherwise distressed or disturbed person can gain some relief from their miseries by engaging in one or another simple activity: by, for example, sewing, drawing, acting, singing, building, carving, cooking, potting, and so on. To sing in a choir might make the difference between feeling unwell or well, as might building shelters for the homeless, meditatively hand-building ceramic sculptures, or working with others on a memorial quilt. While a modest model, it makes a certain sort of strong claim: that activities of this sort not only might complement other helping strategies but might actually be more beneficial than chemicals or talk.

The logic of the model: the model follows a simple principle or guideline, that certain activities are by their nature therapeutic. The "why of it" may be that these activities are social, or meditative, or meaningful, or creative, or work for some other reason—but the "why of it" is much less important than that they garner results.

Alternative 10: The social model

Many pundits argue that personal distress is always a social issue having to do with an individual's experience as powerless and as a pawn of society. You might call this the Marxist view of distress. Others argue that isolation, social distancing, and social fracture are major players in the distress game and solutions come under the headings of intimacy, friendship, community, and even the company of strangers.

In this view, to take one sort of example, sitting on a park bench among other park visitors is healthier and more therapeutic than sitting on a bench in one's own garden, maybe stewing too much or reminiscing too much. To love and be loved, to not be oppressed, to have friends to chat with and commiserate with, to experience human warmth and contact on a regular basis—that's the ticket, in this view.

The logic of the model: the model takes society and the society of others as not just influential and important factors with regard to achieving and maintaining emotional well-being, but as number one factors. Oppression creates distress and loneliness creates distress; and the remedies required are actions in the world, not pills or talk.

Alternative 11: The social work model

The social work model is a variation of the social model and pulls together elements of various models to paint the following picture: your circumstances matter; your support systems matter; your family matters, for better or for worse; your class and status in society matter; and that your individual psychology and personal wellness connect to your social experiences, whether that's living in poverty, suffering from abuse, needing medical help, growing up in foster care, etc. In line with this model is the idea that society at large must create institutions that help individuals—institutions that, as shorthand, might be called "social services." The individual is massively affected by his social conditions; society, in turn, is obliged to help individuals better their conditions.

The logic of the model: society is instrumental in harming individuals and individual distress ought to be viewed primarily through a societal lens. Second, since society harms individuals, it is on society's shoulders to provide help to those individuals who are being harmed by society, help in the form of social services. In this view, individual development, psychology, and personality all matter, and individuals can be helped via other models (like talk, activities, therapeutic communities, etc.), but the addition of institutional help in the form of social service is a necessity.

Alternative 12: The improved circumstances model

The social model and the social work models posit that circumstances matter a lot. The general version of this model is that having money is better than living in poverty, that having food is better than starving, that having loved ones is better than living lonely, that writing a novel and publishing it is better than writing a novel and failing to publish it, that not being beaten is better than being beaten, that good health is better than chronic illness, and so on.

When one friend says to another, "Things will get better," implied in that hope is the idea, "Things will get better and *as a result* you will feel better." We believe that, all things being equal, better circumstances help produce emotional well-being. Yes, we can picture all sorts of exceptions: for instance, the bored aristocrat who has everything and feels empty and terrible or someone so harmed by life that improved circumstances do not make enough of a difference. But as a general rule, we tend to believe that improved circumstances are keys to reducing difficulty and distress.

The logic of the model: the psychiatric or mental disorder model makes believe that human beings are indifferent to and unaffected by their circumstances. They are depressed because they have hormonal or neurotransmitter problems, not because they are living in a box under a bridge or are penniless. The "improved circumstances" model, by contrast, argues that the particular circumstances in which a person finds himself contribute greatly to his emotional well-being or lack of well-being.

Alternative 13: The familial model

The familial model posits the family as profoundly important in both helping and harming—and more than that, even determinative. Family therapy operates on the assumption that a family member's troubles can't be understood without an understanding of that family's rules, roles, and dynamics—that is, without understanding the "family system."

To chat with a child who is the "identified patient" and not inquire about his family life sounds absurd on the face of it. Yet, the psychiatric model allows for that; and the familial model absolutely does not. Common sense tells us that in some cases, the family will prove of great value in helping the sufferer, going "above and beyond" what someone without blood ties would be willing to do. And in other cases, family members may prove the worst culprits. Family life matters—even long after an offending family member has died.

The logic of the model: The model sees family life as a theater of dramas, a Shakespearean world of Lears and Hamlets and Lady Macbeths who are psychologically connected to one another. These dramas play out as rivalries, as estrangements, as abiding differences, and more; and also as the deepest love and affection possible. To look at a person's troubles and not inquire about his or her family life is to miss what may be actually causing those troubles.

Alternative 14: The social group model

The social group model posits the following idea: that we may be harmed or helped by the groups with which we identify; and, whether we are harmed or helped, we are bound to be affected by those identifications, interactions, rules, and constraints. We may be helped when we can make deals based on a handshake, because we have complete trust that this fellow Jew or Mormon or police officer will keep his or her word.

We may be harmed when, for instance, we do not accept the role our group has demanded that we adopt or when our group chastises us for breaking with custom—say by marrying outside the group. In looking at what is causing a person's distress and what might help alleviate that distress, a helper had better not ignore the individual's group affiliations and interactions.

The logic of this model: this model focuses on the power of the group to both provide comfort and cause distress. Unlike the social model, which looks to the broader culture as influential, the social group model argues that the local group—this Mennonite community, this fire station, this monastery, this real estate office, this local village—is where the psychological action is and where a person either flourishes or flounders.

Alternative 15: The developmental model

The developmental model posits one core idea: that a person may simply not be "ready." To take two examples, the youngest child in a class may not be mature enough to cope and so may bounce off walls or act out and end up with an ADHD diagnosis; and an adult suffering a tremendous loss may not be ready to move on for the longest time, meaning that the despair he or she is experiencing is not a clinical matter but predictable and natural.

The phrase that captures the essence of the developmental model is "going through a phase": maybe it's a teenage rebellious phase, a military enlistment that comes with hard drinking, a period of sexual experimentation following the end of a lengthy marriage, etc. While not all distress and difficulty can possibly be explained as a matter of "going through a phase," some no doubt can.

The logic of the model: the model is premised on the idea that "development" is a rich, important, and true aspect of the human experience; that, while meaning many things (including the Jungian idea that human beings tend to un-develop over time, arriving them at a predictable mid-life crisis), ought to be considered when looking at a given individual's distress, difficulties, and current level of functioning.

Alternative 16: The home nursing model

Highly impractical, but well worth thinking about, is the home nursing model. Here we picture the distressed person having his or her personal angel who is always available and who helps in multiple ways. This "mental health home nurse" is available for chatting; provides human warmth and contact; knows to join her charge in a little knitting or a walk outside; suggests actions for her ward to take; and functions as a combination therapist, coach, social worker, and cruise director. Of course, no such helpers currently exist, none are being trained, and few people could afford the luxury of such a full-time, live-in helper. But if this person were conceptualized as part-time help, appearing even only once every few days, then we begin to see the outline of something at once valuable and not completely impractical.

The logic of the model: that it is theoretically possible for helpers to be trained in many non-psychiatric helping methods and that these new helpers might make a significant contribution to the emotional well-being and mental health of their charges. This may be a fanciful vision; or it might not be.

We can look at **Alternatives 17, 18, 19, and 20** together. They are the humanistic model, the witnessing model, the talking group model, and the 12-step model. The core tenet of the humanistic model is that people already have answers and only need a safe environment and a warm, supportive listener in order to access those answers. The witnessing model holds that if you listen to others who are truthfully and forthrightly describing their difficulties, you will become more truthful and forthright yourself and more able to face your own challenges. The talking group model makes use of ideas one and two and suggests that a certain sort of group, the support group, whether led by a therapist, a pastoral counselor, a coach, or someone else, is a valuable way for troubled individuals to feel safe, feel heard, and bear witness. These ideas of safety (including the safety that comes with anonymity), authentic speaking, bearing witness, and the "talking group" model come together in Alternative 20, the well-known 12-step model.

For brevity's sake, we can also look at numbers 21-24 together. **Alternative model number 21** is the *spiritual or religious model*. This model posits that the support and comfort afforded by spiritual beliefs (for instance, in a heaven) and the community afforded by like-minded believers promote emotional well-being. **Number 22** is the *existential model*, which posits that human beings are emotionally healthier if they've found meaning, or can make meaning, and if they feel that their life has purpose or multiple purposes; and, conversely, that they can't really feel well if they have meaning and purpose shortfalls. Related to this model is **number 23**, the *philosophy of life model*, which posits that having, practicing, and living a coherent philosophy of life makes for mental health: that is, living like a Stoic or a Buddhist provides a sense of coherence and well-being. Related to these three is **number 24**, the *indigenous model*, that is, the idea that indigenous cultures, with their rituals, ceremonies, belief systems, and community feeling, meet their members spiritual and existential—and therefore emotional—needs.

Last for now, **alternative model 25**, is the eclectic model. This is a commonsense model that best matches our understanding of what is really needed, namely help appropriate for the situation. Sometimes you need talk. Sometimes you need social services. Sometimes you need a psychological approach that helps you understand your motives. Sometimes you need help from others—from family, from friends, from the dedicated helpers at a therapeutic community. Sometimes you need the cheerleading and goal-setting of a coach. Sometimes you need to take strong or difficult action. Sometimes you need an existential helping hand that brings you back from the precipice of meaninglessness. Sometimes you need a new philosophy that brightens or broadens your world view. A helper who could provide you with all of this or who could point you in the direction of all of this—well, that person is desperately wanted.

And what about "models of the future"? Of course, they are coming—and many of them are either here already or are right around the corner. What are we to make of "therapy apps" and "coaching via text messages" and other technology-driven, device-based helping? What is artificial intelligence about to bring? How soon will we be sitting across from helpful robots? But let's leave all of that to one side. The main takeaway I want to leave you with is that the psychiatric model, while "in our face" by virtue of its expert patina and its connections to Big Pharma, is only one way to look at what promotes mental health and emotional well-being—and maybe the very worst way. If a psychiatrist wants to say, "We're all you've got," you're entitled to flat-out laugh. And you might take that arrogant and unjustified notion of his as reason enough to march right out the door.

A Mental Health Concerns Classification System: A Revolutionary Alternative to the *DSM*

Jeffrey Rubin

Abstract: *Most individuals seeking to access mental health services must have their concerns translated into medical sounding, psychopathologizing terms such as mental disorders, and mental illnesses. Mental health service providers, to be reimbursed for their services by insurance providers, are required to select from a variety of these psychopathologizing terms and then place its code on the service user's health insurance form. The reasons for this psychopathologizing and its shortcomings are presented in this article, along with a proposal for a revolutionary, scientific, humanistic, practical alternative. This alternative is described and involves creating a manual for a classification system that replaces psychopathologizing with mental health concerns that potentially serve an adaptive function. It is argued that, in contrast to the pathologizing approaches, this alternative would increase the self-efficacy of individuals struggling with these concerns, improve their outcomes, provide a new preferred choice to both mental health service users and professionals, stimulate fresh perspectives, and open new avenues of research.*

Most folks who seek mental health services because their behavior, thoughts, or feelings have begun to concern them find that mental health service providers will translate their concerns into mental disorder terminology. Synonyms for "mental illness" are "mental disorder," "mental disease," and "psychopathology." In this chapter, we examine the main reasons for this translation, the problems this process creates, and a proposal for eliminating these problems that is scientifically defensible, practical, humanistic, and health promoting.

The Reasons Why Mental Health Concerns are Pathologized

Szasz (1961) reviews the history and several main reasons for pathologizing mental health concerns. In brief, for centuries medical doctors had been treating patients who came to them with various physical complaints. Occasionally, a patient would come in with a complaint and the doctor, upon examination, found nothing physically wrong. This frequently led to the doctor referring the patient to the clergy, but some doctors were intrigued by these types of complaints.

They began to develop theories about what was causing them and trying out various interventions to see if they helped. When writing articles about these efforts, they drew on the language with which they were most familiar. Terms like "pathology," "disorder," and "disease" commonly used in their practices were utilized, but they simply began to make distinctions between physical pathologies and psychopathologies, between physical disorders and mental disorders, and between physical diseases and mental diseases.

By the twentieth century, a new medical profession had sprung up that specialized in treating these concerns. They called themselves psychiatrists and formed professional organizations. Psychologists, counselors, social workers, and psychiatric nurses also began to organize. Complicating their efforts, many different approaches were being used to classify the various concerns that interested them.

Although their overarching concept usually were the various synonyms for mental disorders, the subcategories of these classification systems differed in what was labelled, their defining features, and their etiology. Moreover, some systems included only a handful of diagnostic categories; others included hundreds. By mid-century, the World Health Organization (WHO) and the American Psychiatric Association (APA) recognized that the existence of so many approaches was confusing and began attempts to create a common classification system upon which the profession might agree.

APA has been calling its version the *Diagnostic and Statistical Manual of Mental Disorders* (DSM). The WHO, in contrast, has been including its versions in a separate section of its *International Classification of Diseases* (ICD). To address various criticisms, every few years the APA and WHO put out their latest updated versions. In recent years, the ICD has become very similar to the DSM, and they now share the same diagnostic codes used by administrators in mental health clinics, hospitals, and insurance companies (APA, 2013, p. 13).

While these classification systems were being revised every few years, the public and mental health professionals began to advocate that mental health services be covered by health insurance policies. Consequently, in 2008 the United States Congress with the support of its president, passed the "mental health parity law" that requires coverage of services for mental health, behavioral health, and substance-use disorders to be comparable to physical health coverage. The codes for each "mental disorder" that appears in the DSM and ICD proved convenient for the insurance industry's recordkeeping.

Even before this law was passed, the pharmaceutical industry has had a huge financial interest in promoting the idea that psychological concerns were real "illnesses" that require drug treatments just like physical illnesses. Cosgrove and colleagues (2023) make a compelling case that this can be seen by how the industry is exerting a great deal of influence on psychiatric research and practice, resulting in publications and news reports that exaggerate claims of its drug treatments' effectiveness while minimizing harms.

For example, Cosgrove and colleagues (2009) explain that the Clinical Practice Guidelines (CPG) for mental health services are developed, endorsed, and disseminated through APA as the standard of care for health care providers. The confidence in the benefits of these drug treatments, if free of industry influence, would be more convincing but they caution that:

> Ninety percent of the authors of 3 major guidelines in psychiatry had financial ties to companies that manufacture drugs which were explicitly or implicitly identified in the guidelines as recommended therapies for the respective mental illnesses. None of the financial

associations of the authors were disclosed in the CPG (Cosgrove et al., 2009, p. 228).

The industry also has a compelling financial interest in the DSM revision processes. The vaguer the definitions of the various mental disorders, the easier it is for people to be labeled as having a disorder, and thus become qualified for drug treatments that qualify for reimbursement. Reflecting this interest, it has been shown that, as an example, one hundred percent of the members of the DSM-IV revision panels on "Mood Disorders" and "Schizophrenia and Other Psychotic Disorders" had financial ties to drug companies (Cosgrove et al., 2006).

Joining the pharmaceutical industry in promoting that these mental health concerns are illnesses are some parent groups and people labeled as having a mental disorder. The idea that certain actions that violate societal norms are mental illnesses like any other illnesses can be attractive because of the belief it eliminates guilt and shame. The analogy often used is just as parents are not properly blamed for their offspring contracting diabetes, they are not properly blamed for their offspring contracting a mental illness. Similarly, many folks who did some serious wrongs when they were in the throes of alcohol addiction found some relief from guilt and shame by apperceiving their addiction as an illness.

While all of this was going on, there were science-minded people who became interested in scientifically studying various psychological concerns. Scientists using the scientific method do basically three things:

1. Observe their domain of interest in both natural and experimental settings.
2. They then share their observations with other scientists and other interested parties.
3. To make this sharing process efficient, they create a classification system specifically for their area of interest that has an overarching concept, and, below this, various sub-concepts. For example, scientists interested in birds use the concept of birds as its overarching concept, and various types of birds such as blue jades, orioles, and eagles, as sub-concepts. Classification systems

structured this way make it vastly more efficient to retrieve specific information about a subject. If I want to find information about recent observations regarding eagles, I do not have to search through all books in a library until I find some that contain this information. By simply looking for the word "eagles" in either the index of non-fiction books with titles about birds or placing it in a search engine, relevant information is retrieved.

Because those in the practice of providing mental health services had already created their classification system, scientists interested in the domain that became known as "psychopathology" adopted the same classification system. By doing so, they found its various short phrase classification terms such as major depressive disorder, anxiety disorder, and so on (convenient for book titles, indexes, and search engines). When used in this way, they found much of the information they wanted to share was readily retrievable by other psychopathologists and interested parties.

So, in sum, mental health service providers, the pharmaceutical industry, some parents of those labeled as mentally ill, some labeled as mentally ill, and scientists of psychopathology have found translating mental health concerns into mental disorder jargon helpful in the following ways:

1. It provides a common language for mental health professionals to communicate about those utilizing their services.
2. It furthers the pharmaceutical industry's interest in selling drugs.
3. Apperceiving some behavior that violates social norms as illnesses appears to diminish feelings of guilt and shame.
4. Third-party payers and administrators of mental health services have found that its coding system works well as part of a practical method for their record keeping. With the aid of these codes, people manage to access mental health services, mental health service providers manage to get paid, and for-profit health companies tend to make a profit.
5. Its various classification terms, such as major depressive disorder, anxiety disorder, and so on, are short phrases that provide an efficient method for accessing information.

Despite these benefits, as we shall now see, many have pointed out that the DSM/ICD classification system has several serious shortcomings, some well-known, and others, less so.

The Well Recognized Shortcomings of the DSM/ICD Approach

Critics of the DSM/ICD approach have pointed to several of its weaknesses, and these have been discussed extensively in the literature. Here, I briefly describe the major ones before focusing on two that have not received the attention they deserve.

The shortcomings of the pathologizing approach that have been widely discussed are,

1. It is stigmatizing to mental health service users (Corrigan, 2004; Johnstone, 2014; Rubin, 2000; Taylor, 1984).
2. It privileges the clinician's perspective over that of the mental health service user (Fatemi, 2015; Johnstone, 2014; Miller et al., 2014).
3. It is a monopoly with all the drawbacks associated with such institutions (Raskin & Gayle, 2015).
4. It has serious reliability and validity problems (Insel, 2013; Rubin, 2018).
5. By pathologizing psychological concerns, it promotes the use of psychiatric drugs that in many situations worsen outcomes (Breggin, 2007; Whitaker, 2011).
6. By focusing on what's wrong with the individual, it tends to miss the complex relational context and malfunctioning social structures (Robbins et al., 2017).

Two Problems Created with the Use of the DSM/ICD Approach Not Often Recognized

The "diagnosis" and "disorder" concepts as used in the DSM/ICD are vague enough to be very misleading. To bring this to light, we shall first examine the "diagnosis" concept.

The Misleading Use of the "Diagnosis" Concept

The use of the diagnosis concept in both the DSM and ICD is misleading for two reasons. The first has to do with whether a mental disorder diagnosis indicates a cause has been determined for the expressed concern that led to the seeking of professional help. The second has to do with how a "clinically significant disturbance" is determined during the diagnosis process.

Does a mental disorder diagnosis indicate causality has been determined?

Both the DSM and ICD claim they are *diagnostic* systems. When used in the medical profession, a diagnosis can suggest that the cause of the disease has been determined. That is not the meaning being used in the DSM and ICD.

Consider the definition of a mental disorder in the most recent version of the ICD, the ICD-11 (World Health Organization, 2023):

> Mental, behavioural and neurodevelopmental disorders are syndromes characterised by clinically significant disturbance in an individual's cognition, emotional regulation, or behaviour that reflects a dysfunction in the psychological, biological, or developmental processes that underlie mental and behavioural functioning. These disturbances are usually associated with distress or impairment in personal, family, social, educational, occupational, or other important areas of functioning.

There are a lot of problems with this vague definition that we will soon see, but, for now, notice the word, "syndrome" in the first sentence. The DSM's definition of mental disorders also states in its first sentence they are syndromes (APA, 2013, p. 20). What does that mean?

According to the United States' National Library of Medicine (Calvo et al., 2003) which refers to itself as the National Center for Biotechnology Information, it states:

The improper use of the terms "syndrome", "disease" and their relations to "diagnosis" is one of the difficulties with which medical informaticians must deal, especially when developing expert systems to support diagnoses. Although ubiquitous in medical and lay discourse, the term "disease" has no unambiguous, generally accepted definition. However, most of those using this term allow themselves the comfortable delusion that everyone knows what it means.... A **syndrome** is a recognizable complex of symptoms and physical findings which indicate a specific condition for which a direct cause is not necessarily understood...Once medical science identifies a causative agent or process with a fairly high degree of certainty, physicians may then refer to the process as a **disease**, not a syndrome...

Medical literature, even that from governmental organizations and institutions authorized to implement standards, is plagued with misleading assertions such as "a syndrome is a disease ...", "a syndrome indicates a particular disease..." and "Lyme disease syndrome" (It is inappropriate to apply "syndrome" to Lyme disease because its causative agent is known).

Clearly, the National Library of Medicine is advocating that to improve specificity, "syndrome" should only be used to describe a condition when medical science has *not* identified the cause of a condition. It is crucial to fully understand this point if the reader is to follow the rest of the arguments in this article, so I will provide a few examples to make the point as salient as possible.

Imagine you have trouble starting your car. You bring it to Fred, your friendly local mechanic. On hearing your concern, he provides an initial theory of what is causing this—perhaps your car needs a new starter. This is the initial "theoretical" diagnosis. Then, Fred inspects the starter and finds that it is in fine shape. Thus, his original theory of what is wrong proves incorrect.

He then theorizes that your spark plugs are dirty. He looks and finds that they are indeed dirty. He cleans them up, puts them back in their proper place, and the car starts right up. In the end, he "diagnosed" what was wrong with your car—it had dirty spark plugs.

Now, let us say that Fred, instead, had just asked you a few questions. Then, before finding out what was the cause of why your car had not been starting, he told you that the problem is that your car has "Major Non-starting Disorder." This statement is very different than "diagnosing" your car's problem unless we want to dramatically expand the definition of diagnosis.

The DSM and ICD, by claiming they are manuals for making diagnoses, is too vague about the difference between the following three types of statements:

1. "My theory is your car is not starting because it has a broken starter."
2. "The cause for your car not starting is it has dirty spark plugs."
3. "Your car has 'Major Non-starting Disorder.'"

These three statements refer to distinctly different meanings. Statement one indicates someone has made an educated guess at what may be causing the problem. Statement two indicates that the reason for the problem has been identified. Statement three just translates the problem into jargon.

Now, let us look at an example of a medical doctor using the "diagnosis" concept to indicate the cause of the concern has been determined. Matt, after being tackled in a football game arrives at the hospital hopping on his right leg and explains to a medical doctor that he is unable to put any weight on his left leg without feeling excruciating pain. The doctor asks a few questions, learns about the football game tackle, and theorizes that Matt might have broken a bone. He decides to take an x-ray of Matt's left leg. Minutes later, he sees in the x-ray that Matt has a left leg fractured fibula. The doctor then declares his or her diagnosis—a left leg fractured fibula.

Here, the "diagnosis" concept represents the idea that the doctor has identified what is causing the patient's complaint. Prior to identifying the cause, the doctor offered an initial theory of the cause. Using the "diagnosis" concept without clearly stating that it is just a theory would be a misleading use of the concept. If the doctor, prior to taking the x-ray, told the patient, "My diagnosis is, you have 'Major Inability to Stand Disorder'," this would be a very different use of the "diagnosis" concept because it simply translates the expressed concern into jargon.

A theory of a cause, a proven cause, and jargon for an expressed concern are three distinct things. To refer to all three as a diagnosis makes it more difficult to see this difference and leads to the following common misconception.

On one fine spring day, I was sitting on a Central Park bench and two women were sitting one bench to my right reading their newspapers. Suddenly, one of them cried out,

- "Sophie, can you believe this! The story I'm reading here, oh my God! This young boy, seventeen years old mind you, the same age as my Jonathan, he's struggling with ideas about suicide. Seventeen years old, his whole life before him and he wants to kill himself. What would lead a boy to this?"
- "Such a young boy, Bessie?"
- "Yes. My God!"
- "He must have some type of mental illness."
- "Oh, you're right, Sophie. I just glanced at the next paragraph, and a psychiatrist explains that the boy has been diagnosed as having major depressive disorder."

With this explanation, the two women nodded to one another and continued to another story, seemingly satisfied that they now understood the reason the boy was dealing with this suicidal issue.

The notion that when a psychiatrist says someone has some type of mental illness it has offered a valid explanation for why the person is struggling with personal difficulties is terribly misleading, while too often cutting off the search for deeper meaning. Contrast this abbreviated understanding by Bessie and Sophie with what happens when seeing Shakespeare's Hamlet about a suicidal boy the same age as the one in the story Bessie was reading. As Shakespeare's story unfolds, the audience is presented with a character that has motivations, conflicts, frustrations, disturbing situations, and powerful emotions. In the end, the audience is left with some insights into why the character of Hamlet might struggle with feelings of suicide.

Even a play, which lasts but two or three hours, can only provide in its narrative a simplified account of what real life stories are all about. And yet in today's world, many people believe an adequate explanation has been provided when a mental health service provider labels someone as having a mental disorder diagnosis, typically within twenty to sixty minutes. However, in time, some come to understand that they were misled. This is illustrated by a comment of a service user that appears in Johnstone (2014):

> By the time I was entering my second decade of service use, the medical model, which I had initially found reassuring, seemed increasingly unsatisfactory, without the capacity to encompass the complexity of my interior or exterior life and give it positive value. As a result, I began to actively explore frameworks that better met my needs. (p. 63)

As a further example of how the public is misled by use of the term "diagnosis" in the manner used in the DSM and ICD, surveys suggest that 80% or more of the general public have now become convinced that when someone is diagnosed with Major Depressive Disorder, the cause has been determined and they know what it is—a chemical imbalance (Pescosolido et al., 2010; Pilkington et al., 2013). Many general practitioners also subscribe to this view (Read, et al., 2019) and popular websites commonly cite the theory (Demasi & Gøtzsche, 2020).

This theory claims that the imbalance involves low serotonin levels in the brain. Despite this belief, Moncrieff and colleagues (2022), in a recent article titled "The serotonin theory of depression: a systematic umbrella review of the evidence," concluded, "Our comprehensive review of the major strands of research on serotonin shows there is no convincing evidence that depression is associated with, or caused by, lower serotonin concentrations or activity" (p. 3253).

In the DSM and ICD, other than post-traumatic stress disorder (which presumes the cause of this set of emotions, moods, and behaviors has been experiencing a traumatic event), what causes the other "mental disorders" is largely ignored. There is a sound reason for this.

The problem the DSM/ICD approach would have if it did take a position on the causes of the various "disorders" is it would dramatically reduce the number of people who would use it because people have very different views on this. Some lean toward faulty cognitive styles as being causative. In contrast, behaviorist, psychoanalyst, humanistic psychologists, narrative psychologists, and interpersonal psychologists, to name just a few, have very different perspectives on the causes of mental health concerns.

Rather than making a different classifying system for each perspective, it made sense to create a system that can be used more generally by all these various perspectives. It is for this reason that the DSM/ICD approach shies away from discussing causation in any firm manner.

So, in sum, to follow the rest of the arguments in this chapter, it is crucial to keep the following points in mind. The DSM and ICD provide descriptions of various sets of emotions, moods, and behavioral concerns for which people seek mental health services. Each set is labeled a particular disorder. Although both manuals are largely silent regarding making the case that the cause for any of these sets has been determined, their use of the term "diagnosis" misleads many people in this regard.

What is the meaning of the phrase "clinically significant disturbance" as used in the DSM and ICD definition of a mental disorder?

To answer this question, it will help to take another look at the definition of a mental disorder as defined in the ICD-11 (2023):

> Mental, behavioural and neurodevelopmental disorders are syndromes characterised by clinically significant disturbance in an individual's cognition, emotional regulation, or behaviour that reflects a dysfunction in the psychological, biological, or developmental processes that underlie mental and behavioural functioning. These disturbances are usually associated with distress or impairment in personal, family, social, educational, occupational, or other important areas of functioning.

Every individual at various times in his or her life has experienced some disturbance in one or more of the processes mentioned in this definition. As we see in the above definition, distinguishing between such experiences from the special case in which a mental disorder diagnosis is warranted requires a mental health service provider to declare the disturbance is "clinically significant." How does the mental health professional make this determination?

I have been a PhD level psychologist for over forty years and have observed the following: The vast majority of mental health service providers accept clients who have third-party mental health insurance coverage. When a person seeking such mental health services makes an appointment and then shows up, that person ends up leaving the appointment with a mental disorder diagnosis. This intuitively makes perfect sense because mental health professionals are in the business of increasing the number of their clients. Given that they have over 300 vaguely described "mental disorders" to choose from, and the only way they will get paid for their services is to declare that the person seeking services has a "clinically significant" disturbance, who can doubt that no one is turned away.

The DSM and ICD definitions of "clinical significance" should be clearly defined as *the point* that occurs after someone makes an appointment for third-party payer services and then shows up. By not doing so, the public is misled to think some special expertise is being utilized. The professional status of the service provider leads the public to think something more serious has been established. Although it is true that some expressed concerns are more serious than others, a mental disorder diagnosis is not indicative of this.

In sum, above we examined how the diagnosis concept as used in the DSM and ICD is misleading. It confounds differences between theory of cause, cause clearly determined, and jargon for an expressed concern. It also unfairly implies that people with a mental disorder diagnosis have more serious disturbances than that of the general population, and only a properly trained mental service provider can distinguish when a concern is serious enough to be diagnosed as a mental disorder.

We now move on to examine a not often recognized problem with the "mental disorder" concept.

The Mental Disorder Concept Can Discourage Active Coping

The mental disorder conceptualization of the types of concerns classified under that heading often fails to motivate active coping beyond taking a pill. Moreover, it fails to honor the labeled person's perspective. In contrast, framing these concerns as a potentially healthy functional signal can lead to less self-stigma and greater self-efficacy in making healthy life-style improvements.

This viewpoint began as early as 1896. William James, in his Lowell Lectures on Exceptional Mental States (which were reconstructed by Eugene Taylor in 1984 from James's notes), stated that experiences that are commonly viewed as unhealthy or morbid are really "an essential part of every character" and give life "a truer sense of values" (Taylor, 1984, p. 15). James went on from there to note that medical writers tend to,

> [R]epresent the line of mental health as a very narrow crack, which one must tread with bated breath, between foul friends on the one side and gulfs of despair on the other…. There is no purely objective standard of sound health. Any peculiarity that is of use to a man is a point of soundness in him, and what makes a man sound for one function may make him unsound for another…. The trouble is that such writers use the descriptive names of symptoms merely as an artifice for giving objective authority to their personal dislikes. The medical terms become mere appreciative clubs to knock a man down with…. The only sort of being, in fact, who can remain as the typical normal man, after all the individuals with degenerative symptoms have been rejected, must be a perfect nullity. Who shall absolutely say that the morbid has no revelations about the meaning of life? That the healthy minded view so-called is all? (Taylor, 1984, pp. 163-165)

Later, James (1902/1961) discussed Tolstoy's experience with severe, suicidal depression which took place at a time when Tolstoy's outer circumstances seemed excellent. In time, his melancholy stimulated a gnawing questioning that eventually led to one insight after another. As James (1902/1961) described it,

> His trouble had not been with life in general, not with the common life of common men, but with the life of the upper, intellectual, artistic classes, the life that he had personally always led, the cerebral life, the life of conventionality, artificiality, and personal ambition. He had lived wrongly and had to change. (pp.156-157)

Then, one day in early spring, while he was alone in the forest listening to its mysterious noises, he was filled with a sense of deeper meaning. After that, Tolstoy wrote "things cleared up within me and about me better than ever, and the light has never wholly died away" (as quoted in James, 1902/1961, p. 157). According to Tolstoy, his suicidal feelings disappeared, and he went on to live a productive life until passing away at the age of 82 of natural causes.

James then discussed individuals who view themselves as "healthy-minded." These individuals believe that those who worry are "morbid-minded" and "diseased" (pp. 78-114). James responded to this name-calling by stating that those referred to as morbid-minded have argued that "the world's meaning most comes home to us when we lay them most to heart" (p. 116). After describing the argument between the so-called "healthy-minded" and the "morbid-minded," James then states:

> In our attitude, not yet abandoned, of impartial onlookers, what are we to say of this quarrel? It seems to me that we are bound to say that morbid-mindedness ranges over the wider scale of experience, and that its survey is the one that overlaps. The method of averting one's attention from evil and living in the light of good is splendid as long as it will work. It will work with many persons; it will work far more generally than most of us are ready to suppose; and within the sphere of its successful operation there is nothing to be said against it as a religious solution. But it breaks down importantly as soon as melancholy comes; and even though one be quite free from melancholy one's self, there is no doubt that healthy-mindedness is inadequate as a philosophical doctrine, because the evil facts which

it refuses positively to account for are a genuine portion of reality; and may after all be the best key to life's significance, and possibly the only openers of our eyes to the deepest levels of truth. (p. 140)

In more recent times, more and more people are beginning to view "mental disorders" as possibly helpful. For example, Joshua Wolf Shenk (2005), in his biography of Abraham Lincoln, makes the case that his depression fueled his greatness. Similarly, David Yaffe (2017) has written a biography about the music legend, Joni Mitchell, titled *Reckless Daughter. There, he writes of her frequent bouts of depression.* In a review of the biography, Matt Mullin (2017, para. 1) provides the following quote of hers,

Depression can be the sand that makes the pearl. Most of my best work came out of it. If you get rid of the demons and the disturbing things, then the angels fly off, too. There is the possibility, in that mire, of an epiphany.

Schroder and colleagues (2023) recently carried out a relevant study. As the authors describe it,

We describe the historical development of popular messages about depression and draw from the fields of evolutionary psychiatry and social cognition to describe the alternative framework that depression is a "signal" that serves a purpose. We then present data from a pre-registered, online randomized-controlled study in which participants with self-reported depression histories viewed a series of videos that explained depression as a "disease like any other" with known biopsychosocial risk factors (BPS condition), or as a signal that serves an adaptive function (Signal condition) …. The Signal condition led to less self-stigma, greater offset efficacy, and more adaptive beliefs about depression. (p. 1)

In short, the DSM/ICD approach, with its focus on the concepts of "diagnosis," "mental disorder," and "dysfunctions" in individuals accessing mental health services distracts from human strengths within a cultural context (Miller et al., 2014). These shortcomings, along with the others mentioned above, have led to a great deal of dissatisfaction with this pathologizing approach as we will see in the next section.

Dissatisfaction with the DSM/ICD

Raskin and Gayle (2015) recently surveyed psychologists who regularly use the DSM. The authors summarized their results as follows:

> Although more than 90% of psychologists report using the DSM, they are dissatisfied with numerous aspects of it and support developing alternatives to it—something that psychologists over 30 years ago supported, as well. The finding that almost all psychologists use the DSM despite serious concerns about it raises ethical issues because professionals are ethically bound to only use instruments in which they are scientifically confident. (p. 1)

The main reason that they continue to use it is for third-party insurance reimbursement. Although the survey specifically looked at how clinicians view the DSM, as pointed out above the DSM approach is very similar to that of the ICD.

Supplementing the survey findings involving psychologists, Holzman (2015) carried out a series of surveys in New York City with non-mental health service providers. Forty percent felt that psychiatric diagnosis was not valuable. For the 60% that felt that psychiatric diagnoses could be valuable, most said the main reason was that it was the only way to access services. Moreover, 90% of them had reservations about how valuable it was. Typical comments were that it was only sometimes helpful, there was a danger of misdiagnosis, there was racism involved in diagnosis, and it leads to stigma and overmedication.

As we evaluate the implications of the above surveys, it is important to bear in mind that the views of the people surveyed developed in the context of a multibillion-dollar advertisement campaign by the pharmaceutical companies over many years, designed to convince people that emotional concerns are diagnosable illnesses requiring medication treatment. The views of those surveyed might have been dramatically different if there was a viable alternative that could tap into third-party payer systems and received comparable promotion campaigns.

The surveys do clearly indicate that some do value the current DSM/ICD approach. With the alternative that we now turn to, those who want to continue to use the DSM/ICD approach would be free to do so. But for all those who would prefer a non-pathologizing approach to accessing mental health services, a fresh new choice would become available. Competition between the two approaches could be a major impetus to improving services for all.

The Classification and Statistical Manual of Mental Health Concerns: 2nd Draft

Criticism is far more useful when, in addition to pointing out the faults of something, it is combined with a clear vision of an alternative that would have fewer faults. Without this vision, supporters of the DSM/ICD approach can just discount all the criticism directed at it believing that it is the only viable approach—and, after all, nothing is perfect. Therefore, having provided a set of faults of the DSM/ICD approach, I now turn to my vision of an alternative that aims to have significantly fewer of them.

I presented the first draft of this alternative five years ago in the *Journal of Humanistic Psychology* (Rubin, 2018). It called for the creation of the *Classification and Statistical Manual of Mental Health Concerns* (CSM) and provided an outline of what it would contain. Having had an opportunity to consider the various suggestions I received for making improvements, I here present an outline of its latest updated version.

Chapter 1: CSM Basics

The first chapter would begin with the following quote from William James's *A Pluralistic Universe* (1909/1977):

> Individuality outruns all classification, yet we insist on classifying everyone we meet under some general head. As these heads usually suggest prejudicial associations to some hearer or other, the life of philosophy largely consists of resentments at the classing, and complaints of being misunderstood. (pp. 3-4)

It is for this reason that the CSM does not seek to classify anyone. Instead, it classifies the expressed concerns of individuals seeking to have their concerns addressed by a mental health service provider. Additionally, the CSM seeks to avoid using terms that simplistically devalue an experience. Such experiences, it emphasizes, may turn out to be indispensable stages in acquiring valued fruits.

The first chapter would then explain that the CSM begins from the perspective of the person seeking services. Then, it would clearly define its main construct:

> A mental health concern occurs when a person seeking mental health services expresses to a mental health service provider a concern about any of these topics: behavior, emotion, mood, addictions, meaning of life, death, dying, managing chronic pain, work, relationships, education, eating, cognition, sleep, and challenging life situations.

This is an observable event that occurs at a specific time and place and, therefore, avoids the reliability and validity problems of the DSM/ICD approach.

Further along in this chapter would be a section explaining the use of the "mental health" concept in the CSM. Mental health, here, is used because we have such enormous organizations as Mental Health America and its state and regional affiliates, the National Institute of Mental Health, programs offering degrees in mental health counseling, and states offering certifications in this field. Psychologists, social workers, counselors, and psychiatrists regularly refer to themselves as providing services under the umbrella of "mental health service providers." For these reasons, the CSM would maintain the concept of "mental health" so it can be comfortably and realistically accommodated into the many large organizations currently using it.

However, this chapter would explain that the CSM uses the term "mental health" in a way that is different from what is implied in the DSM and the ICD. The CSM would explicitly reject the idea that the opposite of mental health is mental illness. Rather, the word "health" in the CSM's "mental health" would be phrased in a manner that indicates that professionals dealing with mental health concerns are part of the allied health professions. The reason for thinking of these professionals as health providers follows.

Many of the concerns that would fall under the CSM's list of related topics have been identified in scientific studies as "physical health risk" factors. For example, people who express a concern about being addicted to alcohol are at increased risk of developing sclerosis of the liver (O'Shea et al., 2010). Those who express concerns about eating more than average may be at greater risk of diabetes and heart disease (Mokdad et al., 2003). Quality of interpersonal relations, lack of sleep, depression with thoughts of suicide, and various other concerns or clusters of concerns can be studied for the degree of physical health risk that they pose.

A major goal of mental health providers under the proposed CSM system is to turn "physical health risk" factors into "physical health protective" factors. The degree to which this is successful can be studied using currently available methodologies. It is in this very specific sense that the mental health concern topics are viewed not merely as mental concerns but also mental *health* concerns. By being explicit about this change in conceptualizing mental health, we have good reason to believe that the CSM proposal holds promise for avoiding most of the negative baggage that comes with this type of terminology.

Chapter 1 would then summarize the additional shortcomings of the current dominant DSM/ICD approach discussed above. The chapter would conclude with an overview of how the CSM provides a valuable alternative for those seeking and providing mental health services.

Chapter 2: Classification of Mental Health Concerns and Codes

The CSM has two classes of expressed mental health concerns: concerns expressed about oneself, and concerns expressed about someone else. An example of the first class is: Sally is seeking mental health services and expresses a concern to a mental health service provider that she has been experiencing a great deal of anxiety when she enters social situations. This might be classified as a "Social Anxiety Concern." An example of the second class is: Bob, a father, on seeking counseling for his son, expresses a concern about his child's frequent angry outbursts. This might be classified as "Childhood Anger Concern."

Each of these two classes of mental health concerns would have under each of its headings a list of specific concerns, along with a numerical code to be used for third-party payer bureaucratic record keeping. The actual expressed concern would be useful for providing those in the mental health profession and others a common language that can serve as an alternative to the common pathologizing language now employed for such purposes. The brief expressed concern terms would also serve as useful terms for article and book titles, and for search engines to retrieve relevant information.

In both sections (concern expressed about oneself and concern expressed about someone else), to keep the number of classified concerns at a manageable number and to protect clients from having to reveal too much deeply personal information on bureaucratic forms, there would be some slightly abstract terms used to summarize a group of very similar concerns. For example, there would not be a separate classification for every conceivable concern expressed about dealing with stressful situations (e.g., I was in a terrible car crash, I was raped, I have been living in a war zone, etc.). All various types of expressed concerns involving stressful situations could be coded under the single label, "Challenging Life Situations."

Nor would there be a separate listing for every expressed concern about someone stating he or she is Jesus Christ, Napoleon, God, and so on. A single listing for this type of concern would suffice, perhaps something like "Identity Disagreement." Likewise, other terms that briefly summarize a host of very similar concerns would be utilized in this part of the CSM.

Two types of data sources would be utilized to identify the list of concerns. The first would come from a large sample of mental health service providers asked to list the various concerns they have been asked to address in their practice in the past year without couching them in psychopathological language, and to stick as closely as possible to the language used by those seeking their services. The second source would come from another survey that would ask the membership of mental health service user organizations to list the various concerns that led them to seek mental health services. They, too, would be asked to avoid psychopathological terminology. At the back of the CSM would be a summary of the findings of the data from these two sources and their related statistics.

Chapter 3: The CSM's Approach to Psychological Formulation

This chapter of the CSM would be devoted to describing good practice guidelines for the use of psychological formulation (The British Psychological Society, 2011), which is an assessment approach that is consistent with the CSM's philosophy of not pathologizing individuals (Johnstone & Dallos, 2013). Psychological formulation provides an approach that expands on the expressed concerns of individuals by developing a narrative of several paragraphs.

It can be defined as the process involving a mental health service user and a mental health service provider co-constructing a hypothesis or "best guess" about the origins of the mental health service user's concerns in the context of his or her relationships, social circumstances, cultural heritage, life events, and the sense that he or she has made of them. Once it has been established what the concerns are, the immediate next question is, "How do we jointly understand these experiences, why they arose, and how we might be able to address them?"

Unlike the term "diagnosis" as employed in the DSM and ICD, this type of psychological formulation is not about making an expert judgment, but about working closely with the individual to develop a shared understanding that will evolve over time. And, unlike the DSM/ICD type of "diagnosis," it draws attention to the service user's resources and strengths in surviving what are nearly always very challenging life situations. It also presents the theory to the service user that many people achieve something valuable for having gone through the challenges they are facing.

The CSM proposal adds an outline to the psychological formulation which would be developed by a series of questions from the clinician:

1. What is the main concern you would like us to address together?

2. When did this concern first begin to surface?

3. When or in what situations is the concern most problematic?

4. When or in what situations is the concern least problematic?

5. In addition to your main concern, what are other concerns that you would like us to address together?

6. Please rate how distressing are each of the concerns that you mentioned on a scale of 1 to 7, with 1 indicating just a little distressing, and 7 being very, very distressing.

7. Personal strengths

8. Functioning: (Rate each of the following on a scale of −7 to +7, with −7 being very much below average for the general population and +7 being very much above average for the general population.)

    a. Sleep

    b. Eating

    c. Work

    d. Education

    e. Relationships

9. Theory of cause or causes

This outline would provide some consistency to the CSM formulation approach while providing ample room to create a narrative that reflects the individuality of each mental health service user.

Chapter 4: Two Programs of Research

The last chapter of the CSM would be devoted to describing two programs of research: one looking at statistical correlations between mental health concerns and physical health problems, and another comparing mental health outcomes for services provided with the use of the CSM versus those services provided with the use of the DSM/ICD approach.

In the first edition of the CSM, the current relevant information would be reviewed along with an action plan to move this research forward. In future editions of the CSM, Chapter 4 would expand as these two research programs gather reportable data.

Arguments for the Practicality of the CSM

In Some Settings Using Expressed Concerns Has Worked Fine

When I was doing my practicum at the University of Minnesota's Counseling Center, we had no need to use the "mental disorder" jargon of the DSM and ICD to communicate. When my advisor asked me to quickly tell him about my morning cases, I would reply with words like, "My 9:00 a.m. case is concerned about feeling depressed, my 10:00 case is concerned about his failing grades, my 11:00 case is concerned about how anxious she is in social situations."

If my advisor wanted to know more about a case, we went into the psychological formulation type of information. This informal way to communicate among the professionals and graduate students at the counseling center flowed smoothly while we provided a wide range of mental health services.

The CSM is Practical Because it Can Be Easily Used by Third-Party Payers

An argument can be made that there is no need to have any classification system. According to this argument, a psychological formulation approach by itself could replace the DSM/ICD approach (Johnstone & Dallos, 2013). But note that currently third-party payer systems in the United States do use the DSM/ICD codes. These payer systems utilize forms that must be filled out whenever someone seeks mental health services under their plan. These forms typically have a little box that reads, "Diagnosis." In that box, mental health professionals must fill in a short DSM/ICD code that corresponds to some specific "mental disorder."

Utilizing just the psychological formulation approach, which involves the creation of several paragraphs, as an alternative to the shorthand DSM/ICD coding, would be far too cumbersome. The CSM approach, like the DSM/ICD approach, provides a short descriptive phrase coupled with a code and is therefore far more workable. With the CSM proposal, all that third-party payer institutions would need to do differently to add value for their customers is to slightly change that little "Diagnosis" box. Instead of just reading "Diagnosis," that box would add two simple words so it would read, "Diagnosis or Concern."

Then, when mental health professionals fill in the box, they would be given the choice to either write in the letters "DSM/ICD" and the code number that corresponds to the so-called diagnosis, or they would write the letters "CSM" and the code number that corresponds to the main expressed mental health concern. Mental health consumers would be given the choice to go to pathologizing mental health service providers or those using the CSM approach. This is all the change that would be required to increase value for a significant number of mental health service users. The cost and effort for third-party payers to make both the pathologizing and CSM approaches available would be minimal.

Moreover, a short word or phrase that could replace terms like "major depressive disorder" or "attention deficit hyperactivity disorder" is necessary for other practical means of communication. For example, if I want to write a title for a research article, it would not be practical to insert several of the formulation paragraphs into the title. The psychological formulation approach would be far more widely used if it had some practical way of providing some standard short terms for conceptualizing an individual's mental health concerns arranged in a scientific classification manual.

Service users that think the pathologizing approach reduces shame and guilt would continue to be free to access this type of service. Those service users who object to being labeled as having a mental disorder would find having the option to access services utilizing a CSM approach more compatible than the DSM/ICD approach. Moreover, service users would find that the CSM approach also provides support for reducing shame and guilt feelings. It does so, not by claiming their concerns are illnesses like any other illnesses, but by being respectful and collaborative.

Some may argue that the CSM is not practical because if everyone could go to a mental health professional merely to have their concerns addressed, then the system would soon be overloaded with clients and third-party payers' costs would soar. Because insurance companies only cover people with more serious conditions known as "mental disorders," so the argument goes, this limits the number of people who can get to see a mental health professional.

However, as explained above, third-party payer executives would readily come to understand, with a little explaining, that mental health service providers now using the current DSM/ICD approach do not turn anyone away who has mental health insurance coverage and comes to their office expressing what the CSM refers to as a mental health concern. Professionals are in the business of increasing the number of their clients.

The CSM is Practical Because it Would Be Atheoretical

Practically, it would be too confusing for third-party payers to use a different coding system for every conceivable theoretical group. A practical alternative must therefore avoid being bound to any single theoretical orientation.

A mental health concern classification system achieves this practical necessity because all mental health service providers, regardless of their theoretical orientation, can agree that people seeking mental health services do express mental health concerns. To agree to utilize just two sets of codes (DSM/ICD and CSM) to accommodate the powerful feelings of those who object to being pathologized would show respect to these mental health service users in a practical manner.

Conclusion

The creation of the CSM could improve mental health services for both mental health service users and providers. It would do so by offering a new choice for those who are dissatisfied with the DSM/ICD approach while also being more scientific and respectful toward mental health service users.

Moreover, the creation of the CSM is designed to increase the self-efficacy of users by providing a framework that highlights the many folks who found that going through their challenging experience led to valued fruits. The CSM would break up the DSM/ICD monopoly and, by doing so, would create new avenues of research for understanding the nature of all the concerns that mental health service providers are asked to address.

References

American Psychiatric Association. (2013). *Diagnostic and statistical manual of mental disorders* (5th ed.). American Psychiatric Publishing.

Breggin, P. R. (2007). *Brain-disabling treatments in psychiatry: Drugs, electroshock, and the psychopharmaceutical complex.* Springer Publishing Company.

Calvo, F., Karras, B. T., Phillips, R., Kimball, A. M., & Wolf, F. (2003). Diagnoses, syndromes, and diseases: a knowledge representation problem. In *AMIA annual symposium proceedings* (Vol. 2003, p. 802). American Medical Informatics Association.

Corrigan P. (2004). How stigma interferes with mental health care. *American Psychologist,* 59, 614-625.

Cosgrove, L., Bursztajn, H. J., Krimsky, S., Anaya, M., & Walker, J. (2009). Conflicts of interest and disclosure in the American Psychiatric Association's Clinical Practice Guidelines. *Psychotherapy and Psychosomatics, 78*(4), 228-232.

Cosgrove, L., D'Ambrozio, G., Herrawi, F., Freeman, M., & Shaughnessy, A. (2023). Why psychiatry needs an honest dose of gentle medicine. *Frontiers in Psychiatry, 14,* 1167910.

Cosgrove, L., Krimsky, S., Vijayaraghavan, M., & Schneider, L. (2006). Financial ties between DSM-IV panel members and the pharmaceutical industry. *Psychotherapy and psychosomatics, 75*(3), 154-160.

Demasi, M., & Gøtzsche, P. C. (2020). Presentation of benefits and harms of antidepressants on websites: A cross-sectional study. *International Journal of Risk & Safety in Medicine, 31*(2), 53-65.

Fatemi S. M. (2015). Questioning the unquestionability of the expert's perspective in psychology. *Journal of Humanistic Psychology,* 55, 263-291.

Holzman L. (2015). *A report on community outreach: Lay opinions on emotional distress and diagnosis.* Retrieved from http://dxsummit.org/archives/2249

Insel T. (2013, April 29). Director's blog: Transforming diagnosis [Blog post]. Retrieved from http://www.nimh.nih.gov/about/director/2013/transforming-diagnosis.shtml

James, W. (1902/1961). *The varieties of religious experience: A study in human nature*. New York: Macmillan.

James, W. (1909/1977). *A pluralistic universe*. Harvard University Press.

Johnstone L. (2014). *A straight talking introduction to psychiatric diagnosis*. Monmouth, England: PCCS Books.

Johnstone L., Dallos R. (2013). *Formulation in psychology and psychotherapy: Making sense of people's problems* (2nd ed.). New York, NY: Routledge.

Miller D. M., Nash T., Fetty D. G. (2014). Fostering community: Explicating commonalities between counseling psychology and humanistic psychology. *Journal of Humanistic Psychology*, 54, 476-493.

Moncrieff, J., Cooper, R. E., Stockmann, T., Amendola, S., Hengartner, M. P., & Horowitz, M. A. (2022). The serotonin theory of depression: a systematic umbrella review of the evidence. *Molecular psychiatry*, 1-14.

Mullin, M. (2017). Joni Mitchell is telling her side now in a new biography, in Interview, Magazine, https://www.interviewmagazine.com/music/joni-mitchell-reckless-daughter.

Mokdad A. H., Ford E. S., Bowman B. A., Dietz W. H., Vinicor F., Bales V. S., Marks J. S. (2003). Prevalence of obesity, diabetes, and obesity-related health risk factors, 2001. *Journal of the American Medical Association*, 289, 76-79.

O'Shea R. S., Dasarathy S., McCullough A. J. (2010). Alcoholic liver disease. *Hepatology*, 51, 307-328.

Pescosolido, B. A., Martin, J. K., Long, J. S., Medina, T. R., Phelan, J. C., & Link, B. G. (2010). "A disease like any other"? A decade of change in public reactions to schizophrenia, depression, and alcohol dependence. *American journal of psychiatry*, 167(11), 1321-1330.

Pilkington, P. D., Reavley, N. J., & Jorm, A. F. (2013). The Australian public's beliefs about the causes of depression: Associated factors and changes over 16 years. *Journal of Affective Disorders*, 150(2), 356-362.

Read, J., Renton, J., Harrop, C., Geekie, J., & Dowrick, C. (2020). A survey of UK general practitioners about depression, antidepressants and withdrawal: implementing the 2019 Public Health England report. *Therapeutic Advances in Psychopharmacology, 10*, 2045125320950124.

Regier D. A., Narrow W. E., Clarks D. E., Kraemer H. C., Kuramoto S. J., Kuhl E. A., Kupfer D. J. (2013). DSM-5 field trials in the United States and Canada, Part II: Test-retest reliability of selected categorical diagnoses. *American Journal of Psychiatry, 170*, 59-70.

Raskin J. D., Gayle M. C. (2015). *DSM-5*: Do psychologists really want an alternative? *Journal of Humanistic Psychology, 56*, 439-456.

Robbins, B. D., Kamens, S. R., and Elkins, D. N. (2017). DSM-5 reform efforts by the Society for Humanistic Psychology. *J. Humanist. Psychol. 57*, 602–624. doi: 10.1177/0022167817698617

Rubin J. (2000). William James and the pathologizing of human experience. *Journal of Humanistic Psychology, 40*, 176-226.

Rubin, J. (2018). The classification and statistical manual of mental health concerns: A proposed practical scientific alternative to the DSM and ICD. *Journal of humanistic psychology, 58*(1), 93-114.

Schroder, H. S., Devendorf, A., & Zikmund-Fisher, B. J. (2023). Framing depression as a functional signal, not a disease: Rationale and initial randomized controlled trial. *Social Science & Medicine*, 115995.

Shenk, J. W. (2005). *Lincoln's melancholy: How depression challenged a president and fueled his greatness.* Houghton Mifflin Harcourt.

Szasz T. S. (1961). *The myth of mental illness: Foundations of a theory of personal conduct.* New York: Hoeber-Harper.

Taylor E. (1984). *William James on exceptional mental states: The 1896 Lowell lectures.* Amherst: University of Massachusetts Press.

The British Psychological Society. (2011). *Good practice guidelines on the use of psychological formulation.* Retrieved from http://www.bps.org.uk/system/files/Public%20files/DCP/cat-842.pdf

Whitaker, R. (2011). *Anatomy of an epidemic: Magic bullets, psychiatric drugs, and the astonishing rise of mental illness in America.* Crown.

World Health Organization. (1992). *The ICD-10 classification of mental and behavioural disorders*. Retrieved from http://www.who.int/classifications/icd/en/bluebook.pdf

World Health Organization. (2001). *International Classification of Functioning, Disability and Health (ICF)*. Geneva, Switzerland: Author.

World Health Organization. (2023). *The ICD-11*. Retrieved from https://icd.who.int/en.

Yaffe, D. (2017). *Reckless Daughter*. New York: Sarah Crichton Books.

Toward a Descriptive Problem-Based Taxonomy for Mental Health: A Proposed Organizing Framework

Arnoldo Cantú

Abstract: *Psychiatric diagnoses found in the Diagnostic and Statistical Manual of Mental Disorders (DSM) and International Classification of Diseases (ICD) are pervasive in the field of mental health to help individuals access services such as psychotherapy. In the United States, they are used for insurance reimbursement purposes and by providers in client–clinician encounters. Psychiatric disorders have been critiqued for contributing to iatrogenic harm in addition to fundamental concerns about their validity and reliability. However, current practice of requiring psychiatric diagnoses within health care systems occurs due to federal regulations and does not allow for the formal use of alternative taxonomies, forcing clinicians and clients into the biomedical model. This chapter will explicate technicalities dictating the use of psychiatric diagnoses. It will introduce an organizing framework borrowing from the field of social work suggesting how the field can move away from the biomedical model given the regulations at play. This chapter proposes the interdisciplinary development of an alternative nonmedicalized, psychosocial, and codified descriptive problem-based taxonomy that can decouple psychiatric diagnosis from the eligibility for and provision of mental health services.*

Acknowledgement: A version of this chapter was originally published as Cantú, A. (2023). Toward a descriptive problem-based taxonomy for mental health: A nonmedicalized way out of the biomedical model. *Journal of Humanistic Psychology*, 1–24. https://doi.org/10.1177/00221678231167612. It is reprinted here with permission.

Introduction

Psychiatric diagnoses are ubiquitous in the field of mental health and help individuals gain and maintain access to services such as counseling and psychotherapy. They are frequently used for third-party insurance reimbursement purposes and are regularly applied by psychotherapists (e.g., clinical social workers, clinical psychologists, and licensed professional counselors) when meeting with a client. They can be found in the American Psychiatric Association's (APA) *Diagnostic and Statistical Manual of Mental Disorders, Fifth Edition, Text Revision* (DSM-5-TR) (American Psychiatric Association [APA], 2022). They are also in the World Health Organization's (WHO) *International Classification of Diseases (ICD)* (2019).

The biomedical model of mental health, under which the *DSM* tends to be subsumed, posits that human suffering stems primarily from biological factors within the individual that are then conceptualized as mental disorders (Fritscher, 2020). The *DSM* and current practice of requiring psychiatric diagnoses within contemporary health care forcibly pigeonhole clinicians and clients alike into the biomedical model due to regulations set forth by Department of Health and Human Services' (DHHS) Centers for Medicare & Medicaid Services (CMS).

However, the *DSM* and psychiatric diagnoses remain shrouded in controversy with critics pointing to fundamental concerns about their validity (Insel, 2013), low reliability rates (Freedman et al., 2013), their role in medicalizing everyday experiences (Fawcett et al., 2020), and contribution to iatrogenic harm (Cornwall, 2013; Walsh & Foster, 2020). Given the ingrained biomedical model guiding mental health services for the past several decades, this chapter first explicates the key stakeholders maintaining the *DSM*'s embedded nature in United States health care.

This is followed by a practical suggestion as to how the field of mental health and psychotherapy can shift away from the biomedical model. Influenced by ecosystems theory suggesting people and their environments reciprocally affect one another (Tyler, 2020), and social work's three levels of practice (i.e., the micro-, mezzo-, and macro-levels) (USC School of Social Work, 2018), this chapter proposes the interdisciplinary development of an alternative nonmedicalized, psychosocial, and codified descriptive problem-based taxonomy.

Envisioning it as a plausible option to supplement the *DSM* in health care, a proposed system of this kind can ultimately decouple diagnosis from the eligibility for and provision of mental health services. Accessing mental health services should not be predicated on being diagnosed with a scientifically questionable psychiatric diagnosis, but by simply having real-life problems named and described.

Mental Health Care Coding, Billing, and Federal Regulations

To set the stage with a fact not well-known to many, there is currently no such thing as an official *DSM* diagnostic code. A statement in the *Diagnostic and Statistical Manual of Mental Disorders, Fifth Edition (DSM-5)* (APA, 2013a, p. 23) corroborates how each disorder within the manual is accompanied by a diagnostic code established by the WHO. The WHO (2019) developed the *ICD*, of which one of its chapters is titled "Mental, Behavioral, or Neurodevelopmental Disorders."

Initial editions of the *DSM* were markedly different compared with the *ICD* until more recent editions of the *DSM* were eventually aligned with the aforementioned *ICD* chapter (American Psychological Association, 2009; APA, n.d.). Accordingly, the *DSM-5* (APA, 2013a, p. 29) states the manual "contains the diagnostic criteria approved for routine clinical use along with the *ICD*-9-CM codes (*ICD*-10 codes are shown parenthetically) . . . These codes are adapted from *ICD*-9-CM and *ICD*-10-CM and *were neither reviewed nor approved as official DSM-5 diagnoses* [emphasis added]."

Interestingly, the first three editions of the *DSM* up until the influential *DSM-III* also noted using codes from the *ICD* as shown below:

- DSM-I: "The number in parenthesis in the right hand margin is the appropriate code number from the International Statistical Classification" (APA, 1952, p. 2).

- DSM-II: "The APA Committee on Nomenclature and Statistics found it necessary to add a fifth digit to the ICD code to obtain still further detail within each four-digit ICD category for the mental disorders..." (APA, 1968, p. 64).
- DSM-III: "All official DSM-III codes and terms are included in the ICD-9-CM [Clinical Modification]...unofficial non-ICD-9-CM codes are provided in parentheses for use when greater specificity is necessary" (APA, 1980, p. 15).

Copies of the *DSM* can be found in the offices of clinicians across the United States. When a client enters the office of a therapist for the first time, what the clinician typically conducts is some sort of diagnostic evaluation or assessment—asking questions to help gather facts about the nature of the client's presenting problem. Following this interaction, if health care coverage is to be utilized, the clinician is then prompted to think about what psychiatric diagnoses the client meets the criteria for. The clinician will usually consult the latest version of the *DSM* to find an appropriate diagnosis and its associated *ICD* code. This occurs because, in general, insurance companies cover only medically necessary services and will require a psychiatric diagnosis before they pay claims (Whelan, 2022).

After selecting a diagnosis, clinicians will then identify the kind of service they would like to have reimbursed. In the United States, current procedural terminology (CPT) codes are essential components of health insurance billing processes (Boyles, 2019). Clinicians ensure CPT codes on insurance claim forms reflect the kind of service they provided (e.g., CPT code 90791 is a Psychiatric Diagnostic Evaluation) (Coleman, 2017). CPT codes in conjunction with *ICD* codes paint a complete picture for health insurance companies: the CPT code explains the kind of service provided and the *ICD* code describes the diagnosis and justification for treatment or service. This process, in effect, *pigeonholes* clinicians into diagnosing clients with a mental disorder listed in the *DSM* if the individual wishes to use their health care coverage.

This restriction requiring the provision of a psychiatric diagnosis occurs due to regulations set forth by DHHS' CMS. CMS has specific components (Centers for Medicare & Medicaid Services [CMS], 2014) and rules

associated with CPT codes (CMS, 2018) designated for psychotherapy—
with most insurance payers sharing these requirements—one of which is the
documentation of a mental health diagnosis in the client's medical record
(CMS, 2015). With CPT and *ICD* codes being used concurrently, the *DSM's*
ICD codes are used to facilitate "a cross-walk to the new coding system . . .
for all U.S. health care providers and systems, *as recommended by . . . the*
Centers for Medicare and Medicaid Services (CMS) [emphasis added]" (APA,
2013b, para. 6; see also APA, 2013a, p. 23; O'Connor, 2014). (The newest
manual reiterates the use of *ICD-10-CM* codes for *DSM-5-TR* disorders as
being required by CMS [APA, 2022]).

As a result, if an individual is seeking mental health services and plans to
use their insurance, CMS regulations force clinicians and clients into the
DSM's biomedical model of mental health with no formally endorsed
taxonomic alternatives. For example, the American Psychoanalytic
Association publishes its *Psychodynamic Diagnostic Manual*, but it does not
authorize insurance reimbursement (McWilliams, 2008). The National
Association of Social Workers (NASW) also made an attempt to no avail
with Karls and Wandrei's (1994) *Person-In-Environment System: The PIE*
Classification System for Social Functioning Problems.

The message typically conveyed to clients—and that some clinicians
confidently proclaim—is the person in front of them has now been
diagnosed with a mental disorder that can be found in the *DSM* and will be
billed accordingly—when, truthfully, an *ICD* code is being billed and
documented in the individual's psychotherapy notes or medical record.

Notably, there is a section in the *DSM-5* (with *ICD* coding) titled "Other
Conditions That May Be a Focus of Clinical Attention" containing
psychosocial problems that "may be a focus of clinical attention or that
may otherwise affect the diagnosis, course, prognosis, or treatment of a
patient's mental disorder" (APA, 2013a, p. 715; see also Ingle, 2021).
Regrettably, the use of these psychosocial problems (i.e., Z- and T-codes) as
a "primary diagnosis" to help individuals gain access to services is
typically not reimbursable by insurance companies (Desantis, n.d.;
TherapyNotes, LLC, 2018). As such, instead of a child, for example, being
able to access mental health services following the experience of sexual

abuse (e.g., Child Sexual Abuse, Confirmed, T74.22XA), the child will most likely need to be diagnosed with a mental illness first to receive help.

Forced Into Questionable and Harmful Model

Recalling that CMS regulations force clinicians and service users into the *DSM*'s biomedical model of mental health, what results is a vulnerable segment of the population being needlessly pathologized at the expense of discounting contextual and environmental factors that can contribute to a client's difficulties. Proponents of using mental disorders stress the utility and need for using psychiatric diagnoses, asserting a correct diagnosis is crucial to pursuing appropriate treatment. In addition, some people are reassured by psychiatric diagnoses as a way to have their distressing experiences validated (Avdi, 2019).

Others have argued that psychiatric diagnoses have limited utility for prognosis with outcomes seeming more dependent on contextual and psychosocial factors (Kinderman, 2019). Psychiatric diagnoses suffer from low reliability rates (Regier et al., 2013; Vanheule et al., 2014) and, perhaps more concerningly, a lack of scientific verification as to their validity (Kirk et al., 2013). Their use has been associated with "othering" people—that is, a form of "stigmatic thinking" (Walsh & Foster, 2020).

They lend themselves to people experiencing worsened self- blame, self-efficacy, and prognostic pessimism (Kemp et al., 2014), in addition to a lessened belief in the effectiveness of psychotherapy and less empathy in clinicians (Lebowitz & Ahn, 2014). Others have argued that psychiatric diagnoses and the biomedical model converge in creating "long-term patients" (Timimi, 2021). At its core, the biomedical model promotes a deficits-based lens by attempting to define psychopathology, abnormality, and illness.

Why Is This Important?

What is the relevancy of technical regulations and bureaucratic decision-making when people (e.g., clinicians, researchers, and psychiatric survivors) are continuing to push for meaningful change within the field of mental health—an overall shift away from the biomedical model given its precarious foundation (see, for example, Carney, 2014; Kamens et al., 2017; Kinderman et al., 2017; Robbins et al., 2017; Ruby, 2017)? How is knowing about coding, billing, and policy vital when a different message can be manufactured to a client, helping them formulate a different account of their problems without medicalized language? Why not advocate for CMS and/or private insurance companies to allow Z- and T-codes to be billed as primary diagnoses when they already exist, regardless of whether they are found in the *DSM* or *ICD*?

The importance of all this is twofold. First, because despite continued criticisms of the *DSM* since the influential *DSM-III* was published in 1980, a medicalized lexicon used to describe people's emotional, behavioral, and psychological difficulties dominates research, professional, and everyday discourse to this day. It can be argued this is due to the *DSM*'s embedded use—piggybacking onto the *ICD*—within contemporary American health care supported by federal regulations. As such, advocating for changes within the policy arena, coupled with a viable alternative, is the key for making meaningful change if the *DSM* is to be eventually supplanted.

Second, although advocating for Z- and T- codes (psychosocial problems) to be billed as primary diagnoses as another way to access mental health services could be seen as progress, one could presume granting that would still allow the *DSM*'s commanding presence in the field of mental health to remain unchecked. Since these codified psychosocial problems are found in copies of the *DSM* in clinicians' offices around the United States, this would allow their continued co-existence alongside scientifically questionable psychiatric diagnoses.

The *DSM* and biomedical model of mental health can be seen as a runaway freight train using their momentum accumulated since 1980. Consequently, any scenario in which the manual's content and biomedical model continues to have a predominant platform will continue to make it challenging to enact large-scale change in opposition of (or to circumvent) it. Developing an alternative distinctly separate from the *DSM* and *implementable* into the structure of contemporary health care is paramount.

Toward a Descriptive Problem-Based Taxonomy

For the field of mental health and psychotherapy to pivot away from the biomedical model, this chapter proposes the interdisciplinary development (i.e., a collaborative effort by psychologists, social workers, psychiatrists, and related disciplines) of an alternative nonmedicalized, psychosocial, and descriptive problem-based taxonomy. This would be a system that would effectively drop the language of disorder (see Kinderman et al., 2012; van Hulst et al., 2021) and instead describe people's problems. After all, people typically enter mental health services when they are experiencing some sort of *problem* in their lives. That should be sufficient reason to gain access to services.

Undergirding the accumulation of problems can be viewpoints of the public, service users, clinicians, and psychiatric survivors through conceptualizations of their own difficulties (e.g., Adame, 2006; Adame et al., 2017; Dhar, 2022; Toikko, 2016). It would also be vital to incorporate literature delineating some of the social and environmental causes of distress (e.g., Florence & Pūras, 2020; Manning, 2020; WHO, 2008).

This proposed taxonomy's practical and nonmedical bent is influenced by Kinderman (2015) demonstrating how one can easily describe and list people's problems; Rubin (2017) proposing how human concerns can be investigated and systematically classified (sometimes as problems); Gomory et al. (2017) putting forth a problem-solving model; and Maisel (2015) delineating a "life formulation model" (pp. 172–180).

A Case for the Multilevel Framework

Warranting a psychosocial focus in this taxonomy is inspired by ecosystems theory's assumption of people and their environment having a bidirectional impact (Tyler, 2020). Ecosystems theory posits an individual is embedded in larger systems (e.g., school, work, family, and neighborhood), all of which can affect one another (Miley et al., 2012; Nazar, 2020). Since we do not live in a vacuum, we should appropriately capture factors outside of our ontological selves shaping our well-being to provide a more complete picture. Doing so could also capture vital epidemiological data to help with policymaking and programmatic efforts geared toward human welfare (e.g., American Hospital Association, 2020).

This proposed descriptive and problem-based taxonomy synthesizes and builds upon the aforementioned literature by being structured and overlayed onto the field of social work's three levels of analysis and practice framework to aid in organizing problems: the *micro-, mezzo-,* and *macro-*levels (USC School of Social Work, 2018). DeCarlo (2018) outlines the *micro-*level to comprise the individual; the *mezzo-*level to include groups and communities; and the *macro-*level to include institutions, policy, and culture. Echoing ecosystems theory, the three levels can interact and influence one another—dynamics that should be captured and recorded when an individual seeks help within the mental health system.

Utilizing social work's levels of practice as this taxonomy's framework is fitting for three reasons: it lends itself to being practical, it is arguably atheoretical, and it is a stable and well-established framework living in the field of social work. This framework has the flexibility to not only name a variety of individual problems but also capture and organize contextual and environmental problems in a descriptive fashion (as will be shown in the next section) that may be influencing one's well-being. In conjunction with being amendable to codification (one of the benefits of the *DSM* [Raskin et al., 2022]), a system of this kind can be adapted to fit into the billing structure of contemporary health care.

This framework sidesteps presuming the causes of distress (as it is only describing problems) and, in a way, can be an alternative to exist alongside the *DSM* as another tool for granting access to services. In addition, it does not align with any particular theoretical viewpoint, but simply describes and honors people's identified problems while superimposing them onto an established organizing framework. By contrast, it is possible other alternatives have not become embedded into contemporary health care because they are either conceptual (i.e., Power Threat Meaning Framework [Johnstone & Boyle, 2018]), not atheoretical (i.e., Psychodynamic Diagnostic Manual [Lingiardi & McWilliams, 2017]), cumbersome (i.e., Person-in-environment System [Karls & Wandrei, 1994]), or retain assumptions about "psychopathology" (i.e., Research Domain Criteria

[National Institute of Mental Health, n.d.] and the Hierarchical Taxonomy Of Psychopathology [Kotov et al., 2017]). It is also unclear which alternatives, if any, have moved past development and onto formal advocacy for incorporation into the United States health care structure.

Finally, this multilevel framework is a foundational tenet taught in schools of social work across the country (Council on Social Work Education, 2022; Hepworth et al., 2013). It was discussed in the field no later than approximately five decades ago (Hopps & Lowe, 2012; Minahan & Pincus, 1977). It helps practitioners and researchers reliably guide practice and interventions; assess, analyze, and place problems that people experience in context (i.e., across small-to-large systems); and engage in policy and advocacy work (Miley et al., 2012). As such, given its longevity as a framework and universal teachings to all social work students, it is safe to assume this framework will remain firmly anchored in the field—and the field of mental health given that social workers make up one of the largest segments of the workforce (National Association of Social Workers, n.d.).

Redressing the Psychosocial

Keeping in mind how the *DSM* and biomedical model tend to convert contextual and environmental problems as medical—relocating them within the individual and typically followed by medical intervention (Moncrieff, 2010)—this proposed taxonomy would strike a balance, placing an emphasis on psychosocial issues as much as individual problems. It would recognize and help sort complex human phenomena along a continuum of normality intertwined with the various systems they (i.e., clients and service users) are part of.

Recognizing the practicality of the *DSM* and *ICD*, the empirical research collecting and describing phenomenological data for this proposed taxonomy would require subsequent codification and classification of identified problems to build a databank (and, eventually, a sort of reference book or online repository freely accessible like the *ICD*) followed by field testing. This system would be subject to ongoing revision considering the dynamic interplay between human beings and their environment. Knowing the technicalities and regulations at play, this can be a system with an end goal of being endorsed by CMS to be used by multiple professions in lieu of *ICD* codes (and *DSM* diagnoses) when billing a CPT code.

A descriptive problem-based taxonomy would deal less with questions asking, "What's wrong with you?" and more with "What happened to you? What's happening in your life right now?" Helping people identify and describe their problems can validate how most reactions to life stressors can be seen as understandable responses—and that help can still be offered. This proposed system would not stop insurance companies from requiring a billing code; however, it could allow us to ask, "Would we rather have a questionable and controversial diagnosis be billed so we can get help? Or a comprehensible human problem?"

Some will argue that a model of this nature already exists: the biopsychosocial (BPS) model (Engel, 1977). However, a revitalized focus on the "psychosocial" aspect can provide a more balanced view of possible factors contributing to people's difficulties that the biomedical model has subjugated (Read, 2005). In addition, the BPS model has been critiqued for being too general, vague, and lacking specific content (Bolton & Gillett, 2019). Others have suggested the BPS model is all-encompassing yet imprecise, lacking guidance for clinicians (Ghaemi, 2012).

To be sure, the BPS model has been a helpful clinical and teaching tool throughout mental health. However, serving as a "tool" has been the extent of its use, whereas the *DSM* and its biomedical model of mental health have been used as clinical and teaching tools in addition to being *firmly embedded* into the structure of contemporary health care.

Draft of Proposed Taxonomy

A project of this kind would be a complex venture. However, once developed, field tested, and accepted by regulatory agencies, a descriptive problem-based taxonomy can be one way out of being pigeonholed into using psychiatric diagnoses to offer or receive help given the policies outlined earlier. We can build out a list of codifiable common problems people experience at the micro-, mezzo-, and macro-levels (see also Lacasse & Gambrill, 2015).

Examples of problems are listed below with pretend codes; corresponding varying hypothetical domains are italicized below. To address criticism referring to the BPS's lack of specific content and vagueness, the proposed taxonomy can look like the following:

- Micro (e.g., the individual) problems:
  - *Behavioral, emotional, and psychological problems*:
    - BEP 1.1 - saddened mood
    - BEP 1.2 - self-harm
    - BEP 1.3 - substance use
    - BEP 1.4 - negative core beliefs
    - BEP 1.5 - suicidal ideation
    - BEP 1.6 - significant weight loss/gain
    - BEP 1.7 - disrupted sleep
    - BEP 1.8 - loss of interest/pleasure in things
  - *Cognitive concerns*:
    - CC 2.1 - intellectual delay
    - CC 2.2 - cognitive disability
    - CC 2.3 - developmental delay
    - CC 2.4 - learning difficulty
    - CC 2.5 - difficulty focusing
  - *Perceptual issues*:
    - PI 3.1 - hearing voices
  - *Spiritual/existential concerns*:
    - SE 4.1 - death anxiety
    - SE 4.2 - loss of meaning in life
- Mezzo (e.g., groups and communities) problems:
  - *Interpersonal/relational problems*:
    - IR 1.1 - lack of familial support
    - IR 1.2 - domestic violence
    - IR 1.3 – loneliness
    - IR 1.4 – trauma
    - IR 1.5 – bullying
- Macro (e.g., institutions, policy, and culture) problems:
  - *Environmental/social factors*:
    - ES 1.1 - foster care

- ES 1.2 - poverty
- ES 1.3 - housing instability
- ES 1.4 - academic problem
- ES 1.5 - acculturation issues
- ES 1.6 - crime in neighborhood

Case Example and Application of Model

A case example in how the proposed taxonomy can be implemented follows:

> A tired older teenager presents by himself to a school-based therapist with concerns about having "depression" over the past month following an incident at school during which he was severely beaten by neighborhood peers. He also expresses having thoughts of killing himself due to recent poor academic performance. He struggles to focus, wonders what's wrong with him, and his recurrent use of social media points him into thinking he may be suffering from depression. He is unsure what the purpose of his life is now and staying up all night thinking about it—and if he will run into the neighborhood bullies again—has not been helping.

A psychiatric interview through the lens of the *DSM* may yield a billing a diagnostic evaluation (CPT code 90791) for Major Depressive Disorder, Single Episode, Moderate (*ICD* code F32.1), which in turn the adolescent may be informed to be a likely contributor or cause of his recent difficulties:

- Symptoms of MDD, Single Episode, Moderate (F32.1):
  - o Depressed mood most of the day, nearly every day
  - o Markedly diminished interest in please in all, or almost all, activities most of the day and nearly every day
  - o Insomnia or hypersomnia nearly every day
  - o Fatigue or loss of energy nearly every day
  - o Diminished ability to think or concentrate nearly every day
  - o Recurrent thoughts of death

An assessment through the lens of a descriptive problem-based model can yield a list of codifiable psychosocial problems resembling the following, and can be mutually prioritized for urgency by both the adolescent and therapist (with just a few needing to be billed):

- Problems at the micro-, mezzo-, and macro-levels:
  - Micro (e.g., the individual) problems:
    - BEP 1.5 – suicidal ideation
    - BEP 1.1 – saddened mood
    - BEP 1.7 – disrupted sleep
    - BEP 1.8 – loss of interest/pleasure in things
  - Mezzo (e.g., groups and communities) problems:
    - IR 1.4 – trauma
    - IR 1.5 – bullying
    - IR 1.1 – lack of familial/social support
  - Macro (e.g., institutions, policy, and culture) problems:
    - ES 1.4 – school/academic problem
    - ES 1.6 – crime in neighborhood

Benefits of Proposed Model

Using the brief and oversimplified example above, a problem-based taxonomy for describing people's emotional, behavioral, and psychological difficulties with an emphasis on contextual issues can provide the suffering individual—and helping professional—a richer, more humane, and accurate running narrative of the problems. This can help prevent both clients and clinicians from assuming that the cause of one's difficulties lies solely within the person in the form of a mental disorder or mental illness.

"Treatment" can evolve from being a technical, protocol-based, and diagnosis-specific endeavor to a more person-centered and humanistic vocation in which clinician and client work together to identify problems across varying domains and their possible solutions. Maisel (2015) describes the uncertain and dynamic exploratory process as follows:

She [the therapist] will travel with the person suffering through difficult territory where neither knows for sure what they will find or even what exactly they are looking for. She will own a personal menu of tactics that allow her to offer support, frame issues, hold the person across from her accountable, and do the sorts of things that good helpers know to do. A willing person and a savvy helper enter into a certain sort of collaboration, use everyday language like "sadness," "anxiety," and "boredom," and work together to choose and even create language that serves the sufferer. To put it simply, our human experience specialist would do no particular thing except try to be of help. (pp. 124–125)

A clinician may not always know the causes of problems for a client. To complicate things further, even if there is an understanding of the client's issues and needs, one can experience great uncertainty in knowing what therapeutic models, strategies, or framework will yield the results a clinician and client envision (Maisel, 2017). However, despite not knowing the causes of problems or indicated interventions with certainty, a clinician can still be of help with "a personal menu of tactics" (Maisel, 2015, p. 125) while accepting being unsure as to whether they will work.

To accomplish this, both clinician and client should be able to enter an open-ended therapeutic experience—not predicated on diagnosis and abstaining from complete adherence to protocol- based treatments—and allow for technique and choice to *organically arise* from each unique clinical encounter (Yalom, 2017). Yalom (2017) writes:

At its very core, the flow of therapy should be spontaneous, forever following unanticipated riverbeds; it is grotesquely distorted by being packaged . . . to deliver a uniform course of therapy. One of the true abominations spawned by the managed-care movement is the ever greater reliance on protocol therapy. (p. 34)

Using a descriptive problem-based approach, a clinician can walk alongside the client, allow the problems to slowly reveal themselves, collaboratively make sense of them, and let interventions emerge from the grab bag of techniques the clinical encounter is calling for—all while tolerating uncertainty as to whether they will be helpful.

Relatedly, this approach can also generate alternate avenues for interventions not strictly limited to psychotherapy. For example, in the case example previously mentioned, the therapist can encourage more family involvement for the adolescent, request for additional school support, or seek help from law enforcement.

There are many practitioners who already deem the psychiatric diagnosis irrelevant in clinical work by making all efforts to help the client understand how challenges can be viewed as adaptable responses to life stressors along a continuum of normality (e.g., Boyle & Johnstone, 2020). Some will augment that approach with a psychiatric diagnosis, stressing the importance of retaining the *DSM* in practice.

However, some guidelines suggest that a successful psychological formulation will make the use of a psychiatric diagnosis superfluous (Division of Clinical Psychology, 2011). Others may offer what the diagnosis could be at the client's request while subsequently practicing informed consent, advising the individual about the controversy surrounding mental disorders.

Some clinicians find diagnoses that vaguely match their client, ignoring *DSM* rules and diagnostic criteria (Greenberg, 2013; Phillips, 2010). Furthermore, others have reported using "workarounds" in clinical practice via reducing the *DSM* to a few frequently utilized diagnoses, "damping down" or negotiating diagnoses with clients to minimize stigma, and "fudging" codes to ensure insurance reimbursement (Probst, 2012; Whooley, 2010).

It has also been shown that clinicians identify insurance reimbursement as one of the main uses of the *DSM* (Patureau-Hatchett, 2008; Raskin et al., 2022). This highlights the redundancy of psychiatric diagnoses and questions their clinical utility in everyday practice.

Moving Discourse Away from Diagnosis and Deficits

The key difference in being able to draw from a descriptive problem-based taxonomy throughout clinical work is that the question of "What's the diagnosis?" would no longer have to be the elephant in the room—it can eventually become a *nonissue*, the elephant being rendered nonexistent, as a psychiatric diagnosis would no longer have to be billed. Put another way, in the words of psychologist Richard Bentall (2004, p. 141), "Once these complaints have been explained, there is no ghostly disease [or disorder] remaining that also requires an explanation. Complaints are all there is."

The focus would be placed on the person's problems and how to go about addressing them. Inserting a taxonomy of this kind into mental health discourse can also begin to shape how people view themselves and others, slowly shifting the pendulum from a medicalized individual lexicon (e.g., "I have a mental illness called depression") toward a nonmedicalized one (e.g., "I experience these kinds of problems because of what happened to me and what's going on in my life").

Relatedly, with more children entering mental health services and headlines alluding to a mental health crisis among our youth (e.g., Tingley, 2022), it is paramount for our most vulnerable to receive help understanding their challenges in a context-dependent and non-pathologizing framework. This prevents the possibility of incorporating a psychiatric disorder as part of their selves and identities during a crucial time in development that, if unchecked, can lead to long-term existential and ontological harm (see Davis, 2020 and Fay, 2022).

Being psychiatrically diagnosed can lead to a crisis of self-definition and identity (Jutel, 2011). Psychiatric diagnoses can brand people with "sticky" labels that may become equated to the total sum of the person and create a defeatist expectation of hardship in life (Duncan et al., 2004). The affixing of a psychiatric label as a "stamp of identity" (Jenkins & Csordas, 2020, p. 241) can run the risk of limiting possibilities in one's life and a chance at self-actualization. Lucy Johnstone (2022) compiled a disheartening list of negative reactions to being psychiatrically diagnosed (pp. 76–80) in which people experienced a loss of identity and sense of self, stigma, hopelessness, despair, inadequacy, humiliation, shame, and the end of one's life (see also Kemp et al., 2014).

Co-creating the Puzzle

A model like the one proposed can also influence how clinicians and clients co-create an interpretation of the presenting problem(s) while testing the hypothesis and not needing to give a mental disorder primacy for being a cause of one's suffering. For example:

Scenario 1:

Adolescent: "Why do I feel this way? Like I have no reason to live—no purpose. I'm sucking at school, I can't sleep, and I worry all day and night about what the future holds for me, if I even make it."

Clinician: "You most likely feel this way and have difficulties because you have major depressive disorder, a kind of mental illness. It's common for people to develop this kind of mental disorder at some point in their life, sometimes after distressing experiences. However, the symptoms you describe sound like you have depression."

Scenario 2:

Adolescent: "Why do I feel this way? Like I have no reason to live—no purpose. I'm sucking at school, I can't sleep, and I worry all day and night about what the future holds for me, if I even make it."

Clinician: "You experienced a life-threatening event, one in which the memories maybe keep replaying and affect your ability to focus in general. Because of that, you've been understandably struggling academically— and maybe now feel directionless and that you'd be better off dead, especially as you feel without any kind of family support. I can see how these kinds of thoughts and sad feelings could also keep you up at night, further contributing to a vicious cycle in which you are exhausted again the following day due to having sleep significantly disrupted."

With a healthy dose of humility, in a clinical interaction—or in any human-to-human chance encounter—we may never be able to find all the pieces to the puzzle that will explain the causes of an individual's problems with complete certainty. We may, at most, be able to find some or most pieces to the puzzle—and for many, that is plenty.

However, we also need to be given the opportunity to do such exploratory work, sometimes at the gradual unfolding pace it requires. Unfortunately, the use of psychiatric diagnoses and labeling people with a mental disorder to offer help provides the allure that all we need is one or two pieces (i.e., diagnoses) to the puzzle to explain the entire, complicated picture. Nothing could be further from the truth.

Discussion

The *DSM* and biomedical model have been shown to contribute to stigma (Read & Magliano, 2019) and iatrogenic harm (Boisvert & Faust, 2002; Fava & Rafanelli, 2019). Most psychiatric diagnoses in the *DSM* have retained intractable concerns for decades (Lacasse, 2013), chief among them being their lack of scientific validity (Lynch, 2018) and low reliability (Carney, 2013). Others argue the biomedical model of mental health has been a significant contributor to poor outcomes (The British Psychological Society, 2022), coupled with billions of dollars and decades-worth of research not yielding convincing scientific evidence to validate its footing (Simons, 2022).

As such, for the field of mental health and psychotherapy to pivot away from the *DSM* and biomedical model, a pragmatic alternative will ultimately need to be incorporated into the structure of contemporary health care as an adjunctive tool for clinicians and clients alike. If the *DSM* will someday cease to be the sole taxonomy, which would allow other classification systems to move the field of mental health forward (Cooper, 2014), the development and implementation of a descriptive problem-based taxonomy is one candidate to help eliminate barriers (e.g., perceived stigma upon being diagnosed with a mental disorder), ensure fairer access to resources, and decouple diagnosis from the eligibility for and provision of mental health services.

This endeavor will not be without its hurdles. To be determined from the initial proposed conceptualization of this descriptive problem-based taxonomy is how to go about assessing individual functioning and severity of problems. One can wonder how comprehensive or concise a system of this kind can or should be. Relatedly, there will also be definitional concerns; that is, some problems may be straightforward (e.g., "saddened mood") while others may be more open to interpretation (e.g., "loss of meaning in life"). That is something that could and should be collaboratively ascertained.

It is also worth pondering if this proposed model would eventually lead to the continued requirement by insurance payers of using psychotherapy protocols to address problems. It has been argued that psychotherapy should not be guided by a technical and medical protocol-based model (Shedler, 2018; Timimi, 2021). One reason is due to research demonstrating that matching a psychotherapy approach with a *DSM* diagnosis does not necessarily lead to improved outcomes.

For example, one study with over 2,000 clients showed that less than one percentage point in clinical outcomes could be attributed to the client's diagnosis (Wampold & Imel, 2015). Further undermining traditional thinking of needing to match diagnosis with a particular protocol, clinicians tend to end up practicing with integrative and pluralistic approaches (Cooper & McLeod, 2010; Zarbo et al., 2016). The eventual hope is payers would not mandate protocol-based services with the use of a framework such as the one proposed in this chapter.

Those challenging the *DSM* and biomedical model will be faced with not only with the influence that large pharmaceutical companies have on the *DSM* (and ensuring its continued existence) (Whitaker & Cosgrove, 2015), but with the cultural authority and power psychiatry retains as a branch of medicine (Davis, 2016; Simons, 2019), whose existence is arguably contingent on the psychiatric diagnosis (Johnstone, 2022). The development of classification systems takes time (e.g., it took at least six years to develop the influential *DSM-III* [APA, n.d.]), as does the changing of larger systems (Waddell et al., 2015).

Some people are also not fond of radical changes, and they may push back on efforts to modify a system that has influenced their identity and has brought them validation. However, we should be able to support one another without being forced to enter a fraudulent and deceitful system (Newnes, 2015; Whitaker, 2022). Incremental and gradual changes will be key.

As mentioned earlier in this chapter, it is important to reiterate that a project of this kind will require a *collaborative effort* by psychologists, social workers, psychiatrists, licensed professional counselors, and related disciplines. With sufficient empirical backing and advocacy by our associated professional organizations, it is possible a system like the one proposed in this chapter can eventually become endorsed by CMS just as they have recommended the *ICD* (and, by proxy, the *DSM*) to be used in health care. To start, however, a practical and implementable organizing framework needs to be agreed upon.

We can also surmise how daunting the task can be in developing a comprehensive taxonomy to help describe an infinite number of problems people experience within dynamic environments and systems. Again, a complex endeavor—but people are complex. And what the *DSM* loses for the sake of simplicity is the richness that can be gained by a more all-encompassing model. Preserving the richness of people's lives is how we honor their story, maintain their dignity, and help bolster their sense of self-worth.

It can be argued that the default setting of the human experience is to consist of challenges and suffering. Dysfunction is normal and having problems is to be expected throughout a lifetime. As such, when struggling we deserve to enter systems of care that will lift us up rather than tell us what, at our existential core, is wrong or "disordered" with us while we are already suffering.

We deserve to understand our challenges within a context-dependent and non-pathologizing framework that explains our struggles as differences along the continuum of normality. A renewed and practical focus on psychosocial problems of human existence can be one way to do that—a way out of being pigeonholed into the biomedical model.

References

Adame, A. L. (2006). *Recovered voices, recovered lives: A narrative analysis of psychiatric survivors' experiences of recovery* [MA Thesis, Miami University].

Adame, A. L., Bassman, R., Morsey, M., & Yates, K. (2017). *Exploring identities of psychiatric survivor therapists: Beyond us and them.* Palgrave Macmillan.

American Hospital Association. (2020, January 24). *CMS releases first data on Z code use in Medicare.* https://www.aha.org/news/headline/2020-01-24-cms-releases-first-data-z-code-use-medicare

American Psychiatric Association. (n.d.). *DSM history.* https://www.psychiatry.org/psychiatrists/practice/dsm/history-of-the-dsm

American Psychiatric Association. (1952). *Diagnostic and statistical manual of mental disorders.*

American Psychiatric Association. (1968). *Diagnostic and statistical manual of mental disorders* (2nd ed.).

American Psychiatric Association. (1980). *Diagnostic and statistical manual of mental disorders* (3rd ed.).

American Psychiatric Association. (2013a). *Diagnostic and statistical manual of mental disorders* (5th ed.). American Psychiatric Publishing.

American Psychiatric Association. (2013b, May 3). *Insurance implications of DSM-5* [Press release]. https://www.psychiatry.org/File%20Library/Psychiatrists/Practice/*DSM*/APA_*DSM*_Insurance-Implications-of-*DSM*-5.pdf

American Psychiatric Association. (2022). *Diagnostic and statistical manual of mental disorders* (5th ed., text rev.). American Psychiatric Publishing.

American Psychological Association. (2009, October). *ICD vs. DSM.* https://www.apa.org/monitor/2009/10/icd-dsm

Avdi, E. (2019). Negotiating diagnostic talk in psychotherapy. In J. N. Lester & M. O'Reilly (Eds.), *The Palgrave encyclopedia of critical perspectives on mental health* (pp. 1–17). Springer Publishing.

Bentall, R. (2004). *Madness explained: Psychosis and human nature.* Penguin. Boisvert, C. M., & Faust, D. (2002). Iatrogenic symptoms in psychotherapy. *American Journal of Psychotherapy, 56*(2), 244–259. https://doi.org/10.1176/appi.psycho-therapy.2002.56.2.244

Bolton, D., & Gillett, G. (2019). *The biopsychosocial model of health and disease: New philosophical and scientific developments.* Palgrave Macmillan.

Boyle, M., & Johnstone, L. (2020). *A straight talking introduction to the power threat meaning framework: An alternative to psychiatric diagnosis.* PCCS Books.

Boyles, O. (2019, February 27). CPT code basics: What you should know. *ICANotes*. https://www.icanotes.com/2019/02/27/cpt-code-basics-what-you-should-know/

The British Psychological Society. (2022, August 16). *The medical model has presided over four decades of flat-lining outcomes.* https://www.bps.org.uk/psychol-ogist/medical-model-has-presided-over-four-decades-flat-lining-outcomes

Carney, J. (2013, May 3). The *DSM*-5 field trials: Inter-Rater reliability ratings take a nose dive. *Mad in America*. https://www.madinamerica.com/2013/03/the-dsm-5-field-trials-inter-rater-reliability-ratings-take-a-nose-dive/

Carney, J. (2014). Where are the social workers? One social worker's road to active opposition to the new *DSM. Ethical Human Psychology and Psychiatry, 16*(1), 63–79. https://doi.org/10.1891/1559-4343.16.1.63

Centers for Medicare & Medicaid Services. (2014, June). *Fact sheet: Outpatient psychiatry & psychology services.* https://downloads.cms.gov/medicare-coverage-database/lcd_attachments/31887_33/Outpatient_Psych_Fact_Sheet09.18.14.pdf

Centers for Medicare & Medicaid Services. (2015, October 1). *Psychiatric diagnostic evaluation and psychotherapy services (L33252).* https://www.cms.gov/medi-care-coverage-database/view/lcd.aspx?lcdId=33252&ver=29

Centers for Medicare & Medicaid Services. (2018, October 3). *Billing and coding: Psychiatric diagnostic evaluation and psychotherapy services (A57520).* https://www.cms.gov/medicare-coverage-database/view/article.aspx?articleid=57520&ver=23&

Coleman, M. (2017). *Most frequently used CPT* codes by clinical social workers*. National Association of Social Workers. https://www.socialworkers.org/ includes/newIncludes/homepage/PRA-NL-27117.CPT-Codes-PP.pdf

Cooper, M., & McLeod, J. (2010). Pluralism: Towards a new paradigm for therapy. *Therapy Today, 21*(9). https://www.bacp.co.uk/bacp-journals/therapy-today/2010/november-2010/

Cooper, R. (2014). *Diagnosing the diagnostic and statistical manual of mental disorders.* Routledge.

Cornwall, M. (2013, September 7). Does the psychiatric diagnosis process qualify as a degradation ceremony? *Mad in America.* https://www.madinamerica.com/2013/09/psychiatric-diagnosis-process-qualify-degradation-ceremony/

Council on Social Work Education. (2022). *2022 EPAS.* Retrieved February 18, 2023, from https://www.cswe.org/accreditation/standards/2022-epas/

Davis, J. E. (2016). Reductionist medicine and its cultural authority. In J. E. Davis & A. M. Gonzalez (Eds.), *To fix or to heal: Patient care, public health, and the limits of biomedicine* (pp. 33–62). NYU Press. https://doi.org/10.18574/nyu/9781479878246.003.0002

Davis, J. E. (2020). *Chemically imbalanced: Everyday suffering, medication, and our troubled quest for self-mastery.* University of Chicago Press.

DeCarlo, M. (2018). *Scientific inquiry in social work.* Pressbooks. https://scientificinquiryinsocialwork.pressbooks.com/

Desantis, G. (n.d.). An introduction to *ICD*-10 z codes. *TenEleven.* https://10e11.com/blog/an-introduction-to-icd-10-z-codes/

Dhar, A. (2022, September 14). Is service-user research possible in mental health? An interview with Diana Rose. *Mad in America.* https://www.madinamerica. com/2022/09/service-user-research-diana-rose/?mc_cid=91f1af17fc&mc_eid=22edfddc75

Division of Clinical Psychology. (2011, December). Good practice guidelines on the use of psychological formulation. *The British Psychological Society.* https://shop.bps.org.uk/good-practice-guidelines-on-the-use-of-psychological-formulation

Duncan, B. L., Miller, S. D., & Sparks, J. A. (2004). *The heroic client: A revolutionary way to improve effectiveness through client-directed, outcome-Informed therapy.* Jossey-Bass.

Engel, G. L. (1977). The need for a new medical model: A challenge for biomedicine. *Science, 196*(4286), 129–136. https://doi.org/10.1126/science.847460

Fava, G., & Rafanelli, C. (2019). Iatrogenic factors in psychopathology. *Psychotherapy and Psychosomatics, 88*(3), 129–140. https://doi.org/10.1159/000500151

Fawcett, B., Weber, Z., & Bannister, H. (2020). *The medicalisation of everyday life: A critical perspective*. Red Globe Press.

Fay, S. (2022). *Pathological: The true story of six misdiagnoses*. HarperOne.

Florence, A., & Pūras, D. (Hosts). (2020, May 27). Bringing human rights to mental health care: An interview with UN Envoy Dainius Pūras [Audio podcast episode]. *Mad in America*. https://www.madinamerica.com/2020/05/bringing-human-rights-mental-health-care-interview-dainius-puras/

Freedman, R., Lewis, D. A., Michels, R., Pine, D. S., Schultz, S. K., Tamminga, C. A., Gabbard, G. O., Gau, S. S. F., Javitt, D. C., Oquendo, M. A., Shrout, P. E., Vieta, E., & Yager, J. (2013). The initial field trials of *DSM*-5: New blooms and old thorns. *American Journal of Psychiatry, 170*(1), 1–5. https://doi.org/10.1176/appi.ajp.2012.12091189

Fritscher, L. (2020, March 10). How the medical model for mental disorders works in psychology. *Verywell Mind*. https://www.verywellmind.com/medical-model-2671617

Ghaemi, S. N. (2012). *The rise and fall of the biopsychosocial model: Reconciling art and science in psychiatry*. Johns Hopkins University Press.

Gomory, T., Dunleavy, D. J., & Lieber, A. S. (2017). The solving problems in everyday living model: Toward a demedicalized, education-based approach to "mental health." *Journal of Humanistic Psychology, 61*(1), 132–151. https://doi.org/10.1177/0022167817722430

Greenberg, G. (2013). *The book of woe: The DSM and the unmaking of psychiatry*. Plume.

Hepworth, D. H., Rooney, R. H., Rooney, G. D., & Strom-Gottfried, K. (2013). *Direct social work practice: Theory and skills* (9th ed.). Brooks/Cole.

Hopps, J. G., & Lowe, T. B. (2012). Social work practice in the new millennium. In C. N. Dulmus & K. M Sowers. (Eds.), *The profession of social work: Guided by history, led by evidence* (pp. 51–89). John Wiley & Sons.

Ingle, M. (2021, July 24). Why not diagnose social conditions instead of individual symptoms? *Mad in America*. https://www.madinamerica.com/2021/07/not-diag-nose-social-conditions-instead-individual-symptoms/

Insel, T. (2013, April 29). *Transforming diagnosis. [Blog].*
https://psychrights.org/2013/130429NIMHTransformingDiagnosis.htm

Jenkins, J. H., & Csordas, T. J. (2020). *Troubled in the land of enchantment.*
University of California Press.

Johnstone, L. (2022). *A straight talking introduction to psychiatric diagnosis* (2nd
ed.). PCCS Books.

Johnstone, L., & Boyle, M., (with Cromby, J., Dillon, J., Harper, D.,
Kinderman, P., Longden, E., Pilgrim, D., & Read, J.). (2018). *The power
threat meaning frame- work: Behaviour, as an alternative to functional psychiatric
diagnosis.* British Psychological Society.

Jutel, A. G. (2011). *Putting a name to it: Diagnosis in contemporary society.* Johns
Hopkins University Press.

Kamens, S. R., Elkins, D. N., & Robbins, B. D. (2017). Open letter to the
DSM-5. Journal of Humanistic Psychology, 57(6), 675–687.
https://doi.org/10.1177/0022167817698261

Karls, J. M., & Wandrei, K. E. (Eds.). (1994). *Person-in-Environment system:
The PIE classification system for social functioning problems.* NASW Press.

Kemp, J. J., Lickel, J. J., & Deacon, B. J. (2014). Effects of a chemical
imbalance causal explanation on individuals' perceptions of their
depressive symptoms. *Behaviour Research and Therapy, 56,* 47–52.
https://doi.org/10.1016/j.brat.2014.02.009

Kinderman, P. (2015). Imagine there's no diagnosis, it's easy if you try.
Psychopathology Review, a2(1), 154–161. https://doi.org/10.5127/pr.036714

Kinderman, P. (2019). *A manifesto for mental health: Why we need a revolution in
mental health care.* Palgrave Macmillan.

Kinderman, P., Allsopp, K., & Cooke, A. (2017). Responses to the publication
of the American Psychiatric Association's *DSM-5. Journal of Humanistic
Psychology, 57*(6), 625–649. https://doi.org/10.1177/0022167817698262

Kinderman, P., Read, J., Moncrieff, J., & Bentall, R. P. (2012). Drop the
language of disorder. *Evidence Based Mental Health, 16*(1), 2–3.
https://doi.org/10.1136/eb-2012-100987

Kirk, S. A., Gomory, T., & Cohen, D. (2013). *Mad science: Psychiatric coercion,
diagnosis, and drugs.* Routledge.

Kotov, R., Krueger, R. F., Watson, D. I., Achenbach, T. M., Althoff, R. R., Bagby, R. M., Brown, T. M., Carpenter, W. T., Caspi, A., Clark, L. A., Eaton, N. R., Forbes, M. K., Forbush, K. T., Goldberg, D. E., Hasin, D. S., Hyman, S. E., Ivanova, M. Y., Lynam, D. R., Markon, K. E., . . .Zimmerman, M. (2017). The hierarchical taxonomy of psychopathology (HiTOP): A dimensional alternative to traditional nosologies. *Journal of Abnormal Psychology, 126*(4), 454–477. https://doi.org/10.1037/abn0000258

Lacasse, J. R. (2013). After *DSM*-5: A critical mental health research agenda for the 21st century. *Research on Social Work Practice, 24*(1), 5–10. https://doi.org/10.1177/1049731513510048

Lacasse, J. R., & Gambrill, E. (2015). Making assessment decisions: Macro, mezzo, and micro perspectives. In B. Probst (Ed.), *Critical thinking in clinical assessment and diagnosis* (pp. 69–84). Springer.

Lebowitz, M. S., & Ahn, W. K. (2014). Effects of biological explanations for mental disorders on clinicians' empathy. *Proceedings of the National Academy of Sciences, 111*(50), 17786–17790. https://doi.org/10.1073/pnas.1414058111

Lingiardi, V., & McWilliams, N. (Eds.). (2017). *Psychodynamic diagnostic manual: PDM-2* (2nd ed.). Guilford Press.

Lynch, T. (2018). The validity of the *DSM*: An overview. *The Irish Journal of Counselling and Psychotherapy, 18*(2), 5–10.

Maisel, E. R. (2015). *The future of mental health: Deconstructing the mental disorder paradigm*. Routledge.

Maisel, E. R. (2017). *Humane helping: Focusing less on disorders and more on life's challenges*. Routledge.

Manning, J. (2020). *Suicide: The social causes of self-destruction*. University of Virginia Press.

McWilliams, N. (2008, May 1). The psychodynamic diagnostic manual: A clinically useful complement to *DSM*. *Psychiatric Times.* https://www.psychiatrictimes.com/view/psychodynamic-diagnostic-manual-clinically-useful-complement-dsm

Miley, K. K., O'Melia, M., & DuBois, B. (2012). *Generalist social work practice: An empowering approach*. Pearson.

Minahan, A., & Pincus, A. (1977). Conceptual framework for social work practice. *Social Work, 22*(5), 347–352. https://doi.org/10.1093/sw/22.5.347

Moncrieff, J. (2010). Psychiatric diagnosis as a political device. *Social Theory & Health, 8*(4), 370–382. https://doi.org/10.1057/sth.2009.11

National Association of Social Workers. (n.d.). *NASW—National Association of Social Workers.* https://www.socialworkers.org/News/Facts/Social-Workers

National Institute of Mental Health. (n.d.). *About RDoC.* NIMH. https://www.nimh.nih.gov/research/research-funded-by-nimh/rdoc/about-rdoc

Nazar, N. (2020). The ecosystem approach in health social work. *Mental Health: Global Challenges Journal, 4*(2), 16–18. https://doi.org/10.32437/mhgcj.v4i2.90

Newnes, C. (2015). *Inscription, diagnosis, deception and the mental health industry: How psy governs us all.* Palgrave Macmillan.

O'Connor, S. (2014, April 9). *ICD* and *DSM* coding: What's the difference? *Advanced Data Systems Corporation.* https://www.adsc.com/blog/icd-and-dsm-coding-whats-the-difference

Patureau-Hatchett, M. (2008). *Counselors' perceptions of training, theoretical orientation, cultural and gender bias, and use of the Diagnostic and Statistical Manual of Mental Disorders-IV-Text Revision* (Doctoral dissertation). http://scholarworks.uno.edu/td/847/

Phillips, J. (2010). Another *DSM* on the shelf? *Association for the Advancement of Philosophy and Psychiatry Bulletin, 17*(2), 70–71.

Probst, B. (2012). "Walking the tightrope": Clinical social workers' use of diagnostic and environmental perspectives. *Clinical Social Work Journal, 41*(2), 184–191. https://doi.org/10.1007/s10615-012-0394-1

Raskin, J. D., Maynard, D., & Gayle, M. C. (2022). Psychologist attitudes toward *DSM*-5 and its alternatives. *Professional Psychology: Research and Practice, 53*(6), 553–563. https://doi.org/10.1037/pro0000480

Read, J. (2005). The bio-bio-bio model of madness. *The Psychologist, 18*(10), 596–597. https://thepsychologist.bps.org.uk/volume-18/edition-10/bio-bio-bio-model-madness

Read, J., & Magliano, L. (2019). "Schizophrenia"—The least scientific and most damaging of psychiatric labels. In J. Watson (Ed.), *Drop the disorder! Challenging the culture of psychiatric diagnosis* (pp. 88–109). PCCS Books.

Regier, D. A., Narrow, W. E., Clarke, D. E., Kraemer, H. C., Kuramoto, S. J., Kuhl, E. A., & Kupfer, D. J. (2013). *DSM-5 field trials in the United States and Canada, part II: Test-retest reliability of selected categorical diagnoses. American Journal of Psychiatry, 170*(1), 59–70. https://doi.org/10.1176/appi.ajp.2012.12070999

Robbins, B. D., Kamens, S. R., & Elkins, D. N. (2017). *DSM-5 reform efforts by the society for humanistic psychology. Journal of Humanistic Psychology, 57*(6), 602–624. https://doi.org/10.1177/0022167817698617

Rubin, J. (2017). The classification and statistical manual of mental health concerns: A proposed practical scientific alternative to the *DSM* and *ICD. Journal of Humanistic Psychology, 58*(1), 93–114. https://doi.org/10.1177/0022167817718079

Ruby, C. (2017, February 4). ISEPP calling for organizations to join in petition. *Mad in America.* https://www.madinamerica.com/2017/02/isepp-calling-organizations-join-petition/

Shedler, J. (2018). Where is the evidence for "evidence-based" therapy? *Psychiatric Clinics of North America, 41*(2), 319–329. https://doi.org/10.1016/j.psc.2018.02.001

Simons, P. (2019, March 15). Mad science, psychiatric coercion and the therapeutic State: An interview with Dr. David Cohen. *Mad in America.* https://www.madinamerica.com/2019/05/mad-science-psychiatric-coercion-therapeutic-state-interview-dr-david-cohen/

Simons, P. (2022, September 5). Influential neuroscientist reviews decades of failure. *Mad in America.* https://www.madinamerica.com/2022/09/influential-neuroscientist-failure/

TherapyNotes, LLC. (2018, July 11). How and when to use z codes. *TherapyNotes.* https://blog.therapynotes.com/how-and-when-to-use-z-codes

Timimi, S. (2021, January 11). Insane medicine, chapter 8: Treatment traps and how to get out of them (part 1). *Mad in America.* https://www.madinamerica.com/2021/01/insane-medicine-chapter-8-part-1/

Tingley, K. (2022, March 24). There's a mental-health crisis among American children. Why? *The New York Times*. https://www.nytimes.com/2022/03/23/magazine/mental-health-crisis-kids.html

Toikko, T. (2016). Becoming an expert by experience: An analysis of service users' learning process. *Social Work in Mental Health, 14*(3), 292–312.

Tyler, S. (2020). *Human behavior and the social environment I*. University of Arkansas Libraries. https://uark.pressbooks.pub/hbse1/

USC School of Social Work. (2018, February 27). *Do you know the difference between micro-, mezzo- and macro-level social work?*. https://dworakpeck.usc.edu/news/do-you-know-the-difference-between-micro-mezzo-and-macro-level-social-work

Vanheule, S., Desmet, M., Meganck, R., Inslegers, R., Willemsen, J., De Schryver, M., & Devisch, I. (2014). Reliability in psychiatric diagnosis with the *DSM*: Old wine in new barrels. *Psychotherapy and Psychosomatics, 83*(5), 313–314. https://doi.org/10.1159/000358809

van Hulst, B., Werkhoven, S., & Durston, S. (2021). We need to rename ADHD. *Scientific American*. https://www.scientificamerican.com/article/we-need-to-rename-adhd/

Waddell, S., Waddock, S., Cornell, S., Dentoni, D., McLachlan, M., & Meszoely, G. (2015). Large systems change: An emerging field of transformation and transitions. *Journal of Corporate Citizenship, 2015*(58), 5–30. https://doi.org/10.9774/gleaf.4700.2015.ju.00003

Walsh, D., & Foster, J. (2020). A contagious other? Exploring the public's appraisals of contact with "mental illness." *International Journal of Environmental Research and Public Health, 17*(6), 2005. https://doi.org/10.3390/ijerph17062005

Wampold, B. E., & Imel, Z. E. (2015). *The great psychotherapy debate: The evidence for what makes psychotherapy work* (2nd ed.). Routledge.

Whelan, C. (2022, July 14). How to know if your insurance covers therapy. *Healthline*. https://www.healthline.com/health/does-insurance-cover-therapy

Whitaker, R. (2022, August 13). Psychiatry, fraud, and the case for a class-action lawsuit. *Mad in America*. https://www.madinamerica.com/2022/08/psychiatry-fraud-and-the-case-for-a-class-action-lawsuit/

Whitaker, R., & Cosgrove, L. (2015). *Psychiatry under the influence: Institutional corruption, social injury, and prescriptions for reform.* Palgrave Macmillan.

Whooley, O. (2010). Diagnostic ambivalence: Psychiatric workarounds and the diagnostic and statistical manual of mental disorders. *Sociology of Health & Illness, 32*(3), 452–469. https://doi.org/10.1111/j.1467-9566.2010.01230.x

World Health Organization. (2008). *Closing the gap in a generation: Health equity through action on the social determinants of health.* World Health Organization. https://www.ncbi.nlm.nih.gov/nlmcatalog/101488674

World Health Organization. (2019). *International Classification of Diseases, Eleventh Revision (ICD-11).* World Health Organization.

Yalom, I. D. (2017). *The gift of therapy: An open letter to a new generation of therapists and their patients.* Harper Perennial.

Zarbo, C., Tasca, G. A., Cattafi, F., & Compare, A. (2016). Integrative psychotherapy works. *Frontiers in Psychology, 6,* 2021. https://doi.org/10.3389/fpsyg.2015.02021

Súmptōma: From Discrimination Through Destruction to Transfiguration

Todd DuBose

Abstract: *If we were to discriminate against any person the way we do symptoms, we would be charged with hate crimes. From a medically-modeled perspective, symptoms are pathogens to excise and jettison. In this chapter, I employ a critical-hermeneutical-phenomenological destruction of assumed and implicit ideologies and value allegiances taken for granted in the medically-modeled paradigm regarding the very notion of "symptom." I will expose how this discrimination occurs and is held in place such that no manner of de-stigmatization is even possible if symptoms continue to be pathologized in numerous ways. Moreover, I will show that symptoms are pathologized because they have been perpetually and systematically misunderstood and concealed from their showings as events or enacted "sayings" of significance. I will then offer a concrete example of Disruptive Mood Dysregulation Disorder to show possibilities of moving from discrimination through destruction to transfiguration by way of a hermeneutical-phenomenological alternative to diagnostics that is distinct from the dominant medically-modeled hegemony.*

Introduction

Discrimination is commonly understood in at least two ways (Harper, n.d.-a). One is to negate, ostracize, demote, or demean a person's, group's, or, as I will argue here, an ideology's difference simply due to the difference; it is a practice of pathologization as degradation and subsequent segregation, if not annihilation. If "pathologization" was a process of discerning what *pathos* originally meant—that is, suffering and joy—then stigmatization would be assuaged.

But this is not what happens. The very structure of medical modeling positions pathologization as pathogen-ization; this facilitates stigmatization when symptoms are equated with pathogens. If one is symptomatic, one is "less than," contaminated, with the word "symptom" being the postmodern world for sin.

Another understanding of discrimination is as a process of differentiation or discernment of differences as simply different—not less than, nor better than, just different. The former use of the word discrimination presumes something deviant, ill, or broken in relation to something normed, centric, healthy, or elite. The latter definition has no norm or centrism; hence, difference is relative to just other differences. Difference is not "deficient" any more than "other" is freakish from the familiar other.

My hope in this chapter is to take the latter approach to expose the supremacist hegemony of the former approach in diagnostic and therapeutic care while offering an alternative model of care to this medically-modeled, algorithmic engineering way of caring beginning with an analysis of the concept "symptom." I will call the alternative model of care "the phenomenological way," which views "symptoms" not as pathogens or illness but as "sayings" of lived meaning.

Without getting into extensive pages of what I mean by the phenomenological way, I will briefly describe it here and then show it in practice as we explore the concept "symptom," and a concrete example of a symptom that was added to the 5th edition of the *Diagnostic and Statistical Manual for Mental Disorders* (2013): Disruptive Mood Dysregulation Disorder (DMDD).

By "phenomenology" I mean a post- or late-Heideggerian hermeneutical phenomenology of the inconspicuous (Alvis, 2017; Heidegger, 2012; McNeill, 2020; Vallega-Neu, 2012) in concert with a critical-theoretical eye to how phenomena, as lived in the world (world as web of meaning) and not just as experienced in consciousness, are covered or veiled by common language, values, and assumptions or lived ideologies. This is, of course, influenced by the Frankfurt school of critical theory as well as Michel Foucault's critique of power, knowledge, and institutions, particularly regarding madness (Foucault, 1988). The hermeneutical aspect of this phenomenological way is a radical hermeneutics of John Caputo, combining Heideggerian phenomenology and Derridean deconstruction that maintains an incessant reinterpretability in discerning contexts and incomparable uniqueness, resisting any reduction or closure of knowledge (Caputo, 1987, 2000, 2006).

In a very condensed description of a very complex process, Being as *Existenz* (existential, rather than biological as existen*ce*) is experienced inconspicuously in any and every way of being in the world. The inapparent is indirect and only shyly shows itself as it cannot be gasped or objectified without losing itself. The moment we name it is the moment we lose it. It is not an object for analysis by an observing subject. It is experienced, registered—sometimes non-dually, sometimes glimpsed momentarily—but nonetheless are enactments of significance disclosing the meaning of Being for a being.

When we think we "see" it, we have objectified it and have in hand a re-presentation of an experience that has already slipped away, rather than the experience itself. What is "seen" is not seen with the eyes, or heard with the ears, but harkened, *heeded*, experienced as intangible lived meaning (Schurmann, p. 179). It is invisible; science cannot study it (Heidegger, 2001; Henry, 2012). It is not invisible as non-existent as it is experienced; it just cannot be measured, objectified, thingified, or bottled for production.

Although immeasurable, lived meaning is nonetheless evidential as it is present in every moment of our lives, including moments of despair and meaninglessness (DuBose, 2016). It is the most important "evidence" to and for us but cannot be accessed through calculative or procedural thinking; only through the poetic and meditative opening of phenomenology—that is to say, only by "letting it be" without why (McNeil, 2020, pp. 54-56; Schurmann, 1987, p. 20). Without why does not mean that a comportment or way of being is without lived meaning—just the opposite. Without why means without explanation, justification, or commodifiable (i.e., sellable for efficient production) so that it can unfold more freely and completely—a completion that, of course, never fully arrives, never fully exhausted.

One would understandably wonder how we can think such a process that cannot be seen, objectified, or fully known. Much has to do with how we look for what. When someone laughs, the conspicuous presencing of that comportment is recognizable as a behavior, even in its variance. The laughter can be seen, but what is funny to the one laughing is invisible. They will tell us, but even then "funny" is not something we see. We perhaps see mouths open, heads thrown back—some kind of vocalization associated with what we call a laugh. But prescribing this comportment does not equal funny. We also don't know the inapparent links to other experiences in the laugher's life story such that what they are laughing at may have originally been frightening or sad.

Just because we cannot see it, grasp it, know it (cognitively) does not mean it doesn't exist or isn't meaningful. I argue the direct opposite: It is the intangible that matters most in the tangible, the happening (intangible) in the happening (tangible behaviors, physical materialism). The critical-hermeneutical-phenomenologist heeds what is being said (verbally, by comportment) that matters most at that moment to that person saying, and as shown and disclosed in how they are saying it, and what they want me to "get" in the way they want me to get it.

We are heeding lived meaning, not illness or health, which are imposed valuations covering what the lived meaning is trying to say. To heed lived meaning requires "seeing" what is invisibly weaving its inconspicuous presencing in, around and through conspicuous obviousness. One can measure neurotransmitters all day and still not see fear, anger, hurt, sadness, worry, or love though no one would deny any of these experiences. Nevertheless, as phenomena, as events, they do not "have a number" as aren't considered evidence by the medical model, thus jettisoning what matters most to the realms of the khora space outside the city walls. That is where the critical-hermeneutical-phenomenologist lives.

The hermeneut enhances this opening with a clearing to unfold rather than reducing it with deductive interpretations. Discerning the particular and nuanced differentiations of specific contexts and situations in which they occur does not get in the way of letting something be but allows it to *be* even more so. The phenomenologist, however, checks to see if the hermeneut is bracketing enough while the hermeneut real-izes that showings are never general or generic—only specific. The hermeneut de-*construct*-s and re-*context*-ualizes the birth of the specific and unique while the critical theorist, on the other hand, checks for blind spots in the hermeneutical phenomenologist's interpretive unfolding, lest the process of "interpretive unfolding" slouch into an oxymoronic canceling of itself.

To do so, says the critical theorists, we need to see what ideologies are employed to show phenomena as *they* want it shown, and how they may want it shown, in service of self-interested political agendas. This is hermeneutical violence, an eisegesis that reads back into and disseminates information to ensure self-serving agendas such as withholding or not communicating adverse side effects on medications, leaving out evidence or conceptualizations that do not fit with traditional scientific research, or simply telling the public that something is for their own good when it can do harm so as to accelerate marketing over the caution of what the research is and could show.

The ideologies explored are not separate from, above or beyond empiricism—they are embedded *in* the very empiricism assumed to be objectively unbiased. Ideologies are the intangibles in tangible empiricism. I don't first think about a value and then apply it. Whatever I am empirically doing (walking to the car) is an enactment *of* my lived values (to go towards a desired destination for some conviction of task). A phenomenologist exposes coverings of phenomena that mislead or cloak without imposing a replacement hegemony of dominant values—medical model out, phenomenological way in, and the only way. Doing this would mitigate against the very point of phenomenological openness.

The medical model is not a pathogen itself—just a different model from the phenomenological way. The phenomenologist is just saying that it has its place and function, but understanding lived meaning is not it. Using medically-modeled, natural science methodology to understand lived meaning is like cooking spaghetti with a vacuum cleaner—bad fit between task and tool. Neither would one clean a house with a wooden spoon, unless one sees the house as a bowl of spaghetti. Then, only a phenomenologist would help us understand how that is for this particular chef. Hence, all three (critical-hermeneutical-phenomenology) tri-constitute each other or, as I argue, any one of them is excellently what it is when being all three. So, from this point on when I refer to "the phenomenology way," this is what I mean.

Now on to the de-construct-ion, re-context-ualization and transfiguration of the symptom. Caputo states our task ahead quite well, echoing both Heidegger and Derrida: "To deconstruct something...is to release the event that is harbored by the name, to see to it that the event is not trapped by the name" (Caputo, 2006, p. 28). Our current, consensus, medically-modeled approach to naming traps events.

De-construct-ing and Re-context-ualizing *Súmptōma*

Symptoms, from a medically-modeled perspective and as the average citizen's view would see them, are understood as either causes or outcomes of illnesses—pathogens to be eliminated. We collect those symptoms into clusters, categorize and classify them with taxonomies, algorithmically employ the pre-established "treatment" paired with each classification/ categorization, and then terminate such symptoms with extreme prejudice.

A medical model does not mourn a symptom's death but celebrates it. Symptoms are talked about with disdain, contempt, impatience, irritation, and with intent to banish them as quickly as possible. Here is the rub, a devastating rub: As long as we refer to symptoms in this way, we will never be able to destigmatize suffering. In order to not stigmatize symptoms, we have to free it from how it became stigmatized in the first place and, as I will suggest below, transfigure the word symptom into its original sense of a "saying" about a "befalling."

The ancient Greek conceptualization of σύμπτωμα (súmptōma), though, is actually understood as "a happening, an accident, something that 'befalls us'" (Harper, n.d.-b). Although disease or illness can be a part of befalling, they are not the befalling itself. What befalls us, and our falling into what befalls us, can be due to chance or fate. Fate and chance, though, are not opposed to one another and neither is "without choice or agency."

Fate, here, is not pre-determined even though it is "to allot" or "to assign." It is how one finds oneself in relation to an infinite amount of variables, one of which are our choices and decisions—that simultaneously occur with other variables out of our hands—to create the convergence of a radically incomparable event-as-happening. Disease or illness may be one of those factors in the event but is not the event itself. Nor does disease cause the event. The event is the lived meaning of the befalling. Therefore, a befalling is an event—not a thing, neither a chemical (balanced or not) nor a behavior (maladaptive or not) nor a thought (distorted or not).

One may find oneself frightened, or exhausted, or enraged, or disoriented, or in conflict, or grieving, or loved. These are *events of meaning* in the world, but each of these abstractions are lived experiences and very specific to those involved in the befalling. How one *lives* an occurrence's meaning is their "saying," not just what they verbally communicate about it but also how they comport through it. The meaning of the occurrence shapes the very nature of the occurrence.

If I am a dog lover and a dog comes charging at me, I may be very excited. But if afraid of dogs, this occurrence is quite a different occurrence. There is no occurrence or event without meaning. For the phenomenologist, the befalling as well as the meaning therein is a process of *aletheia*, the unfolding of truth as progressively shown and experienced in "unconcealed" ways (Heidegger, 1992). Taxonomical categorization, unwittingly, conceals.

The symptom-as-saying looks for the inconspicuous in the conspicuous, the intangible in the tangible, such as in what is now a familiar example offered by Heidegger regarding tears: Tears are not the tangible water emitted from tear ducts, but the intangible and immeasurable sadness therein (Heidegger, 2001, p. 81). Hermeneutical violence ignores the intangible due to its immeasurability, but in doing so ignores what is arguably the most important "evidence" for each of us: lived meaning.

Hence, a symptom is *not* a pathogen, but an occurrence, an event, a happening, a befalling, which is also a saying. "A saying is a showing, means a showing" (Heidegger, 2001, p. 185). Attending to a symptom as saying is to heed the meaning of what has befallen someone, which today we may call a difficulty or challenge or concern in living. We heed the intangible, inconspicuous breaking in of lived meaning in the conspicuous presencing before us, with us.

The saying discloses how the befalling is taken up as well as how it "sits" with someone. The saying is also about Being itself, and how one is meaningfully living the existentials present although, again, invisible, in the befalling: uncertainty, unknowing, agency, language, temporality, spatiality, mortality, co-existence, among other givens. This process is incomparably unique and relative to circumstance and to what matters to those in the befalling.

Hence, we cannot essentialize experiences required for taxonomical categorization. This is one of the difficulties with codes and manuals: the loss of the specific, and neither diagnostics nor ethics are general—only and always specific. Specificity works against the algorithmic pull toward "if this, then that." Part of the radically incomparable event of befalling is the unpredictability, unrepeatability, irreversibility, and indeterminacy of each event. We "see patterns" only when we inattend to the rigor of nuance and complexity. A taxonomical approach moves in the opposite direction of the phenomenological way, of attending to the divine within (*therapeia*, *therapeutikos*); that is, of the lived meaning within, of *aletheia*. *The phenomenological way heeds sayings, rather than treats symptoms.*

So, what is someone saying during extreme experiences heretofore called psychosis about being courageous in an unfamiliar and threatening world? What is being said about life pressing down on someone like an immovable bolder heretofore called depression? What are rapid heart rates, sweaty palms, hyperventilation heretofore called anxiety saying about time running out, or threats to what matters most, or the unknowing or uncertainty about what is coming?

What is being said about having to continually check to see if one locked the front door, or needing to correctly step three times in a prescribed place, over and over and over again to avert disaster heretofore called obsessive compulsive disorder? What is being said in what heretofore has been called attention deficit and hyperactivity disorder about being in a world that calls from every angle in each moment, where one fears missing out on life's beauty, or fears not attending to what is around lest one be hurt?

What is the suicidal event, the *sine qua non* pathologized event, saying about self-care or liberation or a cost analysis of suffering and relief, or the unfairness of life? What does the blade say when dragged across one's body over and over again in what has heretofore been pathologized as self-harm? These "symptoms" and others are not illnesses, but sayings of existential matterings, accessed by the heeding critical-hermeneutical-phenomenologist. Let's explore specifically a saying that has pathologized most recently childhood rage: Disruptive Mood Dysregulation Disorder.

De-construct-ing and Re-contextualizing Dys-regulated Dys-ruption

Disruptive Mood Dysregulation Disorder (DMDD) was a new diagnosis added to the 5th edition of the *Diagnostic and Statistical Manual for Mental Disorders* in 2013. It was added partially and seemingly due to pressure applied to psychiatry to walk back the prior tendency to over-diagnose children with bipolar disorder that still wanted a way to pathologize childhood dysregulation or, as I see it, childhood rage.

Situating the medicalization of childhood rage as DMDD requires seeing this event against a larger backdrop of medicalizing pathos (passion) in general, and the irritability-anger-rage continuum in particular. Although children take the brunt of the DMDD diagnosis, adults are even more pathologized as personality disordered or sociopathic if they exhibit dysregulated and disordered comportment as they are expected to behave and act maturely and socially acceptable (e.g., remaining calm, reasonable, using one's words to communicate what is dysregulating them).

Erica Burman is accurate to critique developmental psychology's alignment with privileging patriarchal values of reason and autonomy over emotion and dependency (Burman, 2016). The same could be said of privileging Apollonian comportment of reason and moderation over Dionysian intensity unchained. But the latter is not an illness or disease—

only a preferred comportment—though both are practiced at different times for different reasons.

Michel Foucault's entire canon is premised on the point that we have historically put out of sight what has disturbed us, lest we see it in ourselves. We then created, as Foucault's continues to argue, various institutionalizations of imposed regimes of truth to manage this disturbance through a series of power relations and practices. These are practices of surveillance, controlling classification of confessional information, the suppression and abuse of bodies and desire and passion, even down to the minutia of prescribing how and what one can even experience what one experiences (e.g., what is allowed to be felt and expressed, in what ways, by whom, as decided by whom, in which circumstances) (Foucault, 1988).

Symptoms, from these and similar perspectives, are not discovered as ontologically pathological; they are *constructed* to be so for various socio-politico-economic needs of those in power. These are examples of the critical dimension of phenomenology—not naysaying but loosening grips of implicit ideologies framing particular experiences that mislead, deter, and divert a phenomenon's unfolding.

The phenomenological way, instead, heeds the rage and asks what yelling is saying regarding what is not being heeded when speaking softly, or what the fists are saying that swing to be heeded when words are ignored, or what the gun is saying when fists and words are unheeded, or what the bombs are saying when all else is unheeded. Although counterproductive to heed comportments not preferred, it is exactly by doing so that they are often disarmed though, paradoxically, without the aim to do so. Heeding does not have a hidden agenda of manipulating one way of being in the world over another except to provide a clearing to heed.

The phenomenological way disarms the violence by respecting (heeding) what it has to say, not violently getting rid of violence. Once a respectful heeding occurs, in my experience of thirty-five years of working with violence, the need for the violence more than likely dissipates, tips its hat, and heads out the back door. The violence carries inconspicuously lived meanings that those pathologizing it will never understand (e.g., the hurt, mourning, helplessness, needing to feel power, the fear of being attacked, etc.).

Granted, hurt people do not automatically get a pass to hurt people, and the distancing of violence invites veils and concealment due to fears, revengeful counter-rage, concerns for safety, and moral judgements. Practicing the phenomenological way isn't an easy way despite its letting be, without why. Yet it calls for the courage to bracket such judgments and remain horizontal (i.e., heeding any presentation with respect without privileging or negating what "should" be felt, thought, or enacted).

The reduction of all pathos to fears of destructive rage leaves any dysregulated soul "shut up" with this rage much more likely to perpetuate it. No wonder a raging child, or anyone who finds themselves defined as a medicalized pathogen and subsequently readied for processing and treatment, feels much like a chained werewolf before the rise of a full moon.

Therefore, dysregulation-as-saying calls for a bracketing of implicit classifications, values and assumptions that cover and veil a phenomenon's showing as it is, in its own way. The "dys" rather than "dis-" is intentional and means a *different* way of regulating, not an inferior one. Dys-regulation, seen as a pathogen, privileges regulation. Dys-regulation is necessary for any change or re-regulation. There are times we applaud being off the chain, being all in, going for broke, feasting, throwing caution to the wind, all of which are relative to which scale of measurement is being used. What are any of these dys-regulations saying to us?

Devaluing disruption, by default, privileges un-interruption—that people and events should *not* be interrupted. But this is quite relative as well. In an inclusive environment looking for diversity, the arrival of the "other" is not a disruption but a welcomed addition. For the purist enforcing sameness, otherness is always a disruption. In an atmosphere of silence and stillness, the singing dancer is disruptive but not when clubbing.

Not only is disruption relative to circumstance, whether or not disruptions are harmful or helpful is also relative. Disruption can be lifesaving, as in fighting a virus or arresting someone with violent intent or in the paradox of an intentional burn to halt a wildfire. Disruption can also be life-threatening, as in choking off someone's oxygen supply. Revolutions can be interruptions of uninterrupted states of oppression, or they can be dictatorial disturbances of peaceful heterogenous democracies.

Existence is a series of dys-regulated disruptions, from mitosis to Shiva's dance of destruction and creation, to collisions of electrons, to even how agonists and antagonist medications work. The irony is extraordinary that treatment of disruptive dysregulation often uses disruptive and dysregulating chemistry (i.e., psychiatric drugs) to disrupt and dysregulate disruption and dysregulation! The hypocrisy is breathtaking. On the other hand, the alternative of the hermeneutical vertigo of incessant reinterpretability in the phenomenological way keeps us loose and open for the clearing that invites whoever, whatever, whichever guest of experiences that might show themselves in their inconspicuous presencing.

This is why Nikki, a six-year-old, was sent home day after day for angrily standing in her chair during the middle of class and shouting with her fist in the air, "Praise to all princesses." The teacher "just couldn't have this happen" with the amount of information needing to be disseminated given the approaching standardized tests. She, the teacher, added to me in a phone consult with her, "I am the teacher, she is the student, and she will mind or go home—that is what is appropriate." This is not heeding but concealing via prescribing. It is also privileging needed standardized test scores for school funding over relative learning styles, including that of princesses.

The heeding hermeneutical phenomenologist, instead of assigning a category, would ask other questions: Are princesses not being praised in the class, or are unrecognized? Why princesses and not princes, or queens and kings? Why are princesses needing to be praised at school, but seemingly nowhere else? About what should we particularly praise princesses? How shall we praise them? What are the princesses planning to do? Was Nikki elected to lead them, or self-elected, and what would either one mean for Nikki, for the teacher, for the rest of the class?

Who is disrupting, what is disrupted, and for what reasons? Is the revolutionary child being bullied, perhaps by the princes? Are the parents authoritarian? Is the forced curriculum and standardized testing at school suffocating and boring? Is the child gifted and irritably impatient? Is the year (needed for a diagnosis) of rageful explosions here and there (also needed for a diagnosis) being equally met by a co-constituting year of being shamed? What is inconspicuously being said about Being itself in the conspicuous act of standing in that chair and shouting, "Praise to all princesses"?

Existenz is Context

Nikki's dys-regulated dys-ruption can only be understood in light of its fate; that is, its allotment, its assignment, its situated context and the lived meaning said therein and about it. As it turns out, Nikki's parents were divorcing. Her father was dying. She went mute after time and time again being in trouble at school, and helpless about her parents' marriage ending and her father dying.

She came in and played, though, and liked coloring with one of the puppets, Orville. As they drew lines on pads with reverie, trading off drawing one wild line with a wild color per page, Nikki began to laugh. As the session ended, Nikki stood up, brushed her dress off and spoke for the first time in weeks: "In here, I don't get in trouble."

Clearing the space for the saying of her dysregulation, even an electively mute one, she and Orville the puppet wasted paper and marked broad and bright colors with abandon—but without reprimand. It is in the khora space where one does not get in trouble. No taxonomy is needed. No pathology needs to be eliminated. No muting that needs to be engineered to talk. No chair standing that needs to be tranquilized. No causes that need to be identified. Just a clearing and an awareness of the inconspicuous.

There may be preferred comportments over others, at different times, by any of us—but the unwanted or dys-turbing comportments are saying something, saying a lot, about matterings of existential dilemmas they and others face. *Naming and treating is not heeding, but those are our choices of care: one medically-modeled, one phenomenological.* The latter is called to follow the phenomenon wherever it takes us. What then? The phenomenon will show us. That is the phenomenological way.

Conclusion: Traces of transfiguration—A Synopsis and Differentiation of Divergent Ideologies

(1) For the medical model, the symptom is traditionally understood as an illness or pathogen which is a privation or "less than" the ideal of health. Difference or divergence or deviance is viewed in this supremacist ideology as deficient, whereas the phenomenological way remains horizontal such that what is different is not deficient—just different and with its own integrity and meaning. As long as difference is seen as deficient, a supremacist ideology is locked in place that locks in stigmatization. We cannot destigmatize if we pathologize symptoms. The phenomenologist offers an alternative to the word "symptom": "sayings" as showings, not classifications of pathogens.

(2) For the medical model, symptoms are classified in a taxonomical system of categorization which essentializes experiences such that we miss the nuanced particularizes and relativity of various contexts and situations. A phenomenological way attends to the specifics in contexts as lived by providing descriptive, poetic discourse that expands and extends showings with as much attention to nuance as possible, and with glances out of the corner of our eyes to glimpse but not grasp the inconspicuous. As Claude Monet is said to have quipped, *"To see something, you must forget the name of what you are looking at."*

(3) The "if this, then that" algorithmic, calculative stativity and procedural thinking figures and treats with each intervention implying an illness to be corrected or cured, which unwittingly misses or intentionally ignores what the phenomenological way can offer: heeding the symptoms as sayings of lived meaning without explanation, classification, justification, or production.

(4) The medical model privileges the assessor or the analyst/therapist as the authority who "knows" (with calculative and procedural thinking) whereas in the phenomenological way, the authority rests with the

phenomenon itself which beckons us to follow it and heed its meaning. Symptoms-as-sayings are unexpected teachers for the phenomenologist rather than the practitioners who excise pathogens. Again, there is the place for the learned authority of the physician, such as in the vital need for precision in calculating doses of medication and in surgical procedure. But the authority for soul work (an engaged understanding for lived meaning) is the phenomenon calling for the heeding poet.

(5) The symptom, for a medically-modeled practice of care, is reduced to a tangible, operationalizable and manipulable physiology whereas a phenomenological way attends to the intangible lived meaning that is inconspicuously communicated through enactments of significance in specific contexts and circumstances. The intangibles—particularly lived meaning—is arguably what matters most to any of us but cannot be measured or even seen by natural science methodologies. The intangible is a different kind of "evidence," nonetheless, that is only accessed by the phenomenological way.

(6) The medical model views the good life as an efficiently produced, symptom-free life supported by a purification and decontamination ideologies whereas for the phenomenological way, there is no distinction between the good and bad life, healthy or ill life—but, instead, clears space for the meaningful life lived in each moment. The medically-modeled mission to search and destroy pathogens is differentiated from the phenomenological heeding of inconspicuous, lived meaning.

References

Alvis, J. (2017). Making sense of Heidegger's phenomenology of the inconspicuous or inapparent. Continental Philosophy Review (2018) 51:211–238 https://doi.org/10.1007/s11007-017-9422-8

American Psychiatric Association. (2013). *Diagnostic and statistical manual of mental disorders* (5th ed.). Washington, DC

Berman, E. (2016). Deconstructing developmental psychology. Third Edition. London: Routledge.

Caputo, J. (1987). Radical hermeneutics: Repetition, deconstruction and the hermeneutical project. Indiana University Press.

_____. (2000). More radical hermeneutics: On not knowing who we are. Indiana University Press.

_____. (2006). The weakness of God: The theology of the event. Indiana University Press.

DuBose, T. (2016). Out, out bright candle? The meaning of meaninglessness. In Russo-Netzer, P., Schulenberg, S. E., & Batthyany, A. (Eds.). *Clinical perspectives on meaning: Positive and existential psychotherapy.* New York: Springer, pp. 283-295.

Foucault, M. (1988). Madness and civilization: A history of madness in an age of reason. New York: Vintage Books.

Harper, D. (n.d.-a). Etymology of discrimination. Online Etymology Dictionary. Retrieved from https://www.etymonline.com/word/discrimination

Harper, D. (n.d.-b). Etymology of symptom. Online Etymology Dictionary. Retrieved from https://www.etymonline.com/word/symptom

Heidegger, M. (2001). Zollikon Seminars: Protocols, conversations, letters. Boss, M., Ed. Evanston: Northwestern University Press.

_____. (2012). The four seminars. Indiana University Press.

_____. (1992). "Parmenides". *Internet Archive.* Bloomington and Indianapolis: Indiana University Press. p. 14.

Henry, M. (2012). Barbarism. New York: Continuum.

McNeill, W. (2020). The fate of phenomenology; Heidegger's legacy. New York: Rowman & Littlefield.

Schurmann, R. (1987). Heidegger on being and acting; From principles to anarchy. Indiana University Press.

Vallega-Neu, D. (2012). Heidegger's poietic writings: From Contributions to philosophy to The event. Indiana University Press.

Existential Explorations in Ecotherapy: Rethinking Anxiety Perception and Responsibility in the Human-Nature Relationship

Sarah Clayton

Abstract: *This chapter delves into anxiety, a pervasive global mental health concern, and explores potentially overlooked insights. By examining ecotherapy, it is suggested that a more profound and holistic approach to anxiety management may be found. Drawing on Rollo May's existential psychology, we navigate the intricate interplay between ecotherapy, anxiety, and human nature, providing a theoretical foundation for understanding nature's transformative and therapeutic power. Aligning May's perspective with ecotherapy, we view anxiety as inherent to human existence, constructively challenged through the human-nature relationship. This chapter demonstrates how individuals, by actively engaging with nature, can empower themselves and gain control over anxiety-inducing situations. Incorporating May's framework, it highlights how ecotherapy utilises nature's healing power to foster self-exploration and re-examine anxiety within a broader ecological context. In conclusion, May's existential perspective enriches the discourse on anxiety and ecotherapy, portraying anxiety as a transformative force through a meaningful connection with the natural world. This synthesis offers profound insights into existential explorations in ecotherapy, impacting personal well-being, ecological awareness, and the future of therapeutic practices.*

Introduction

Anxiety as a disorder is widely accepted in the field of psychology (Bandelow & Michaelis, 2015; Steinert et al., 2013). However, there are recent advances that pose a challenge to the existence or validity of anxiety as an entirely distinct mental health disorder. Recognising that these arguments are not yet fully supported by mainstream psychotherapeutic practices, the aim of this chapter is to explore the existential argument that anxiety is an inherent and necessary aspect of the human condition (May, 1950) and to go further by suggesting that anxiety can be a driving force for positive individual, societal and global change.

This exploration traverses two disciplines – psychology and ecology – to underscore the potential for anxiety to become a transformative force in the lives of individuals. The intrinsic and intimate connection that humans have with nature dictates that when they engage in a deeper, more meaningful relationship with the natural world, they are able to adopt new perspectives and discover new horizons that transcend the current concept of anxiety as disorder into something more akin to anxiety as a positive force that humans are free to choose.

This chapter does not intend to dispute the often-debilitating experiences for individuals and patients that arise as a consequence of these anxieties. That withstanding, this chapter will explore whether some valuable insights have been missed in current approaches to anxiety management and a deeper and more holistic treatment perspective; that is, one that attempts to heal individuals by guiding perceptions of the human-nature relationship. Helping them navigate anxiety within this ecotherapeutic framework, this framework will contribute to a richer and more nuanced discussion of the topic.

The Evolution of Ecotherapy

The work of Howard Clinebell (1996) and Theodore Rosazk (2001) laid the groundwork for a collection of practices and philosophies that have emerged as the field of ecopsychology. Ecopsychology is concerned with exploring the relationship between individuals and the natural world (Roszak, 2001). Ecotherapy and the term "eco-anxiety" have developed as a means to address the emotional and psychological distress of individuals concerned about contemporary issues over climate change and the destruction and devastation of our natural world (Roszak et al., 1995).

The framework and techniques therapists use in ecotherapeutic practice are diverse and dependent upon the therapist and the goals of therapy as there is no single approach, but rather a collection of practices that all revolve around the central idea that the natural world has the power to heal. Studies have shown that nature is itself therapeutic and exposure to natural environments can reduce stress, anxiety and depression (Jordan & Hinds, 2016; Naor & Mayseless, 2021; Russell, 2012; Stigsdotter et al., 2011). There is now a burgeoning interest in the field of psychology to explore nature as therapy by expanding therapeutic practices out into the natural world.

Ecotherapeutic practices are diverse and innovative in their approach. Currently, therapy has been shown to be effective in a variety of modalities such as wilderness therapy (Bandoroff, 1989), horticultural therapy (Kamioka et al., 2014), adventure therapy (Bowen & Neill, 2013), and nature-based mindfulness practices (Djernis et al., 2019). The unique qualities of each approach to support mental and emotional well-being cannot be underestimated.

Often practiced is the integration of ecotherapy within traditional psychotherapeutic models to enhance the therapeutic process or as a single approach in which nature serves as "co-therapist" (Segal et al., 2020). The natural world is not simply leveraged as a healing resource; rather ecotherapy recognizes that the relationship between humans and the natural world is a reciprocal one (Scull, 2009). Ecotherapy, therefore, seeks to foster a deeper, more meaningful connection between individuals and the natural world with the ultimate aim of contributing to the well-being and sustainability of the human-nature relationship.

The evolution of ecotherapy as a response to the environmental challenges of our current times aims to address both the ecological crisis and consequent mental health challenges. As such, ecotherapy as a practice is able to acknowledge the healing potential of nature to facilitate personal growth, self-awareness, and psychological healing. Ecotherapuetic practices allows anxiety management to move away from therapist as the agent for change and move more towards the individual taking responsibility for the power of their own human-nature connection. This approach to treating the individual—rather than the anxiety—is ideally suited to an existential conceptualization for the management of anxiety. It relates to our current understanding of the human-nature connection and intricate relationship between anxiety, freedom, and responsibility.

The Relevance of Existential Anxiety

Rollo May (1961), an influential thinker and psychotherapist, has left an enduring body of work on the understanding of human experience and the human psyche (e.g., May, 1983; May, 1999; May, 2009). May explored the profound interplay between anxiety, freedom, and responsibility—and it is at this intersection that ecotherapy and psychology converge.

May's existential insights have significant implications for the developing field of ecopsychology. May urges us to take a closer look at the concept of anxiety with an existential lens that posits how anxiety is, inescapably and fundamentally, a part of the human condition. Furthermore, May's seminal work on anxiety (May, 1996) promotes a broader view on the current yet limiting psychological treatments of anxiety. If anxiety is inherently a response to the profound aspects of human existence, then a broader examination of what it means for individuals to exist seems like a reasonable direction for treatment modalities. May's focus is on the abstract realities of what it means to exist in our environment, breaking away from more specific forms of anxiety.

According to this existential perspective, anxiety is inextricably linked to the burden of choice, freedom, and responsibility (May, 1996). Ultimately, existential anxiety arises when the individual understands the responsibility inherent in the freedom to choose and how anxiety manifests as a fear of making wrong decisions. Within the same lens, May argued that a search for meaning is fundamental to human fulfilment. He contended that existential anxiety could emerge when an individual is challenged or confronted with questions of meaning and one's purpose in life (May, 1996).

May's insights into existential anxiety are symbiotic to the practice of ecotherapy and the human-nature relationship. Both seek to treat the individual rather than the specific anxiety, using a holistic approach that transcends the therapist's room. May speaks of broadening perspectives:

> A therapy that is important, as I see it, is a therapy that enlarges a person, makes the unconscious conscious. Enlarges our view, enlarges our experience, makes us more sensitive, enlarges our

intellectual capacities as well as other capacities. (as quoted in
Schneider et al., 2009, p. 420)

It can be argued that ecotherapy, with its central theme being the human-
nature relationship, has the potential to enlarge a person. May argued that
if therapeutic measures are not constructed to change the person—and,
instead, the specific behaviour— then therapy is unlikely to be successful
in the long-term (Schneider et al., 2009). Shifting the emphasis from
individual behaviours to the innate bond between a person and the natural
world appears to be a means of enlarging a person. It addresses the entirety
of a person's being. Consequently, regardless of the behaviours stemming
from anxiety, therapy that promotes the enlarging of an individual's
human-nature relationship can harness their anxiety as a catalyst for
transformation rather than something to fear.

May's insights into existential anxiety are highly relevant to a reevaluation
of the human-nature relationship. As we face environmental challenges
and a shifting sense of purpose in a rapidly changing world, existential
anxiety can be a transformative force when the emphasis is on people
engaging in deeper, more meaningful relationships with the natural world.
Ecotherapy as a therapeutic medium can offer nature as a guiding force to
serve as a catalyst—for individuals to confront and navigate themselves
through anxieties relating to freedom, responsibility, and meaning in a
more profound and transformative way.

May's existential insights can be applied in the context of ecotherapy to
reshape the perception of anxiety and responsibility within the human-
nature relationship. Correspondingly, May's perspective is pivotal to
understanding the universal nature of existential anxiety and how it
manifests in the human condition so we may be able to shed light on its
pervasive influence on the human experience.

Universality of Existential Anxiety

According to May (1996), existential anxiety is a universal human
experience. It is not limited to specific individuals or groups but is an
inherent aspect of being human. Anxiety stems from our confrontation
with the most profound dimensions of existence such as the inevitability of

death, the uncertainty of the future, and the inherent isolation in understanding what it means to be an individual grappling with aloneness. Existential anxiety arises when we come to understand what it means to be human and are confronted with the ultimate questions of meaning and purpose. May identified several key manifestations of existential anxiety; namely, freedom of choice and the realization that we are free to shape our own lives, which can be both liberating and anxiety-inducing.

Another manifestation of existential anxiety, according to May, is fear of the unknown or an uncertain future, both of which can give rise to feelings of unease and apprehension. Similarly, isolation can give rise to existential anxiety resulting from the recognition of an individual's essential aloneness. We are, in May's view, inherently isolated individuals, and the tension between our desire for connection and the reality of isolation can provoke anxiety.

Relevance to Ecotherapy and the Human-Nature Relationship

May's work on existential anxiety is highly pertinent to the human-nature relationship and practice of ecotherapy. The gravity of contemporary environmental challenges looms large and the long shift in our disconnection from the natural world all combine to intensify existential anxiety, particularly in the context of freedom and responsibility. As individuals are challenged with ecological choices and their consequences, existential anxiety can become a central theme.

It is essential to bridge the gap between ecotherapy and existentialism. Ecotherapy offers a unique context for addressing existential anxiety within the therapeutic context and to help reshape the perception of responsibilities in the human-nature relationship. While these remain two distinct fields of thought, there are interconnected domains that converge— and are pivotal both to our reevaluation of the human-nature relationship and the perception of anxiety and responsibility this gives rise to.

Existentialism revolves around the pursuit of meaning and purpose in life, which can frequently entail existential crises. Likewise, ecotherapy is dedicated to the quest for making meaning by cultivating a more profound and meaningful connection with nature. The intersection of existentialism and ecotherapy is evident in the realms of personal agency and choice. The convergence of freedom and responsibility aligns seamlessly with the ecotherapist's emphasis on an individual's choice in their interactions with the environment and subsequent responsibilities they bear for the natural world.

Existentialism in Ecotherapeutic Practice

There are several avenues in the field of ecotherapy where existential principles are put into practice. Ecotherapy encourages individuals to embrace their freedom in nature and recognize the choices they make in their relationships with their environment. This approach strongly resonates with ideals of existentialism where the concept of freedom inevitably carries the weight of responsibility (May, 1958). Our current ecological crises call for decisive action and compel individuals to reflect upon the idea that with freedom comes responsibility. Cultivating a deep connection with the natural world encourages individuals to reflect on their environment as being an integral part of their humanness.

Ecotherapy provides a structured platform for individuals to delve into their connection with their environment, mirroring the existential journey of self-discovery and finding one's place in the world. This deeper and more meaningful connection has the potential to alleviate feelings of fear and aloneness, leading to true therapeutic transformation.

Reshaping Anxiety and Responsibility

The intersection of ecotherapy and existential psychology provides a profound perspective through which we can explore fundamental aspects of the human experience. This sharing of common ground offers a distinctive opportunity to transform our understanding of anxiety and responsibility, rendering their convergence particularly meaningful.

Ecotherapy provides a platform for individuals to not only grapple with anxiety but also transform it into making responsible and sustainable choices in their relationships with the natural world. This enriches therapeutic practice by giving individuals the scope with which to confront anxiety in a natural setting, allowing for a deeper exploration of the anxiety.

Recognizing the ecological responsibilities we hold within the context of existential freedom can lead to a sense of empowerment and ethical action.

Essentially, the intersection of ecotherapy and existential psychology fosters a more actionable method for healing, transformation, and understanding of the ethical responsibilities that rise from engaging in a meaningful relationship with the natural world. In this journey of existential explorations in ecotherapy, we arrive at the central question that shapes the core of this chapter: can redefining our relationship with nature, guided by the existential wisdom of Rollo May, offer us solace in the face of existential uncertainty?

With this unique collaboration, we stand on the threshold of an enlightening and transformative journey. We have set the stage by acknowledging the environmental challenges of our time, explored Rollo May's insights into existential anxiety, and illuminated the convergence of ecotherapy and existential psychology. The human-nature connection, guided by existential wisdom, can offer solace and inspire ecological responsibility in a world that increasingly incites anxiety and uncertainty.

Practical Insights for Application

Wilderness Therapy

Rollo May's insights into existential anxiety, freedom, and responsibility align closely with the emphasis on immersion in the natural world that forms wilderness therapy. May's philosophy offers a valuable lens through which we can understand how wilderness therapy addresses the existential concerns of individuals. By removing individuals from their comfort zones and placing them in nature, an environment is created whereby existential anxieties can surface more prominently. In the wilderness, the stark realities of life, death, and human vulnerability become palpable, encouraging participants to confront and challenge these anxieties (Bandoroff, 1989).

Wilderness therapy is widely recognised as a natural approach to enhancing physical health and mental well-being. In the UK, a wilderness therapy has been developed from the Japanese practice of Shinrin-Yoku, translated as Forest Bathing. Shinrin-Yoku developed as an antidote to a stress-filled lifestyle (known in Tokyo as *karōshi*, death from overwork; and *hikikomori*, referring to people who shut themselves away for years on end) (Li, 2018).

Wilderness therapies such as forest bathing relate to ideas of our connection with nature, such as that proposed by Erich Fromm. Fromm describes our innate desire for connection to nature as an integral part of our biology — and when we become detached from nature, we abandon the natural part of ourselves, and our emotional and physical health suffer as a result.

The Wilderness Programme in the UK is a registered UK charity providing a residential, non-medical mental health recovery programme specifically designed for adult individuals over the age of 21 years to meet the needs of those dealing with difficulties pertaining to addictions, professional burnout, stress, anxiety, depression, trauma, and other mental health related problems. The programme also supports those who are struggling with aspects of life such as low self-esteem, low confidence, feeling lost or lacking direction.

Wilderness therapy is deeply rooted in hands-on learning and follows experiential educational principles such as those proposed by Gass (1993); that is, learning by doing and reflecting. This philosophy of education puts the emphasis on educators engaging with learnings in direct experiences and focused reflection aimed at enhancing knowledge, skills, values, and an individual's capacity to contribute to their community. In short, it aims to foster personal growth through a deep connection with nature. Moreover, wilderness therapy draws from adventure learning forms including wilderness treatment, adventure-based activity learning, and long-term residential camping (Gillis & Thomsen, 1996). Individuals or groups are placed in real-life settings, fostering problem-solving skills to navigate the environment and address challenges all the while contributing to personal development.

Scientifically proven benefits of immersing in natural environments include boosted immune functioning, reduced blood pressure, lowered stress, and improved mood amongst other beneficial modalities. Regular practice may prove to enhance energy, improve connection with nature, and foster a heightened sense of happiness. Aligned with Rollo May's theory of anxiety and ecopsychology, the Wilderness Programme explores the interplay between human anxiety, nature, and self-discovery. This synthesis emphasises anxiety as an inherent facet of human existence, constructively challenged through the hands-on learning of experiential education in a wilderness setting.

Globally, the concept of Wilderness Therapy has gained momentum with initiatives like Challenge Alaska, Adventure Therapy Europe and Nordic Outdoor Therapy employing its core elements of engaging in adventurous activities with therapeutic intent. Efforts to establish best practices and quality standards have led to the formation of the Outdoor Behavioural Healthcare Centre conducting research on the effectiveness of wilderness therapy. Recent studies highlight the positive outcomes of wilderness and adventure therapy, demonstrating increased credibility in the field.

May's Philosophy and Ecotherapy

In the realm of wilderness therapy, aligned with Rollo May's philosophy on anxiety, we recognize anxiety not as a barrier but an inherent aspect of human existence. Through experiential learning in nature, as exemplified by programs like the Wilderness Programme, anxiety becomes a catalyst for constructive engagement. This approach, resonant with ecopsychology, transforms the human-nature relationship into a source of empowerment, fostering personal growth and resilience. In wilderness therapy, anxiety transcends mere management; it becomes a transformative force shaping our journey toward self-discovery, fulfilment, and connection with the natural world.

May's existential examination emphasizes the importance of reconnecting with the natural world to find comfort and meaning. Wilderness therapy encourages individuals to rediscover their intrinsic connection with the environment, often leading to a more meaningful sense of solace and understanding of the interdependence – and the strong disconnect they arrive with – between humans and the natural world. Individuals undergo significant personal growth during wilderness therapy that manifests as a deeper sense of self-awareness, increased resilience, and a greater capacity to navigate life's existential challenges, thus aligning with May's insights into personal growth and enlargement.

Fundamentally, ecotherapy becomes a practical application of Rollo May's existential philosophy. Individuals encouraged to connect with an immersive experience in the natural world are better able to engage with existential questions, gain solace, and embrace the freedom and responsibility inherent in their choices. Moreover, individuals are encouraged to reevaluate their relationship with nature, embodying May's vision of a more profound and connected human-nature bond (Softas-Nall & Woody, 2017).

May's philosophical insights highlight the relationship between freedom and responsibility. In the context of ecotherapy, individuals gain a heightened sense of freedom as they connect with the environment. They recognize that they have choices in how they interact with nature that carry a sense of responsibility. This realization gradually transforms into a sense of empowerment. Individuals understand the interconnectedness of all living beings and, furthermore, recognize their own role in preserving the balance of nature (Roszak et al., 1995).

Within the framework of ecotherapy, existential anxiety isn't solely a burden; rather, it acts as a catalyst for profound transformation and what Rollo May refers to as enlargement. It presents individuals with the opportunity to shift from passive observers to active agents of their own freedom, acknowledging the inherent connection between freedom and responsibility. This transformation paves the way for a more harmonious and responsible relationship with the natural world.

Ecotherapy empowers individuals to reevaluate their connection with both anxiety and the environment. This transformative journey progresses from perceiving anxiety to accepting it, from acceptance to empowerment, and, finally, from empowerment to taking meaningful action (Schuman-Olivier et al., 2020).

The Contemporary Environmental Landscape and Human-Nature Relationship

We live in unprecedented times marked by rapid environmental crises and ecological upheaval. What is becoming increasingly urgent is the need for change. A unique combination of consequences relating to environmental destruction and uncertainty of the future exposes one to be likely ridded with existential anxiety (Asgarizadeh et al., 2023). Amidst this tumultuous ecological landscape, the burgeoning field of ecotherapy offers us solace.

Where once our inherent human-nature interconnectedness was sacred to us, modern advances in agriculture and industrialization have shattered this powerful relationship resulting in a displaced and exploitative human experience. The field of ecotherapy aims to redress the balance by inviting us to embark on a journey of self-discovery and reconnection, transcending the traditional confines of the therapist's office and offering a framework for healing that embraces nature as co-therapist. With the fusion of an existential lens, ecotherapy not only enlivens our sense of duty towards our planet but also redefines our perception of anxiety.

Presently, our earth is confronted with an array of challenges and transformative changes, igniting, perhaps, a heightened anxiety and urgency in the human-nature relationship. As our awareness of the consequences of environmental deterioration deepens, and we consider the extensive ramifications for the well-being and survival of current and future generations, we are standing at a crossroads seeking a path that guides us toward equilibrium, harmony, and psychological well-bring.

Conclusion and Future Directions

The fusion of Rollo May's existential wisdom with the healing model of ecotherapy stands as a meaningful gateway for the future of psychotherapeutic practices. Through it, individuals embark on a transformative journey towards a deep and meaningful understanding of their place in the world, a re-evaluation of their aloneness, and awareness of their own ability to exert a positive impact in their lives with their human-nature connection.

As we face unprecedented environmental challenges and existential uncertainties, the combination of May's insights and ecotherapeutic practices serve as a guiding source that can illuminate the universal presence of anxiety in the human experience. With this partnership, it can become possible to redefine anxiety as a catalyst for personal growth, empowerment, and individual and social consciousness. Guided by the wisdom of Rollo May, ecotherapy represents not just a therapeutic approach but a profound invitation to realign our relationship with anxiety, to redefine our understanding of freedom and responsivity, and to rekindle our bond with the natural world. May's existential wisdom as it aligns with ecotherapeutic framework is not merely a theoretical concept; it is a profound call to action.

In conclusion, the pressing need to engage with the existential inquiries of our contemporary age demands our enthusiastic acceptance. This entails a bold reevaluation of our perception of anxiety as a potent force for transformation. Through this reexamination, we equip ourselves with a greater capacity to embrace individual freedom, shoulder collective responsibilities, and reestablish intrinsic interdependence between humanness and the natural environment.

This synthesis between existential wisdom and ecotherapy offers a vision for a future characterized by harmony and sustainability. It calls for a future where existential anxiety ceases to be a burden and, rather, emerges as a guiding force and catalyst for positive change. It prompts us to envisage a future in which we relinquish the exploitation of our planet and favor a profound, meaningful connection with the natural world. As we embark on this transformative journey, we celebrate existential anxiety— no longer as a source of fear but a driving force for personal, societal, and ecological metamorphosis.

References

Asgarizadeh, Z., Gifford, R., & Colborne, L. (2023). Predicting climate change anxiety. *Journal of Environmental Psychology, 90*, 102087. https://doi.org/10.1016/j.jenvp.2023.102087

Bandelow, B., & Michaelis, S. (2015). Epidemiology of anxiety disorders in the 21st century. *Dialogues in Clinical Neuroscience, 17*(3), 327–335. https://doi.org/10.31887/dcns.2015.17.3/bbandelow

Bandoroff, S. (1989). Wilderness-Adventure therapy for delinquent and Pre-Delinquent youth: A review of the literature. In *Education Resources Information Center*. Institute of Education Sciences. https://files.eric.ed.gov/fulltext/ED377428.pdf

Bowen, D. J., & Neill, J. T. (2013). A meta-analysis of adventure therapy outcomes and moderators. *The Open Psychology Journal, 6*(1), 28–53. https://doi.org/10.2174/1874350120130802001

Clinebell, H. (1996). *Ecotherapy: Healing ourselves, healing the earth.* Routledge.

Djernis, D., Lerstrup, I., Poulsen, D. V., Stigsdotter, U. K., Dahlgaard, J., & O'Toole, M. S. (2019). A systematic review and meta-analysis of nature-based mindfulness: Effects of moving mindfulness training into an outdoor natural setting. *International Journal of Environmental Research and Public Health, 16*(17), 3202. https://doi.org/10.3390/ijerph16173202

Gass, M. A. (1993). *Adventure therapy: Therapeutic applications of adventure programming.* Kendall/Hunt Publishing Company.

Gillis, H. L., & Thomsen, D. (1996). A research update of adventure therapy (1992-1995): Challenge activities and ropes courses, wilderness expeditions, and residential camping programs. *Research in Outdoor Education, 3*(12). https://files.eric.ed.gov/fulltext/ED413128.pdf

Jordan, M., & Hinds, J. (2016). *Ecotherapy: Theory, research and practice.* Bloomsbury Publishing.

Kamioka, H., Tsutani, K., Yamada, M., Park, H., Okuizumi, H., Honda, T., Okada, S., Park, S., Kitayuguchi, J., Abe, T., Handa, S., & Mutoh, Y. (2014). Effectiveness of horticultural therapy: A systematic review of randomized controlled trials. *Complementary Therapies in Medicine, 22*(5), 930–943. https://doi.org/10.1016/j.ctim.2014.08.009

Li, Q. (2018). *Forest bathing: How trees can help you find health and happiness.* Penguin.

May, R. (1950). *The meaning of anxiety.* Ronald Press Company.

May, R. (1958). Contributions of existential psychotherapy. In R. May, E. Angel, & H. F. Ellenberger (Eds.), *Existence: A new dimension in psychiatry and psychology* (pp. 37–91). Basic Books/Hachette Book Group. https://doi.org/10.1037/11321-002

May, R. (Ed.). (1961). *Existential psychology.* Crown Publishing Group/Random House.

May, R. (1983). *The discovery of being: Writings in existential psychology.* W. W. Norton.

May, R. (1996). *The meaning of anxiety.* W. W. Norton & Company.

May, R. (1999). *Freedom and destiny.* W. W. Norton & Company.

May, R. (2009). *Man's search for himself.* W. W. Norton & Company.

Naor, L., & Mayseless, O. (2021). Therapeutic factors in nature-based therapies: Unraveling the therapeutic benefits of integrating nature in psychotherapy. *Psychotherapy, 58*(4), 576–590. https://doi.org/10.1037/pst0000396

Roszak, T. (2001). *The voice of the earth: An exploration of ecopsychology.* Phanes Press.

Roszak, T., Gomes, M. E., & Kanner, A. D. (Eds.). (1995). *Ecopsychology: Restoring the earth, healing the mind.* Sierra Club Books.

Russell, K. (2012). Therapeutic uses of nature. In S. D. Clayton (Ed.), *The Oxford Handbook of Environmental and Conservation Psychology* (pp. 428–444). Oxford University Press. https://doi.org/10.1093/oxfordhb/9780199733026.013.0023

Schneider, K. J., Galvin, J. P., & Serlin, I. (2009). Rollo May on existential psychotherapy. *Journal of Humanistic Psychology, 49*(4), 419–434. https://doi.org/10.1177/0022167809340241

Schuman-Olivier, Z., Trombka, M., Lovas, D., Brewer, J. A., Vago, D. R., Gawande, R., Dunne, J. P., Lazar, S. W., Loucks, E. B., & Fulwiler, C. E. (2020). Mindfulness and behavior change. *Harvard Review of Psychiatry, 28*(6), 371–394. https://doi.org/10.1097/hrp.0000000000000277

Scull, J. (2009). Tailoring nature therapy to the client. In L. Buzzell & C. Chalquist's (Eds.), *Ecotherapy: Healing with nature in mind* (pp. 140-148). San Francisco, CA: Sierra Club Books.

Segal, D., Harper, N. J., & Rose, K. (2020). Nature-based therapy. In N. J. Harper & W. W. Dobud (Eds.), *Outdoor Therapies: An Introduction to Practices, Possibilities, and Critical Perspectives.* Routledge.

Softas-Nall, S., & Woody, W. D. (2017). The loss of human connection to nature: Revitalizing selfhood and meaning in life through the ideas of Rollo May. *Ecopsychology, 9*(4), 241–252. https://doi.org/10.1089/eco.2017.0020

Steinert, C., Hofmann, M., Leichsenring, F., & Kruse, J. (2013). What do we know today about the prospective long-term course of social anxiety disorder? A systematic literature review. *Journal of Anxiety Disorders, 27*(7), 692–702. https://doi.org/10.1016/j.janxdis.2013.08.002

Stigsdotter, U. K., Pálsdóttir, A. M., Burls, A., Chermaz, A., Ferrini, F., & Grahn, P. (2011). Nature-based therapeutic interventions. In K. Nilsson, M. Sangster, C. Gallis, T. Hartig, S. De Vries, K. Seeland, & J. Schipperijn (Eds.), *Forests, Trees and Human Health* (pp. 309–342). Springer. https://doi.org/10.1007/978-90-481-9806-1_11

Fundamental Flaws of the DSM:
Re-Envisioning Diagnosis as a Holistic,
Human Science

G. Kenneth Bradford

Abstract: *The Diagnostic and Statistical Manual (DSM) of mental disorders derives its authority from the empirical scientific criteria which vouchsafes that authority. It is here evaluated according to the principal empirical scientific criteria of validity and reliability, and it is found to be fundamentally flawed on both counts. Additionally, any diagnostic approach based on the objectivizing principles of empirical science is found to be both ontologically and epistemologically unable to account for the complexity of human subjectivity/intersubjectivity. A revisioning of psychological diagnosis according to specifically human scientific criteria is therefore called for. On this basis, an outline of specific, more appropriate criteria to serve as guidelines for the development of phenomenological and holistic approaches to diagnosis is presented.*

Acknowledgement: "Fundamental flaws of the DSM: Re-envisioning diagnosis in a holistic direction" was first published in *The Journal of Humanistic Psychology, 2010, 50(3), 335-350* and appeared in rewritten form in Bradford, G. K. (2013). *The I of the Other: Mindfulness-based Diagnosis and the Question of Sanity*, Paragon House.

Psychological diagnosis informed by the *Diagnostic and Statistical Manual* (DSM) presumes to make valid and reliable knowledge claims regarding the pathological nature of other minds. As a matter of pragmatics, psychological professionals exercise this bold knowledge and deploy its formidable power on a daily basis. The culture at large relies on this privileged knowledge to distinguish between abnormal mental diseases and normal states of mind. As we know, the import of a clinical diagnosis can be far-reaching not only in terms of dictating medical treatment, but also in terms of shaping a person's identity, both in their own eyes and in the eyes of others. So, it is important to consider, "How accurate is the DSM in making diagnoses?"

In general, psychiatric diagnosis has been problematic for humanistically-oriented psychologies and experientially-keyed psychotherapies for quite some time. Not only have American founders of Humanistic Psychology such as Maslow (1971), Rogers (1961), and Bugental (1965) stridently opposed pathologizing diagnoses, the anti-psychiatry movement (e.g., Laing, 1960 and Szasz, 1974) has been outspoken about the "vocabulary of denigration" (Laing, 1960, p. 27) inherent in pathology-keyed diagnostic discourse. A number of European philosophers and psychologists have not only criticized objectivizing and dehumanizing psychodiagnosis as it is commonly deployed but have addressed the source of the problem in challenging the empirical science paradigm upon which this discourse is based (e.g., Merleau-Ponty, 1942/1963; Husserl, 1954/1970; Binswanger, 1963; Laing, 1960 & 1969; and Boss, 1983).

As early as 1894, Dilthey pointed out that the empirical scientific method that studies the physical world by dissecting an object into its constituent elements is inappropriate for the study of human subjectivity. As Van den Berg (1972) reported, "In [Dilthey's] opinion, the essential characteristic of the psychic aspect of human life is that it is a *totality* not a collection of elements" (p. 126, my emphasis). He goes on to declare, "The aim of psychology is the rendering of a totality....[it] is to observe, to comprehend, then to render explicit...what was at first seen vaguely in the first comprehension" (p. 127).

The way to understand the whole person is to encounter that person as they reveal themselves rather than construing the person according to one's own preconceived categories. Dilthey recognized knowledge that most accurately reveals a whole person proceeds as a process of explicating what is at first only seen vaguely. This holistic, process-based—rather than dissected, content-based—orientation has been generally understood as a phenomenological approach, which was first applied to psychology as early as 1913 by Karl Jaspers.

Since that time, there have been continuing efforts to reconceive psychology as a *human science* by utilizing non-objectivizing, qualitative and holistic approaches sensitive to the complexities of subjective experiencing. (See May et al., 1958; Giorgi, 1970; Boss, 1963/1982 & 1983; Valle & Halling, 1989; Schneider et al., 2001; and Ferrer, 2002.) Even though these ongoing efforts to revise psychology as a subjective and intersubjective human science based on vastly different grounds from empirical, object-based sciences have, to some extent, been heeded in Europe, they have not prevailed in the United States. In the U.S., the dominant power of the empirical science establishment and the diagnostic authority of its handmaiden, the DSM, remains king.

Generally, the various inspired efforts critiquing the DSM do so from outside empirical science proper. There is nothing wrong with this, especially since the most interesting part of human science critiques are often the novel alternatives they offer—be they humanistic, transpersonal, existential, systemic, or feminist. However, the outsider position makes it easier for those who believe that the principles and methods of empirical science are the *only* legitimate science to dismiss alternative critiques as "unscientific."

Thus, in the evolution of the DSM, alternative visions are largely disregarded as the medical diagnostic machine grinds on as a strictly empiricist instrument of classification. This leaves the growing constituency of experience-near therapeutic approaches—everything from psychoanalysis to transpersonal and psychedelic therapies—without a clear, rigorous, and generally accepted diagnostic approach able to account for the uniquely subjective and intersubjective complexities of human experience. Therefore, many such therapists, in spite of serious reservations, fall back on the DSM as the *lingua franca* of the field.

In order to substantially shift this order of things, it is necessary to expose the flaws in the DSM as it currently exists, both from the outside and from inside its empirical paradigm—and in so clearing a space, to more crisply envision a viable human science alternative(s). In this chapter, I critique the DSM according to its own empirical scientific criteria and, finding it fundamentally flawed, propose a revised set of human scientific criteria to guide the development of more holistic, experience-near diagnostic approaches.[i]

Fundamental flaws of the DSM

The DSM is fundamentally flawed in two essential ways. As an instrument of empirical science, its facts—pathological categories—can be considered true only if they are found to be both *valid* and *reliable*. In terms of psychodiagnosis, the test of validity is a measure of whether a particular diagnosis actually exists as it is posited. The test of reliability determines whether a validly established diagnosis can be consistently recognized as the thing it is. For example, a diagnosis of depression is valid if it accurately distinguishes the abnormal disorder "depression"—be it Major Depression, Dysthymia or another Mood Disorder—from each other as well as from normal moody states such as sadness, mopiness, moroseness or grief. The diagnosis is reliable if a particular "depression" is consistently recognized as such by various observers. On both of these crucial empirical standards, the DSM fails.

Regarding reliability, epidemiological research conducted in the 1960's and 70's showed that the diagnoses of major illnesses were unreliable over both time and across cultures (Goldstein & Goldstein, 1978, pp. 138-186). One study comparing psychiatric hospital admissions in New York and London in 1963 found that 77% of all New York admissions were diagnosed as having schizophrenia, whereas only 35% were so diagnosed in London that year. In addition, a mere 7% of New Yorkers were diagnosed with manic-depressive disorders while 32% of the Londoners garnered this diagnosis. This data indicates, quite darkly, an epidemic of schizophrenia in New York, but rather brightly, only scant manic-depression (see Table 1).

Fundamental Flaws of the DSM

	New York	London	Ratio London:New York
Schizophrenia	76.6%	35.3%	0.46
Manic-Depressive Disorders	6.5%	32.3%	5.0
Other diagnoses	16.9%	32.4%	

Table 1: *Original diagnoses of 200 hospital admissions by psychiatrists (excluding alcohol and drug admissions)*

However, when the psychiatric charts of these hospital admissions were re-evaluated by a conjoint team of British and American research psychiatrists, the New York diagnoses were found to be grossly mistaken. Upon re-evaluation, the rate for schizophrenia decreased from 77% to (a more British-like) 39% while the manic-depressive diagnosis dramatically increased from 7% to 35% (close to the British rate). When the conjoint team re-evaluated the London admissions, the British diagnoses did not significantly change (see Table 2).

	New York	London	Ratio London:New York
Schizophrenia	39.4%	37.0%	0.94
Manic-Depressive Disorders	34.5%	30.9%	0.90
Other diagnoses	26.1%	32.1%	

Table 2: *Re-diagnoses of the same patients following a specification of the diagnostic criteria*

This study revealed that American psychiatrists (in the post-WWII era) did not see depression when it sat in front of them just as they did see psychosis where there was none. Based on this cross-cultural comparison, the schizophrenic epidemic in the United States at the time was, seemingly, only happening in the minds of the diagnosticians.

Other studies investigated the reliability of diagnoses made solely in the United States over time. One such study (as quoted in Goldstein & Goldstein, 1978, pp. 149-151) compared original hospital diagnoses made in the 1930's (1932 - 1941) to those made in the decade between 1947 - 1956. This study found that only 28% of hospital admissions were diagnosed as schizophrenia in the 1930s while a full 77% admissions (again) were found to have schizophrenia in the decade following WWII.

As part of this study, the admission charts from both decades were re-diagnosed in 1973, and from that vantage point *both* were found to be in error! The 1973 re-diagnoses found 42% of the 1930s hospital admissions to have schizophrenia, up from the original 28%, while 47% of the 1947 - 1956 admissions were re-diagnosed as schizophrenic, down from the whopping 77% (see Table 3).

	Original hospital diagnosis	Re-diagnosis made in 1973
1932-41 decade	18 (28%)	27 (42%)
1947-56 decade	49 (77%)	30 (47%)

Table 3: *Number of schizophrenia cases out of 64*

Both of these studies found psychiatric diagnoses to be notoriously unreliable. In addition, the discrepancies this research uncovered raised many still-unanswered questions including, "Why might depression-era psychiatry see widespread manic-depression but hardly any schizophrenia, while the post-war era of giddy optimism and rampant materialism saw hardly anyone depressed, but did see in its troubled citizenry an epidemic of schizophrenia?"

Motivated largely by these kinds of revelations, psychiatry attempted to improve the reliability of its diagnoses by completely revising the DSM resulting in the 1980 publication of the DSM-III. Stripping the DSM-II of virtually all personality theory, most notably that of psychoanalysis (including the longstanding distinction between the neuroses and the psychoses), the DSM-III employed strict symptom-focused diagnostic criteria.

One particularly striking change was the complete disappearance of "neurosis" from the DSM-III. This raises the question, "Where did the neuroses go?" Certainly, they had not all been cured—or had they? Or did they ever really exist in the first place, say in the way that a hematoma or tumor exists? Or was neurosis, either deliberately or inadvertently, being suppressed by the psychiatric establishment? Of these questions, the most compelling one to my way of thinking is that which questions the very existence of presumed psychodiagnostic categories such as "neurosis" or "depression."

As based in the medical model, it is presumed that mental illness exists in a similar way as does physical illness. But is it true that psychological disease, including neuroses, exists in the same way as do their physiological disease counterparts? Keep in mind that the medical model is an artifact of empirical science and construes its knowledge by dissecting a whole into its component parts. For instance, recall that physical medicine is above all based on the corpse. It is by dissecting a corpse and gaining an understanding of the separate functions of organs and the different anatomical parts of the body that physical medicine proceeds. This is true both in medical training and research.

Since psychological illness is likewise construed according to this empirical vision, mental functioning is presumed to exist in the same way. But while it is possible to dissect a corpse and see the tumor or hematoma inside of it, *where* in the corpse is the "depression," "anxiety," or "narcissistic personality disorder" to be found? Since the late 20th century, physiological psychology has responded to this conundrum by reporting as empirical "evidence" such objective findings as MRI scans of the brains of chronic schizophrenics which show their brains to be abnormally misshapen; for example, shrunken and darkened in certain areas. But is this the schizophrenia illness itself? Or is a damaged brain a *consequence* of the schizophrenia, like atrophied leg muscles are a consequence of a paraplegic spinal injury?

Obviously, physiological phenomena, which are often observable in and as parts of a physical body, are of a different order than psychological experience, which belong to—and affect—the whole of a human mind(-body). This crucial difference has been consistently ignored by empirical scientific psychology, and apparently the fundamental question concerning the actual nature of psychological—as distinct from physical—phenomena has never seriously been considered in the development of the DSM. Since empiricism has not taken the time to understand the nature of its subject matter (i.e., psychological experience), empirical misunderstandings have continued to proliferate.

For instance, while "neuroses" suddenly disappeared from diagnostic formulae in the DSM-III, in their place mental "disorders" suddenly appeared. But where did *they* come from? And what does "disorder" actually mean anyway? Obviously, it presumes an "orderliness" to mental life that can go awry. But what exactly is a baseline mental orderliness? And who is it that determines this? Since no cogent explanations are given, either of mental order or disorder, how can anyone assume that "disorders"—as a valid explanatory framework—are any more credible than "neuroses" for accurately portraying psychological states?

Even though the new language and symptom-only focus of the DSM-III did nothing to improve its ontological or epistemological soundness, it did improve its reliability. This is so since an assessment that takes into consideration the complex social, historical, and psychodynamic factors influencing a person's state of mind (as in the DSM-II) is open to a greater range of interpretation than is the simple identification of symptoms that ignores those complexities. The DSM-IVs and -5s are but a continuation and elaboration of the symptom-focused -III. Unfortunately for psychodiagnosis, attaining good reliability is based on having first established the validity of a diagnosis; since a diagnosis must first be deemed valid in order for its reliability to make sense. On this more fundamental point, the DSM fails even more decisively.

As Horwitz and Wakefield (2007) spell out in their thorough study of psychodiagnosis, symptom-based criteria alone fail to produce valid diagnoses since psychological symptoms are always context-dependent.

There are always contextual complexities such as age, sex, race, social, cultural, and economic factors as well as physiological and environmental contingencies that call for a more nuanced, complex appraisal than the DSM permits. In a study of depression, they found that the DSM is unable to distinguish between depressive disorders and normal sorrow since many, if not most, of the symptoms belonging to each are shared by both. This finding should be particularly disturbing to those who put their faith in "evidence-based" scientific findings since a distinguishing feature beginning with the DSM-IV-TR revision is that it is more empirically evidence-based.

Horwitz and Wakefield observe that there are powerful vested interests motivated to perpetuate what has become an obfuscation of normal sadness into the mental disorder of depression. These interests include the juggernaut of the pharmaceutical industry, the academic research community funded by grants privileging empirical research, the American Medical Association (AMA), psychological service providers, a growing self-help market, the National Alliance on Mental Illness (NAMI), and, perhaps most importantly, the public itself.

The truth is that we, the people, do not want to suffer the inevitable confusions, anxieties and despair that come with living a mortal life—not to mention the exacerbated anxieties that come from living life within a materialistic and increasingly frantic techno-centric society suffering from the disintegration of the family, the community, the environment and traditional religious institutions.

For instance, if a child is having social problems at school and home, cannot sustain attention on tasks or follow directions without getting distracted, is agitated and often irritating or downright aggressive, does he have an "Attention-Deficit Disorder" and is, thus, in need of medication and placement in "special" education? And/or is he over-stimulated and, perhaps, neurologically infected by the 24/7 anxiety-ridden fever of the furiously-paced, techno-centric, disembodied, and often impersonal culture he finds himself swept up in? Is it the individual child who is sick and mentally "disordered"?

Or, again, if I have lost a love of my life, feel hopeless and despairing and, because of that, am sleeping long hours or suffering insomnia, feeling hopeless, am unable to enjoy the life I once loved, and am unsure whether I want to go on living at all, am I "clinically depressed" — thus in need of medication and, perhaps, cognitive-behavioral therapy to correct my irrational thoughts? Or am I understandably grief-stricken, thus in need of supportive friends and family, time to mourn a wrenching loss and contemplate its meaning, perhaps with some existentially-robust therapy or spiritual guidance? This is a question of distinguishing a normal life transition from an abnormal mental disease: the basic task of pathology-discriminating diagnosis. Yet, the DSM is unable to validly make this discernment.

In basing psychodiagnosis strictly on an accounting of symptoms and, thereby, categorizing an individual as disordered, the DSM adheres to a basic principle of empirical science that requires the isolation of variables in order to arrive at objective truth—in this case, a specific diagnosis. That is, it is reductionistic. While reliability is improved by narrowing the diagnostic focus to mere symptoms, validity is thereby compromised.

By failing to take the complexities of the social-environmental context into account, Horwitz and Wakefield argue that DSM diagnoses are invalid since they do not exist as they are posited, separate and distinct from the social and otherwise complex human context in which they arise. They conclude their study with the sweeping indictment that the DSM-III/IV [and, in perpetuating the same assumptions, the 5] revision is a failure, thereby making a poor diagnostic manual substantially worse by blurring the distinctions between illness/disordered mental functioning and health/normal mental processes.

Jacobs and Cohen (2010) come to the same conclusion from a slightly different perspective. Since DSM diagnoses purport to have scientific credibility when they lack credible empirical scientific validity, it has to be admitted that the DSM is a brash display of pseudoscience. In addition to this research, the Psychodynamic Diagnostic Manual (PDM), conceived in the early 2000's as an alternative to the DSM for psychodynamically oriented clinicians, cites further research studies. The Editorial Task Force of the comprehensive PDM has handily compiled a collection of key research articles, including meta-analyses, citing additional studies which specifically discuss the reliability and validity problems of the DSM (PDM Task Force, 2006, Part III). The serious research diagnostician will profit by consulting these studies.

As devastating as Horwitz and Wakefield's analysis of depression is to the credibility of the DSM, their work is aimed at its rehabilitation—and this rehab agenda stalls their critique just at the point where it becomes relevant to human science and experiential therapies. And, while the PDM offers a viable alternative to the DSM that *does* take contextual factors into account, it does not go so far as to challenge the tacit assumptions of empirical psychodiagnosis. True to empiricism, in the PDM the researcher-diagnostician retains the privileged position of being (supposedly) an objective observer of a disjunct Other. To this extent, at least, the PDM remains experience-distant. A more thorough critique could and should, in my opinion, be rendered to the "evidence-based" empiricist assumptions which ground the DSM and, often unwittingly, many alternative diagnostic schemas, be they Psychoanalytic, Humanistic or Transpersonal.

Only by stepping outside the objectivizing vision of empiricism and adopting a decidedly subjective/intersubjective approach to the knowing of other minds will the diagnostic theory serving experience-near therapies accord to their non-reductionistic, relationally-robust, and contextually-informed practices.

Criteria for psychological diagnosis revisioned

As difficult as it can be to make a discrimination between normal sadness and depression, for holistically-oriented psychologies the diagnostic task is still more challenging. The question is not only that of making a discernment between pathological and non-pathological mental states, but holistically-oriented clinicians and clergy must also consider the maturational or spiritual potential hidden within a "dark night of the soul." In addition to seeing sadness and loss as a normal part of mortal life, it is also possible to recognize that a wrenching loss may break one's heart open to deeper personal and interpersonal meaning as well as open a door to a more profound ontological presence. It seems to me that what we call wisdom is often a capacity born and bred in firestorms of psychic suffering in which we feel and, perhaps, behave not at all normal or emotionally orderly.

As it happens, we may suffer much longer than we, our family, and our doctor would like from symptoms that perfectly describe the disease of "depression." If this is the case,

> 1) should our "depression" be mitigated through medications so to ease our pain and return us to our "previous level of functioning" or
>
> 2) is it better that our "normal grief" be given a socially-circumscribed period of time to be experienced, after which time we are expected to "move on" or
>
> 3) should our "broken-openness" be deliberately cultivated (Chodron, 1997; Schneider, 2009; Taylor, 2009) so as to increase our capacity for being open and becoming more fully human? Bearing broken-openness that is, in order to more fully embrace the mystery of life and death, and, perhaps, thereby finding a deeper humility and wisdom for ourselves and to share with others?

Or should these "ors" (1, 2, and 3) also be considered "ands"? In order to make this kind of discernment, it is necessary to allow for a far more inclusive diagnostic approach than that permitted by the DSM, specifically, and empirical scientific knowledge, more generally.

An alternative view that recognizes the subject matter of psychology to be human subjectivity/intersubjectivity must be based on wholly different grounds than object-based empiricism. It is not necessary that empirical science and the knowledge it generates needs to be rejected out of hand, but that such knowledge be subordinated to a broader and deeper holistic orientation.

To increase the rigor of a human scientific approach, the fundamental assumptions of the approach should address both ontological and epistemological concerns. Simply put, ontology addresses the *nature* of human subjectivity—the *who* who is being understood. Epistemology details *how* that understanding comes about—*how* one approaches and sees another person influences to a considerable degree *what* knowledge is relevant to know about that person.

The principal challenge in any form of psychodiagnosis is to see the other as accurately as possible as they are, undistorted by the diagnosing clinician's personal or professional projections. As mentioned above, a rigorous approach that has taken this daunting challenge to heart has been phenomenology, so it makes sense to draw upon this intellectually robust and research seasoned tradition (e.g., Merleau-Ponty, 1942/1963 & 1962; Husserl, 1954/1970; May, Angel & Ellenberger, 1958; Laing, 1960 & 1969; Luijpen, 1960; Gadamer, 1960/1982; Binswanger, 1963; Boss, 1963/1982 & 1983; Giorgi, 1970; Van den Berg, 1972; Gendlin 1973a & 1973b; Spinelli, 1989; and Bradford, 2013.).

In contrast to empiricism, the starting point of phenomenology is to see a person, couple, family, or any human grouping for that matter—as a *phenomenon* rather than an object. Instead of positing the existence of an external object world disjunct from an internal observer, phenomenology and related qualitative methods recognize that a relationship of mutual influence exists between self and other, self and world, and subject and object. Approaching human experience as phenomena allows for the privileging of subjectivity and complexities of intersubjectivity.

At the very least, in this way the severe dualistic vision of empiricism (splitting perceived objects from a perceiving subject) is considerably softened, preparing the way for a more inclusive and nuanced understanding. Recognizing the relational nature of all perception and experience, a phenomenon is understood simply as *that which reveals itself.* This approach respects and preserves the mystery of existence, in general, and human subjectivity, in particular. It invites the other to reveal themself as they are, as free as possible from the reducing lens of the observer's biases. Diagnostic understanding thus remains open to consideration of various contextual and psychological complexities.

The following sections identify a few critical shifts that mark a transition from an empirical to a holistic approach which can serve as criteria for the development of alternative diagnostic understandings. This list gathers guidelines proposed from many quarters over the past century.

From content-based to process-based psychology

In regard to the question of being (ontology), drawing upon the thought of Existential-Phenomenology, Buddhist psychology, and a variety of non-dualistic wisdom traditions, the nature of human being—the essential subject matter of psychology—is seen to be fundamentally free. Subjectivity is not a fixed thing, but is fundamentally motile, malleable, and open-ended.[ii] Human nature is such that we are free to become stuck, to get unstuck or to remain open, to be conditioned, deconditioned or unconditioned, reactive or responsive, constrained or spontaneous, dignified in living a responsible and free life or to find ourselves (as B. F. Skinner [1971] found us) beyond freedom and dignity.

Human consciousness exists not in a fixed, isolated mind, but in a river of time wherein we are free to live the same year in the same way over and over again or to live each day anew. The inherent freedom of human *being* calls for a process-based psychology, in which the more accurate understanding of a person sees that person as an ongoing work-in-progress—a phenomenon not of fixity but of plasticity.

This does not mean a person is destined to change an old habit, but that a person *might* change. Knowledge of an Other would thus recognize the Other as a being that is more like a verb rather than a noun. In contrast, empirical scientific ontology is content-based. It conceives of others nominatively as discrete, objective entities. This recognition suggests that holding to any fixed diagnostic categorization in a basic sense misunderstands and also underestimates its subject matter.

It is more appropriate to think diagnostically in dynamic terms such as habit patterns, cognitive and behavioral practices, and temporarily fixated tendencies rather than in static terms such as states, types, or other nominative categories. That is, in being respectful of the fluid intelligence of human nature, to think outside rather than inside boxes. This sanity recognizes that any and all conceptual boxes, like planets, only exist in an inconceivably vast space—consciousness—which allows them to arise, persist, and pass away.

From objectivity to intersubjectivity

As we know, empirical science begins by making a sharp separation between the observed object (*res extensa*) and the subject observing that object (*res cogitans*), removing as far as possible any subjective influence that might interfere with the object being investigated. By design, this kind of science privileges the objectivity of the observer. In contrast, human science approaches begin by respecting the mutual influence between human subjects, allowing connections and complexities to emerge between observer and observed, thereby privileging the intersubjectivity of the encounter.

Intersubjectivity is here understood in two senses. In the ordinary sense, it refers to the contextual recognition that a therapeutic or psychological assessment situation is always an interaction between (at least) two subjectivities, each of which bring their respective life experiences and independent unconscious organizing principles to bear on the exchange. With this understanding, the therapist or diagnostician no longer assumes himself to be a neutral, detached observer who exercises little or no influence on a patient. Instead, the therapist is enjoined to take into account both what he sees in the other person and how he himself is being impacted by that person, which is very likely to shape (perhaps unconsciously) what he sees or fails to see.

In a second, more subtle sense, intersubjectivity recognizes the field or inter-ness within which distinct subjectivities interact (Bradford, 2007). The conditional place where two subjects meet is influenced by the respective conditions and history each person brings to the exchange. But at the same time, there is an underlying, subtle, ontologically unconditional place in which two human beings can meet or fail to meet. Whether or not it is recognized as such, this more basic, most intimate dimension of interpersonal exchange occurs in and as the in-between space or, as Winnicott (1971) referred to it, "potential space" that is essential to any exchange, even as it is conceptually indefinable.

Allowing for the inter-ness of subjectivity opens the way for a therapist or spiritual guide and client or spiritual seeker to respect and, perhaps, recognize the unconditioned presence and essential freedom of human being.[iii] Granted, consideration of the ontological freedom of inter-subjectivity—which can allow for the emergence of mystery, awe and unconditional openness—may have limited application in much psychology and therapy. Still, for those compelled or graced to seek deeper truth about themselves, this potentiality opens a door that is most relevant (Bradford, 2021; Prendergast & Bradford, 2007; Schneider, 2004 & 2009; Welwood, 2000).

From prediction and control to spontaneity and freedom

In regard to epistemological differences between empiricism and holism, several critical distinctions can be made. Perhaps most importantly, the prime directive of empirical science is to enhance the "prediction and control" of nature, thus necessitating a decisive separation between man and nature, self and world, mind and body, et cetera. On the other hand, the prime directive of holistic psychologies is to enhance a person's inclusive capacity to be fully human. While "fully human" may be understood in various ways, here it refers to the capacity to be more completely present in the world and with the whole of one's experience. Full presence involves the capability of being both *open* and *responsive* (to others, the world, oneself). Instead of valuing prediction and control of nature, others and oneself, holistic psychologies value the freedom of spontaneity and the deepening of trust in the openness and, at times, *un*predictable responsivity of human interaction.

Again, the point is not that self-control or the making of reasoned predictions are rejected, but it is recognized that they arise from and remain rooted in a broader, more spacious context and capacity for presence. With this understanding, mental health professionals are challenged to discriminate between genuine openness and spontaneous responsiveness on the one hand, and contrived presence, reactivity and defensiveness on the other. Whether a person may be stuck in a diagnosable depression, anxiety, compulsion, or something else is secondary to the primary discernment of noticing to what extent they are open and "in the flow" of their life or closed-up, defended and stuck. This kind of experiential-relationally observed discernment need not be pathologizing, but sympathetic in a "human, all too human" way. More importantly, it empowers a person to get out of whatever pathological box they may have been put it, or put themselves in, and to be open to...something else.

From de-contextualized to context-based assessment

The empirical scientific method is based on isolating (de-contextualizing) variables in order to test a specific hypothesis. This is done in order to eliminate extraneous variables that might interfere with determining the significance of the specific variable being researched. In contrast, human scientific approaches seek to comprehend the totality of a person within their life situation. The assumption here is not that a person exists as an isolatable mind, but that one is always a being-in-the-world, inextricably influenced by the social and natural contexts in which they are embedded.

This approach reverses the empiricist mandate by requiring the *inclusion* of variables in any viable psychological assessment. In addition to the various dimensions of social context which should be considered, such as culture and subculture, race, ethnicity, age, sex, socioeconomic factors, relationship complexities, politics and religion, it may also be relevant to consider still other contextual influences. These might include such factors as the climate and season, geography, physical condition, dietary habits, et cetera.

From logical deduction to intuition and empathic understanding

The prime cognitive function which empiricism exercises in determining scientific truth is logical deduction. Holistically-informed science certainly respects the exercise of logic, deductive and inductive, but also calls for a much wider exercise of cognizance. Phenomenology explicitly privileges the exercise of *intuition* as the cognitive function most able to comprehend the implicit complexities of human experience (Gurwitsch,1957/1962; Husserl, 1913/1962).

Intuition functions as an inclusive form of knowing by taking into consideration the contextual breadth and depth of a phenomenon, granting free reach and range to inquisitive awareness. Understandings that emerge intuitively are not concept-bound, so are more able to reveal the explicit and implicit complexity of a situated human experience. And in being lighter—more open and fluid—are more in accord with the nature of experience as being in-process.

Empathic attunement is an akin mode of non-conceptual cognition that functions according to and within a relational field. Empathy can be distinguished from intuition as being a more visceral feeling-toned knowing. While conceptual thinking excels as a nominative function, dividing a whole into parts and distinguishing between them, intuition and empathy excel in comprehending the sense of whole experiences. This includes the dynamic inter-relations between people and between parts of oneself.

The key assumption here is that the whole person is always more than the sum of his parts, will always elude conceptual understanding, and that to know a person more completely, it is necessary to think with one's heart as much as one's mind. As Rollo May (1958) noted, "One must have at least a readiness to love the other person, broadly speaking, if one is to be able to understand him" (p. 38).

From impersonal causality to a participatory subject

Within the empiricist worldview, subjectivity—including personality structure and interpersonal relationship—is seen as a result of impersonal causes based in the past. As Boss (1983, Chapter 12) notes, by focusing primarily on past preconditions of a current problematic situation, the causal approach relegates the human subject to a passive status. As a mere effect of predefining causes, a personal condition is ipso facto defined as an impersonal artifact.

Within this mindset, psychological problems readily lend themselves to being conceived by physiological causes such as faulty neurotransmitters or other biochemical imbalances, or as resulting from social or psychological causes, such as deficient or traumatic parenting or other social forces. Of course, the manifold and compelling conditions of life exert tremendous formative influence on human subjectivity. *But interpersonal influence is not the same as impersonal causality.*

A human subject is always involved in personally responding to the life conditions in which they find themself, even if they do not have a good ability to respond. This is often the case with children who are still developing their sense of self-agency as well as adults in oppressive situations in which they have little power to freely respond. In such situations, we then speak of people acting-out or repressing their emotions, in some way impulsively reacting rather than skilfully responding.

Nevertheless, the assumption of having and deploying individual response-ability is a cornerstone for the rule of law, democracy, and the work of psychotherapy. The thing is, empiricist causal thinking cannot account for this basic freedom. As Jacobs and Cohen (2010) observe, "The *DSM's* pathology framework…is about what happens to people based on impersonal processes and mechanisms; it does not address the person's situation as far as he or she is concerned." From a human science perspective, a person's *concern* for his situation, his *participation* in it, is what really matters.

Psychotherapy works, when it does work, because we accept that it is less important *what* happened to us than *how* we took, and continue to take, what happened to us. It is by recognizing our participation in the life we are currently living that we have a chance of changing it. Upon this recognition of the primacy of subjective responsiveness, including accepting the freedom to respond differently, turns the effectiveness of any diagnosis, self-reflection, psychotherapy, or spiritual practice.

Conclusion

While there are expedient reasons to continue to professionally reference the DSM, such as for insurance reimbursement or to communicate with medical personnel, issues of expediency ought not be confounded with scientific issues of validity and reliability. On both clinical and ethical grounds, the DSM fundamentally fails as a valid diagnostic instrument. Given its prominence in the mental health field, this failure needs to be highlighted both in clinical training situations and in everyday clinical practice. In the course of such exposé, the assumptions of empirical science which inform the DSM ought also to be observed and brought into question.

Complementing critiques of empiricism and the DSM, alternative holistic diagnostic approaches and formulae need to be developed according to specifically human scientific guidelines. A suite of four definitive diagnostic guidelines can inform a phenomenologically robust, holistically oriented science of human subjectivity. These include:

1) a recognition and affirmation that the purpose of psychodiagnosis serves not utilitarian efficacies of prediction and control, but an enhancement of the spontaneity and freedom of a human subject;

2) that the knowing of other minds ought not sever those minds from their lived worlds, but understand them within their living contexts and implicit complexities;

3) diagnosis is most true to human nature when it is process-based and understood as transitory, not fixed. This involves recognition that a human subject is not an isolated entity but a being that exists within an intersubjective field, including a diagnostic field that is both open-ended and co-constituted between doctor and patient;

4) a privileging of the cognizant functions of intuition and empathic attunement as diagnostic mediums of knowing as much or more than conceptual knowing.

Just because the basic nature of human being is fluid, unconditionally free and open-ended, that does not mean one knows this, accepts it or can handle it. Hence, the value of experience-near diagnosis and self-understanding to help a person be seen and see themselves as they are rather than as they, and others, think they are.

Simply put, in order to have a most inclusive knowing of other minds, it is necessary to accord to those minds as they display themselves. This challenges diagnosticians to not be experience-distant, safely removed in an objective reserve, but to be inter-subjectively present—willing to open themselves to the otherness of the other and dare to respond skilfully from with that open region.

References

Binswanger, L. (1963). *Being in the world*. Basic Books.

Boss, M. (1982). *Psychoanalysis and Daseinsanalysis*. DaCapo. (Original work published in 1963)

Boss, M. (1983). *Existential foundations of medicine and psychology*. Jason Aronson.

Bradford, G. K. (2007). From neutrality to the play of unconditional presence. In, Prendergast, J. & Bradford, G. K. (Eds). *Listening from the heart of silence: Nondual wisdom and psychotherapy, Vol. 2*. St. Paul: Paragon House.

Bradford, G. K. (2013). *The I of the Other: Mindfulness-based diagnosis and the question of sanity*. St Paul, MN: Paragon House.

Bradford, K. (2021). *Opening Yourself: The psychology and yoga of self-liberation*. Manotick, ON: Sumeru Press.

Bradford, K. (2023). On the essence of freedom. *The Journal of Existential Analysis, 34(1)*, 376-392.

Bugental, J. (1965). *The search for authenticitiy: An existential-analytic approach to psychotherapy*. NY: Holt, Rinehart & Winston.

Chodron, P. (1997). *When things fall apart: Heart advice for difficult times*. Shambhala.

Ferrer, J. N. (2002). *Revisioning transpersonal theory*. SUNY.

Gadamer, H.G. (1982). *Truth and method*. NY: Crossroad. (Original work published in 1960)

Gendlin, E. T. (1973a). *Experiential phenomenology. In, Phenomenology & the social sciences*. (Natanson, M., Ed.). Evanston, IL: Northwestern Univ.

Gendlin, E. T. (1973b). Experiential psychotherapy. In, *Current psychotherapies*. Ed. Corsini. Itasca, IL: Peacock.

Giorgi, A. (1970). *Psychology as a human science: A phenomenologically based approach*. N.Y.: Harper & Row.

Goldstein, M. & Goldstein, I. F. (1978). *How we know: An exploration of the scientific process*. NY: Plenum.

Gurwitsch, A. (1964). *The field of consciousness*. Pittsburgh, PA: Duquense University Press. (Original work published 1957)

Horwitz, A. V. & Wakefield, J. C. (2007). *The loss of sadness: How psychiatry transformed normal sorrow into depressive disorder*. Oxford Univ. Press.

Husserl, E. (1962). *Ideas: General introduction to pure phenomenology*. Translated by W. R. B. Gibson. N.Y.: Collier. (Original work published 1913)

Husserl, E. (1970). *The crisis of European sciences and Transcendental Phenomenology*. Trans. D. Carr. Evanston, IL.: Northwestern University Press. (Original work published 1954)

Jacobs, D. H. & Cohen, D. (2010). Does "psychological dysfunction mean anything?: A critical essay on pathology vs. agency. *Journal of Humanistic Psychology*, 50(3), 312-334.

Laing, R. D. (1960). *The divided self*. Tavistock.

Laing, R. D. (1969). *The politics of the family and other essays*. Vintage.

Luijpen, W. A. (1960). *Existential Phenomenology*. Pittsburgh, PA: Duquense University.

Maslow, A. H. (1971). *The farther reaches of human nature*. Penguin.

May, R. (1958). Contributions of Existential psychology. In, *Existence*. Ed. May, Angel & Ellenberger. N.Y.: Simon & Schuster.

May, R., Angel, E. & Ellenberger, H. F. (1958). *Existence*. NY: Simon & Schuster.

Merleau-Ponty, M. (1962). *The phenomenology of perception*. Translated by C. Smith. Routledge & Kegan Paul.

Merleau-Ponty, M. (1963). *The structure of behavior*. (Trans. A. L. Fisher). Boston: Beacon. (Original work published 1942)

PDM Task Force. (2006). *Psychodynamic diagnostic manual*. Silver Spring, MD: Alliance of Psychoanalytic Organizations.

Prendergast, J. J. & Bradford, G. K. (2007). *Listening from the heart of silence: Nondual wisdom and psychotherapy, Volume 2*. St. Paul, MN: Paragon.

Rogers, C. R. (1961). *On becoming a person: A therapist's view of psychotherapy*. Boston: Houghton Mifflin.

Schneider, K. J., Bugental, J. & Pierson, J. F. (2001). *The handbook of Humanistic Psychology: Leading edges in theory, research, and practice.* London: Sage.

Schneider, K. J. (2004). *Rediscovery of awe: Splendor, mystery, and the fluid center of life.* St. Paul, MN: Paragon.

Schneider, K. J. (2009). *Awakening to awe: Personal stories of profound transformation.* Jason Aronson.

Skinner, B. F. (1971). *Beyond freedom and dignity.* Random House.

Spinelli, E. (1989). *The interpreted world: An introduction to phenomenological psychology.* London: Sage.

Szasz, T. S. (1974). *The myth of mental illness: Foundations of a theory of personal conduct.* Revised Edition. Harper & Row.

Taylor, T. (2009). *A spirituality for brokenness: Discovering your deepest self in difficult times.* Woodstock, VT: Skylight Paths.

Valle, R. & Halling, S. (1989). *Existential-Phenomenological perspectives in psychology.* Plenum.

Van den Berg, J. H. (1972). *A different existence: Principles of phenomenological psychopathology.* Pittsburgh: Duquense Univ. Press.

Welwood, J. (2000). *Toward a psychology of awakening: Buddhism, psychotherapy, and the path of personal and spiritual transformation.* Boston: Shambhala.

Winnicott, D. W. (1971). *Playing and reality.* N.Y.: Tavistock.

---

[i] Please note: "empirical" applied to science is used as a term referring to the scientific method, synonymous with the terms "natural" or "positive" science. Holistic forms of human science are also empirical, but in both a broader and more specific sense of attending to subjectively-lived experience.

[ii] For a more in-depth inquiry into the phenomenology of the self and the nature of subjectivity informed by Buddhist and Existential perspectives, see Bradford, 2021, pp. 53-79.

[iii] For a discussion "On the Essence of Freedom," see Bradford, 2023, pp. 376-392.

Stress and Distress: Understandings and Contradictions

Ian Parker

Abstract: *The psy professions (psychiatry, psychology, psychotherapy and sometimes even psychoanalysis) use competing grids of understanding to make sense of stress and distress. This chapter aims to open up contradictions in different traditional and alternative theoretical attempts to make sense of stress and distress. It challenges dominant views of mental distress in the discipline of psychology which are routinely framed as abnormality or psychopathology. Each of these approaches needs to be linked to the question of liberation.*

Different approaches to "stress and distress" often lead to conflicts between academic psychologists and professionals involved in mental health services. These different ways of understanding it, which are sometimes configured in psychology textbooks as competing "understandings" of stress and distress, also sometimes lead to conflict between professionals and their clients—and even between those who are given a variety of diagnostic labels and accept or refuse to accept what they have been told about themselves.

These conflicts are because we do not really know what stress and distress really is. I use this phrase "stress and distress" here to distinguish it from medical terminology that refers to "mental illness" or popular distancing from experience of others who are different in the term "madness."

Contradictions between understandings of 'stress and distress'

This chapter takes the term "stress and distress" as a shorthand to cover the variety of ways that academics, professionals, and users of mental health services debate how mental health should be understood, and it explores consequences of the *difference* of perspective for liberation. The term "stress and distress" is useful because it spans a number of different approaches, and for all of the problems of playing into stereotypical images of the "mad" (which I address in the course of this chapter).

The term "psychosis," for example, which is favored as a term by many professionals today around which they can discuss the value of different treatment modalities already sounds to me, at least, a little more definite, sure of what we are getting at, and I don't think we can be so sure (Bentall, 2004). The term "mad" is disturbing to some practitioners and some users of mental health services but is claimed and even celebrated by others (Curtis et al., 2000).

A minimal point of agreement between researchers and practitioners within different "understandings" is that there are huge differences between ways of understanding stress and distress, between different approaches to, or "understandings" of stress and distress. That difference of approach is one reason why it is good to have multiple perspectives on it, but I am not so sure that practitioners of the medical model, cognitive-behavioral therapy (CBT), systemic approaches and psychoanalysis (to name four main approaches taken today) agree that their different perspectives are even perspectives on the same thing. Perhaps all that can be agreed upon as a first understanding is that there are big, perhaps irresolvable differences between the perspectives.

Those differences are grounded in the distinctive ontology and epistemology of our own particular favorite approach, and differences over ontology and epistemology have massive consequences for social policy, treatment, and liberation. Ontology is about the nature of being itself, what we understand the things in the world to be—and here what we understand the human being, the human subject to be. Different ontologies carry fundamentally different notions of what human beings are. Epistemology refers to the nature of knowledge, how we think we can develop knowledge about those things that our ontology gives us a model for. Not only are there differences over the nature of things concerned "stress and distress," but over how we can come to know what they are, what the criteria for creating knowledge of them is.

It makes a big difference, for example, if we think that the nature of the human being as a biological organism is the stuff we should be targeting — if that is our ontology — for then we will be developing our knowledge through drug trials. This particular process of knowledge production is an epistemology, a way of getting knowledge about what stress and distress is as a chemical imbalance — deficit, excess, perhaps — that is entirely independent of what someone labeled mad thinks about it.

The knowledge of the mad about who they are, their own expertise, is completely irrelevant to what academic or professional psychologists think they can know about the things in the world that matter to us if we are working in a medical model. A CBT perspective also rests on a particular view of the beings that matter to it — individual thinking beings, albeit with some perceptual or mental processing faults that can be corrected.

The procedures we use to understand what works and what does not work as education or training to help people manage their behavior are things we will come to understand through a certain kind of knowledge of cognitive modeling and processes that are usually independent of what the practitioner thinks about them. The procedures work or they do not work, and they can be evaluated scientifically. It is a perspective which presupposes the nature of its object and the nature of knowledge about that object, ontology, and epistemology (Loewenthal & House, 2010).

Briefly put, a systemic approach usually relies on ontology of structured relationships and that is what matters to that approach. The knowledge it develops of those systems and how to intervene in them is the kind of epistemology in which the observer is part of the equation, part of the system, part of the knowledge. Finally, and with respect to the fourth of the approaches that will be considered in this chapter, psychoanalysis rests on ontology of a human subject divided, torn between what they desire and what they can get, between the unconscious and what they are directly aware of. That perspective means that the knowledge we could have of stress and distress cannot be complete, but is infused with our desire to know, to understand — and, psychoanalysts would argue, suffused with our desire not to understand, not to know (Parker and Pavón-Cuéllar, 2021).

There are, of course, some links between these different approaches, and attempts to stitch over the differences between them. Those links are often what enable academics and practitioners with different perspectives to come together from time to time and try to map out some common ground. Some psychoanalysts, for example, are still very much tied to the medical model while some are trying to make links with CBT. Some systemic practitioners look to psychoanalysis—to what they call the 'intra-psychic' as an account of what is going on inside individual members of social systems—and others link with cognitive-behavioral accounts of systems. But eventually, we notice that there is a deadlock in these meetings of different approaches, a failure to agree.

The connection between the perspectives was where this chapter could have begun, and that would have been a more ostensibly consensual and constructive place to start (Fozooni, 2010). The concern of psychologists who wish to bring a liberation dimension into their work is quite understandably often geared to what proponents of different approaches have in common as a starting point, and with how it might be possible to build an inclusive general approach in which we could all work. But liberation for the ostensibly "mad," for those who are described by psychologists of different kinds, requires a more abrasive approach. The *difference* between perspectives is where we have got to start and then we have to learn to live with that.

A consequence of this is that liberation is predicated not on a harmonious shared vision of what problems in the world are, or how distress at the level of the individual should be understood and treated. Rather, we attend to conflict between academic and professional perspectives, and we work those differences in order to open up a space for those who are subjected to psychology to speak about what is being done to them (Chamberlin, 1990).

A premise of liberation from the standpoint of those who are speaking for themselves is that we do not require them to speak the same language as us as a condition for being heard, and that we acknowledge that there is no common language for describing "stress and distress" inside psychology. Psychology as such is internally contradictory, molded to different political-economic conditions, and recognition of this makes resistance to psychology possible in the form of "critical psychology" and by allied approaches that would not choose to adopt that term because it too is internally contradictory (Parker, 2007).

Difference within the understandings of "stress and distress"

There are big irreconcilable differences inside each of the understandings. The fact that there are irreconcilable differences within each of the understandings is actually good for the rival approaches; advocates of one understanding can then sit back and watch their colleagues tear themselves apart without having to do the work themselves.

In the case of psychoanalysis, there are a multitude of perspectives and very little agreement between adherents of different traditions attempting to comprehend and treat what is usually termed "psychosis." At a most basic level, again at the level of assumptions about ontology and epistemology, there is a huge gulf between the Kleinian psychoanalysts, for example, who see "splitting" and "projection" as evidence that every human subject is a bit mad—has something psychotic as part of them (Young, 1994)—and Lacanian psychoanalysts who argue that there is a specific clinical structure, "psychotic structure" that makes this kind of subject quite different from a neurotic (Lacan, 1981/1993).

Within the Lacanian camp, there is a further division between those who will argue that psychotics do not have an unconscious as such—and then this means that if there is no unconscious, there is no subject (Fink, 1997). This position is in stark contrast with those who will say that this is still a subject who lives their relation to the unconscious as one of the "faces of the normal structure," as Lacan (1961-1962, p. 11) puts it.

Inside the systemic tradition there have been big debates about what it means that someone in a family has been made into the "identified" patient, the one who is ill, but who is made to carry the disorder of the family system as if it is inside them (Selvini-Palazzoli et al., 1980). And out of those debates, the narrative therapy approach would ask how it is that certain kinds of families are themselves treated as problems within wider sets of discourses (White, 1989).

Here there is an opening to a fully social, discursive approach to what pathology is, how it is created, and who is made to carry the can for it (Parker, 1999). Then again you have a countertrend that argues that still there is this narrative operating at a cognitive-behavioral level, inside the individual. There is then a connection with CBT, but that connection again itself begs the question about what CBT really is, to what extent the practitioner reflexively uses the approach to include the impact of shared faulty thinking about the nature of "illness" and health, or whether they do want to keep the treatment in the tracks of a journey from disorder to what is now called "recovery" (Walsh et al., 2008).

Inside the medical tradition, what looks to be quite closed and certain from the outside is a field of debate, of dispute. This dispute ranges from the underlying ground rules about how pathology should be categorized to disputes over what is happening inside those who are given treatment. Most psychiatrists working in the medical model, for example, use the American Psychiatric Association's DSM – *Diagnostic and Statistical Manual of Mental Disorders* – as their bible, but this DSM has not only undergone revision after revision, changing the framework in which it operates, but it is based in one particular psychiatric tradition—that of German psychiatry.

Back in its origins, there was a conception of knowledge in the DSM, an epistemology which specified that those involved should build their understanding of the categories (and who fits into them) by way of observation and accumulation of specific kinds of symptoms (Spiegel, 2005). That approach within psychiatry is significantly different from the French tradition which works with a notion of "structure" that is approached in a quite different way. A different notion of ontology, of the way that structure constitutes different kinds of being, means that these medics bypass the immediate symptoms to grasp the underlying nature of the subject they meet in the clinic (Vanheule, 2012).

When we turn to the question of treatment, we notice an enormous shift in the conception of what is happening when someone is given medication. Up until the 1960s it was commonly understood among doctors, psychiatrists, that the drugs each had their own effects—that they changed the physiology of the person. This is a "drug-centered" view of what happens (Healy, 2002). The impact of the pharmaceutical companies since the 1960s has changed the terms of description of what happens, has shifted psychiatric discourse so that now the drugs are supposed to be targeting underlying disease states correcting imbalances and so on. This is now a "disease-centered" approach to distress that creates and reinforces an ontology of illness, of the "illness" as what exists and what should be dealt with (Healy, 2004).

If we shift the discourse back to talk about what the altered states are that the drugs produce, then we are also led to make use of the accounts of those who experience them (Moncrieff, 2009). Otherwise, there is no need to listen to those accounts—they are beside the point. So, even within the medical approach, there is an argument about the democratizing of the approach, to open it to bring the expertise of those who are given the medication, to weigh up what the drugs do.

Some adherents of these different approaches are quite flexible, trained in more than one model and use more than one understanding to understand their object of study and treatment; and some manage the relation between the competing understandings, and the bickering inside them, well enough. But all too often there is a closing of ranks against outsiders, against those from other perspectives, which seals over the differences in it. But those differences are there *inside* the understandings and they are irresolvable.

There are consequences for those attempting to promote a liberation agenda for those who are treated as "outsiders" to these debates, those to whom the diagnostic labels are applied as if there is agreement between the professionals in mental health teams. Liberation for the mad does not presuppose that there should be a choice for one particular treatment modality over others, but that the diversity of perspectives should be made as transparent as possible (Cresswell & Spandler, 2009).

The internal divisions among academic psychologists and practitioners should be seen as an opportunity for those who are usually silent in the debates to be able to participate openly. Only then do we have the possibility of making those who are given the labels partners in a dialogue with those who design the diagnostic systems. The "critical psychiatry" movement that anticipated "critical psychology" was a lesson in dispute among the professionals as a sign of health, of the possibilities of mental health for everyone else (Ingleby, 1981).

Differences between the understandings and "stress and distress" itself

It should be noticed that like each of the four main understandings I have been talking about – CBT, systemic, psychoanalytic, medical – this particular experiential "understanding" is internally contradictory, and different experts by experience in this fifth understanding will have different competing views. I am not so concerned with the nature of this understanding as such but with the differences between the mainstream understandings and it.

This fifth understanding is the experience of "stress and distress" itself. It is necessary to treat stress and distress as a *model of itself*, not only because that brings in the voice of those who are labeled into the mix of perspectives I am acknowledging here, but because it enables us to examine how expert understandings relate to it.

It is itself also a form of expertise. People are experts on their own lives, though they are not always treated as if they are—and it makes a difference if someone who is "mad" can speak about it or not (Bates, 2006). The problem is that when they speak about it, when they speak about their experience, they are too often heard from within the framework of a particular model. So, everything they say is interpreted, reformulated, and slotted into the way the practitioner sees the world, which is what a framework that specifies what ontology and epistemology we should take seriously is—a worldview.

That is usually the way that these different perspectives view stress and distress when they (the professionals) try to fix it in place so they can cope with it. Stress and distress cannot win in the face of these strategies. I am not suggesting that stress and distress should win, or intending to romanticize stress and distress and to treat this struggle as if it is a zero-sum game. That is not the issue here. The issue is how each perspective on stress and distress does, in practice, try to win and the destructive effect of this attempt to win on liberation.

So, on the one hand, stress and distress are characterized both as too disordered, unreasonable, out of control, and, at the same time it is characterized as too certain, excessively rigid, a caricature of reason. The different perspectives on stress and distress are often difficult to grasp by practitioners working in other approaches precisely because of this mixture of flexibility and certainty.

Each of the perspectives on stress and distress appear to the other perspectives as quite peculiar, incomprehensible or, even at the same time, fixed in a rigid unassailable view of what stress and distress is (Newnes et al., 1999, 2001). One might say that the "psychotic discourse" that psychologists try to pin down is actually operating as a discourse that structures the debates among the professionals (Hook & Parker, 2002).

When people who are labeled as mad speak, "diagnosed as psychotic" professionals might prefer to say, this mixture of flexibility and certainty is itself treated as a problem. For example, when a conference on "hearing voices" was held in Manchester in 1995, we invited people to come and give papers on their theory of what it means to "hear voices." We let some psychiatrists, clinical psychologists, and psychotherapists come and talk about their own pet theories. But most of the papers were from people talking about their own experience and their own mad theories about that, making use of telepathy, computer-understandings, Shamanism and so on (Parker et al., 1995).

The conference ended with a huge row between supporters of different spiritualist churches. It was a good argument, more interesting than what you will hear at most academic and professional conferences. The point is that it was an argument which showed us competing understandings of stress and distress, understandings as coherent and supple as the ones we read in the textbooks and journals. We learnt that stress and distress has its own model of itself, and the other understandings find that difficult to come to terms with though we must come to terms with it.

Liberation is only possible when the expertise of those is theorized about begin to have their own voices heard in all their complexity and contradictoriness. The demand that the "mad" should speak clearly and unequivocally as a condition for being heard is itself quite unreasonable. As with the dominant "understandings" of stress and distress, the internal contradictoriness of the mental health system user and survivor movement is a sign of their incompleteness, of the existence of conceptual and political debate, even of their humanity (Billig, 1987).

Liberation requires that we do not set conditions for participation in mental health services that are unequal, that suppose that those who speak about their experience are consistent. Strands of oppositional "discursive" psychology that is allied to critical psychology have helped us to take seriously what users of services have always insisted—that their strength lies in the diversity of perspectives they bring, including a dialectically-worked diversity to each of the particular perspectives (McLaughlin, 1996).

The different understandings of "stress and distress" need to be able to maintain themselves

We need to take seriously the role of power. Each of the understandings needs sources of power to legitimate their own worldview. It is not enough to have a good theory. To make the theory stick, to make enough people believe in it—especially when it is riddled with contradictions, especially when there are lots of other competing theories trying their best to do it down—you need to be able to maintain it and defend it; the "psy complex" here operates as an apparatus to enclose the identity of those concerned with mental health and to divide these professionals from their objects of inquiry and treatment (Ingleby, 1985).

This is not merely a question of polite debate. With respect to differences of opinion which are about what the world is and how we should understand it, about the nature of being and knowledge, the stakes of the debate are very high including for professionals attempting to mark out a territory against outsiders and against those who seem to work with outsiders (House and Totton, 2011).

The debates resonate at the heart of our competing views of social order and what we want (and what we think other people should want). One only has to understand debates about psychiatry and so-called "anti-psychiatry" to see that we are in one of those kind of debates with high stakes (Brown, 1981). And then you see that discourse should be thought of not as being like conversation but as like war (Foucault, 2006).

For those of us inside our own garrisons, things can seem pretty civilized most of the time, and it is only when we have to do battle with the other understandings that things can turn nasty. Take, for example, the way the pharmaceutical industry sets the agenda for the development of different categories of mental disorder. Many specific categories are formulated, not at all on the basis of what psychiatrists have observed but what new drugs seem to be able to remove.

Once a drug "works," the category it comes to define as if it is targeting an already existing disorder has to be lobbied for, it has to be marketed, doctors have to be persuaded to prescribe it, and critics have to be silenced. Millions of dollars are spent by the drug companies as part of this process, and they have succeeded in blocking appointments in universities of people who have argued against them (Healy, 2007). It is a debate conducted with a ruthless strategy like a war.

And if the medical model as an understanding has its big battalions through sheer financial power, the other understandings have their own sources of support. Many CBT practitioners are unhappy at the way a cognitive-behavioral quick-fix approach to "happiness" has been pushed by governments keen to get people off incapacity benefit for long enough to save money. But even so, this state agenda has succeeded in giving CBT far more power than it had before (Layard, 2006).

If we turn to psychoanalysis, we know that its institutions have notoriously been adept at protecting their own privilege, using patronage of wealthy clients to support it when it has been under threat. It does not always work, but it has been crucial to the battle to protect the label "psychoanalyst" in many countries, and then to exert control over what are seen as lesser therapies (Parker & Revelli, 2008). Systemic approaches have also had to maintain and defend themselves and built a following through networks, journals, and links with social work and welfare systems. Of course, "critical psychology" also has a little niche now in some academic institutions, and for me to make these arguments I need some kind of support and protection (Parker, 2020).

In many countries where there is no system "survivor" or "user" movement, those who are labeled by the mainstream understandings have no voice, or it is a voice that is neutralized and absorbed by whatever system has been generous enough to humor it for their own purposes. In some places now this movement, through the hearing voices groups or asylum support groups, does provide spaces—publications for the voices to have an impact, to join battle (Romme & Escher, 1993). There is some power now to these voices, but still pitifully little and hard-won—and this movement still needs to be fought for to maintain its right to be heard.

The necessary next step for liberation, therefore, is for the mental health system user and survivor movement to develop its own collective forms of organization so that it can defend itself against attack—and so that it can defend individuals who are incarcerated and drugged (Fabris, 2011). This organizational dimension also needs to address the way that forms of power that structure academic and professional practice can also be replicated, as a necessary result of the dominance of those forms of power, inside the user movement itself (Lakeman et al., 2007).

The political struggle for liberation that responds to mainstream understandings of "stress and distress" also needs to be a political struggle inside the liberation movement so that it may reflect on its activity, allow all voices to be heard and renew itself in the face of new threats.

The notion of "stress and distress" itself had to be created and maintained

I want to move on to open up the question of institutional support and power that is given to different perspectives on stress and distress because there is a much wider context to the disagreement between different specific understandings. There are attempts by each approach to set its own ground-rules for the debate, and often the dispute is about the ground-rules themselves. But above and beyond those particular squabbles, there are general ground rules set in place which frame what we think we know about stress and distress (Pilgrim & Rogers, 1993).

This frame is reiterated over and over again in the media so that the term "psychotic," for example, is wrenched out of its specific clinical context and treated as equivalent to "stress and distress." Then other words and phrases cluster around this popular representation of the mad so that it is associated not only with being unreasonable but with something dangerous. Headlines that tell us that someone who "heard voices" was then violent repeat this connection so the readers are led to believe that voices automatically lead to violence, despite the fact that most killings and atrocities in the world are carried out by people who are, to all intents and purposes, quite sane (Blackman & Walkerdine, 2001).

The interconnection between the different professional institutions tends to back up popular representations rather than challenge them, and that is mainly because they want to make a claim on state resources or charitable support to do their work and make the case that there is a serious problem. And there is a problem, but broad-brush ways of evoking it for an audience always plays into those problematic popular representations.

The "conditions of possibility" – that is, the guiding assumptions that make it possible for us to have debates about how to understand and respond to psychosis – are themselves discursive and practical, and go well beyond what we have control over. We cannot get into the newsrooms and editorial teams that commission shock magazine features that misrepresent what we know about stress and distress to change those assumptions, those images. Still less can we get back to the historical conditions of possibility that set the terms of the relation between reason and unreason (Foucault, 2009).

We can see that in some other cultures there are more humane and tolerant approaches to distress. This is not to pretend that all is well in these other places, and that there is always wonderful liberal recognition of difference. But neither should we fall in line with the colonial export of psychiatry or the globalization from the West of other understandings of stress and distress to pretend that there is a prevalence of schizophrenia of a certain percentage there because we have bought the story that there is such a prevalence of it here.

Prevalence varies according to political-economic conditions, and the very way that "stress and distress" is conceptualized varies as well (Warner, 1994). What we can see from cross-cultural psychiatry at least is that ways of marking the difference between reason and unreason take different forms in different places. That then makes our world a very dangerous place for those who come here, and who are distressed and who then describe what would be considered in their culture to be normal experiences (such as the hearing of voices) to a Western psychiatrist (Maher, 2012).

We are still living with the legacy of a system of what have been described by the historian and philosopher Michel Foucault (1977) as "dividing practices" that separate those who can speak about experience, who are reasoning about it, from those who are on the other side of a discursive-practical barrier. And this means that you don't have to be in a locked ward of a hospital to have your account treated as evidence of your place on the other side of reason, outside it, as symptom of disease, as faulty reasoning, as the voice of an index patient or of psychotic structure.

This is why it is a necessary aspect of liberation in relation to "stress and distress" that the relation between what is usually specified as "mad" positioned as the opposite of "sane" is itself addressed. The "deconstructionist" elements of critical psychology tended to assume an activist character precisely because deconstruction operates at the level of underlying conceptual assumptions which structure our place in the world, our subjectivity, and those conceptual assumptions necessarily connect with political questions about who has the right to speak in a social order and who is kept silent.

The attempt to "reconstruct" schizophrenia around psychological rather than psychiatric categories, for example, retained a rationalist and functionalist conception of "stress and distress," and it served to guarantee the position of a particular kind of professional, the psychologist (Bentall,

1990). An attention to the concealed "voices" of those subject to psychiatric labels, in contrast, has assumed a "deconstructive" character that discovers in the "meanings" of stress and distress a texture of experience that is not amenable to "reconstruction"; instead, the process of historical excavation situates the meanings in the context of psychiatric power and resistance to it (Hornstein, 2012).

The "stress and distress" of contemporary social reality

Dividing practices ensure that only if the subject speaks in a certain kind of way about stress and distress will they be assumed to be sane. This supposed sanity locks us into something that is actually itself quite mad. I have intimated that the understandings of stress and distress have something mad about them, just as mad as what they try to speak about. I should also say that this quite explicitly sets me against the main traditions in what is sometimes seen as the "anti-psychiatry" tradition, by which I mean the work of Thomas Szasz (1961). He is seen as an anti-psychiatrist even though he vehemently argues that he is not, and he argues that "anti-psychiatry" is a mirror-image of psychiatry and is effectively is a form of psychiatry (Szasz, 2009).

Actually, he is a nice example of a combination of flexibility and certainty that drives his critics up the wall because they cannot quite get a fix on what his position is. It is a bit clearer what he is against rather than what he is for. Szasz's objection to psychiatric coercion does seem to rely on a particular version of US American psychoanalytic ethics, the assumption that people should be treated as responsible reasonable subjects who can stand on their own two feet and demand their rights (Szasz, 1965). And this means that anyone who tries to do good for them or make them dependent is betraying that kind of subject. Again, there is ontology at work here in this quite particular provincial version of psychoanalysis, an idea about what the human subject is, and an epistemology, an idea about what our knowledge about that subject should look like (Parker, 2012).

But what kind of world is this illusion of independence, of the individual subject who must stand up for themselves, buying into? Well, the stress and distress of the markets that is affecting most of us who are being made to pay for the economic crisis is the least of it. Even the idea that we should listen to what the markets say about the measures that are being taken to get us out of the crisis, which is surely as mad as listening to invisible voices, is at the lower end of the spectrum of what I am concerned with here.

We live in a form of reality that we must each assume to be true, as the only way to live, in order to survive. Each day we exchange tokens that we treat as having a certain fixed value, even though we know at some deeper level that they do not, and this money is one of a number of commodities that are themselves bought and sold.

Our thoughts and feelings, fantasies and desires are reified, turned into things that are marketable, and what we imagine to be deepest about ourselves we also know can be repackaged and sold back to us (Mandel and Novack, 1970). The enclosure of natural resources at the beginning of capitalism that forced us to sell our labor power so that we would then have to buy back what was once ours, but in distorted reified form now, extends to the enclosure of emotion so that what we perform at work in the service sector becomes a kind of "deep acting," emotional labor from which others will extract surplus value (Hochschild, 1983).

When Marx (1844) writes about alienation, he identifies four ways that our subjectivity is distorted under capitalism. We are, first, alienated from our own creative labor, from our own sensuous engagement with material in the world as we make something of it. We are alienated from that creativity when we sell our labor power to others, and we know that what we are producing is owned by someone else, that they determine what we produce and how we produce it. We are, second, alienated from our relations to others as we compete to sell ourselves, to make ourselves subject to that first form of alienation where we lose what we produce at the very moment we produce it. That competition requires suspicion and the sense that if the other gains, then we lose.

We are, third, alienated from our own nature, from our own bodies, knowing that if we fail to take ourselves to the marketplace and sell ourselves at a price lower than our competitors, then we will suffer and, perhaps, starve. And this turns our relation to our body into that of a subject inside a machine who must keep that machine working, and who becomes fearful of it breaking down. Fourth, we are alienated from nature itself, treating it as something to be mastered and exploited, as if it must be treated in much the same way as we have treated ourselves or sold ourselves for others to treat us. This, again, makes us anxious about nature that cannot be mastered, so we are divided from what we are actually part of and divided at a deeper level from ourselves (Kovel, 2007).

This social reality is mad. To refuse it is mad but to accept it, which is the condition of being reasonable today, is itself a form of stress and distress. This is the political-economic matrix of reality in which we either adapt or break down or, in some cases, become part of the caring professions to try and rather hopelessly patch things up. The promotion of "happiness" tied to CBT in the UK is one example of this attempt to patch things up and make individuals take responsibility for their alienation (Layard, 2005). Justice here is for each individual one by one, and it occludes the social dimension (Pilgrim, 2008).

In contrast, those who have been concerned with liberation have shown that incidence of distress is correlated with inequality, and they have been arguing for a shift of focus from individual "happiness" to the conditions in which those who have resources relate to those who do not (Wilkinson & Pickett, 2010). There is a vital connection here with the question of how "social pain" is constituted at different moments in political economic conditions that suppress possibilities of liberation (Willoughby, 2012).

Shared social assumptions about "stress and distress" structure clinical practice

Contemporary globalised versions of reality are suffused with images of psychology (De Vos, 2012), and the images of the human subject as vulnerable structures social work interventions, clinical practice, and even the activities of the liberation movements in the field of mental health (McLaughlin, 2012).

Szasz's image of the subject is one that other forms of psychoanalysis would be very unhappy with—those forms of psychoanalysis for whom, as Lacanians say, desire is desire of the Other (Vanheule, 2011). Szasz's image of the subject would be diametrically opposed by many systemic practitioners for whom the web of relationships is exactly what makes us human and dependent on each other. It would jar with a good proportion of those working in the broad cognitive-behavioral tradition who have adopted that framework precisely because it values the collaborative reasoning that makes each individual choice have the weight it does.

And, apart from being stung by his vociferous denunciation of them as modern witch-doctors, even some medical tradition psychiatrists would object that there is a benign side to their discipline where they offer to the patient a kind of responsibility for managing their illness at the same time as they relieve the mad of the burden of being made absolutely morally responsible for what they do when they are under its influence.

Different approaches to stress and distress each have their own very good reasons to be wary of Szasz's version of "anti-psychiatry" because it seems to be an approach that throws people back to the wolves in the marketplace rather than do something to help them. The problem is that our own practice is bound up with these wider macro-social issues I've been describing. In fact, those wider cultural and political-economic dividing practices and frames for stress and distress are actually replicated in the micro-social world of the clinic and self-help groups.

CBT that is offered as part of State provision of mental health does risk, as we have seen in the UK through the "Increasing Access to Psychological Therapies" programme, by turning the reflexive work of puzzling through how choices are made into an instrumental and quite cynical agenda for moving people off benefits, forcing them into work they find difficult to cope with and exposing them to pressures that will eventually lead them back into the mental health system again (Ferguson, 2008). The economic pressures that are already hitting people in the economy are relayed down to them in a different kind of way by professionals subject to "targets," administrative tick-box procedures and cuts in services.

This then means that any sustained engagement with a family structure, let alone support that people might need in tackling community-organizational pressures (the kind of things that a systemic therapist might want to include in their frame of reference when they work with relatives and an extended system) is made difficult. Instead, the practitioner has to justify "short-term" or "brief" interventions which they hope will not merely put sticking plaster over the problem, but which usually amount to little more than that.

In the case of psychoanalysis, provision in the public-sector is subject to the same pressures including bending to demands to measure how much happier the client is after every session. For those psychoanalysts working "independently" (as they like to put it), their private practice means that the worried well who can pay for treatment skews the whole of the practice toward catering to the self-indulgent and shunting off what is seen as the really serious pathology to the other practitioners or, worse, to the psychiatrists (in which case all the drug options start to look attractive to the hard-pressed professional).

And for service-users, the alternative to complete recovery, in which case they may be left with no support at all, might be to turn themselves into entrepreneurs who become professional users, paid for telling their story again and again, and thus reinforcing an identity tied to the mental health system (Cresswell, 2005).

Conclusion: What is to be done?

Spaces to speak or work creatively away from what is now becoming a dominant therapeutic ideology are necessary for new approaches to develop. Those spaces include the work of the democratic psychiatry movement, which I think is different from "anti-psychiatry." It was inspired by the Italian reforms thirty years or so ago that closed the mental hospital in Trieste and set up cooperatives to help people get back into everyday life (Basaglia, 1987). Some activists from France visited and protested, scrawling on the walls that this approach had released the patients only to then put them into the chains of work (Ramon, 1988).

Those alternative traditions operated with a different conception of labor (Holland, 2012). Where there is an approach, there is always a critique. Now "democratic psychiatry" is a phrase still alive in the work of *Asylum: Magazine of Radical Mental Health* (previously the "magazine for democratic psychiatry"), for example, and that ethos is alive in the Hearing Voices Network, the Paranoia Network, Intervoice, the Soteria House groups, Mindfreedom, Mad Pride and so on (McLaughlin, 2003). The more the merrier; this is where the voices in and against stress and distress itself are flourishing, and these alternatives sustain people against the big battalions of medical psychiatry and the other smaller armies of bad professionals, including psychologists (Parker, 2014).

You could say that one consequence of the argument that I've made is that we should acknowledge these issues and be reflexive in our work, whatever it is. That seems to be a little minimal and could leave things just they are. Another consequence—a maximum demand, if you like—could be that you have to get together and collectively act now to overthrow capitalism, which seems overly ambitious (but really, to be honest, I think that is quite necessary).

The space between those two options has been worked by those in the user and survivor movement (Spandler, 2006). There was a serious attempt to avoid the worst of each of the two options. By that I mean that reflexive agonizing can be annoying and paralyzing, what smug professionals can sometimes already do quite well as an excuse for doing nothing. And some attempts to overthrow capitalism, and some of the States that pretended to be post-capitalist, have been quite authoritarian, and have had a very bad record on treatment of the mad.

There is a danger, for example, that a "Marxist" rebuttal of psychiatry simply takes the opportunity to instate another closed and fixed notion of reason and unreason that divides the mad from those who are permitted to speak (Robinson, 1997). Liberation entails operating between those two options, working with those who are on different points of the dimension depending on their own political views, a way of operating so that the possibility is opened for moving from a quite minimal respect for the experience of stress and distress to tackling the conditions that make it so miserable.

References

Basaglia, F. (1987). *Psychiatry Inside Out: Selected writings of Franco Basaglia.* New York: Columbia University Press.

Bates, Y. (Ed.) (2006). *Shouldn't I Be Feeling Better By Now? Client Views of Therapy.* London: Palgrave Macmillan.

Bentall, R. (2004). *Stress and distress Explained: Psychosis and Human Nature.* Harmondsworth: Penguin.

Bentall, R. P. (Ed.) (1990). *Reconstructing Schizophrenia.* London and New York: Routledge.

Billig, M. (1987). *Arguing* and *Thinking: A Rhetorical Approach* to *Social Psychology.* Cambridge: Cambridge University Press.

Blackman, L. & Walkerdine, V. (2001). *Mass Hysteria: Critical Psychology and Media Studies.* Palgrave: London.

Brown, P. (1981). Antipsychiatry and the left. In I. Parker (Ed.) (2011). *Critical Psychology: Critical Concepts in Psychology, Volume 2, Contradictions in Psychology and Elements of Resistance* (pp. 226-243). London and New York: Routledge.

Chamberlin, J. (1990). The ex-patients' movement: Where we've been and where we're going. In I. Parker (ed.) (2011) *Critical Psychology: Critical Concepts in Psychology, Volume 2, Contradictions in Psychology and Elements of Resistance* (pp. 244-257). London and New York: Routledge.

Cresswell, M. & Spandler, H. (2009). Psychopolitics: Peter Sedgwick's legacy for the politics of mental health. In I. Parker (ed.) (2011) *Critical Psychology: Critical Concepts in Psychology, Volume 2, Contradictions in Psychology and Elements of Resistance* (pp. 131-149). London and New York: Routledge.

Cresswell, M. (2005). Self-Harm "Survivors" and Psychiatry in England, 1988–1996. *Social Theory and Health,* 3(4), 259-285.

Curtis, T., Dellar, R., Leslie, E. & Watson, B. (Eds.). (2000). *Mad Pride: A Celebration of Mad Culture.* London: Spare Change Books.

De Vos, J. (2012). *Psychologisation in Times of Globalisation*. London and New York: Routledge.

Fabris, E. (2011). *Tranquil Prisons: Chemical Incarceration under Community Treatment Orders*. Toronto: University of Toronto Press.

Ferguson, I. (2008). Neoliberalism, Happiness and Wellbeing. *International Socialism*, 117, 123-43.

Fink, B. (1997). *A Clinical Introduction to Lacanian Psychoanalysis: Theory and Technique*. Cambridge, MA: Harvard University Press.

Foucault, M. (1977). *Language, Counter-Memory, Practice: Selected Essays and Interviews*. Oxford: Blackwell

Foucault, M. (2006). *Psychiatric Power: Lectures at the Collège de France, 1973–1974*. London: Palgrave Macmillan.

Foucault, M. (2009). *History of Stress and distress*. London and New York: Routledge.

Fozooni, B. (2010). Cognitive Analytic Therapy: A sympathetic critique. *Psychotherapy and Politics International*, 8(2), 128-145.olland, E. (2011). *Nomad Citizenship: Free-Market Communism and the Slow-Motion General Strike*. Minneapolis, MN: University of Minnesota Press.

Healy, D. (2002). *The Creation of Psychopharmacology*. Cambridge, MA: Harvard University Press.

Healy, D. (2004). *Let Them Eat Prozac: The Unhealthy Relationship Between the Pharmaceutical Industry and Depression*. New York: New York University Press.

Healy, D. (2007). The engineers of human souls & academia. In I. Parker (ed.) (2011) *Critical Psychology: Critical Concepts in Psychology, Volume 3, Psychologisation and Psychological Culture* (pp. 193-204). London and New York: Routledge.

Hochschild, A. R. (1983). *The Managed Heart: Commercialisation of Human Feeling*. Berkeley, CA: University of California Press.

Hook, D. & Parker, I. (2002). Deconstruction, psychopathology and dialectics. *South African Journal of Psychology*, 32(2), 49-54.

Hornstein, G. A. (2012). *Agnes's jacket: A Psychologist's search for the meanings of stress and distress* (UK ed.). Ross-on-Wye: PCCS Books.

House, R. & Totton, N. (Eds.) (2011). *Implausible Professions: Arguments for Pluralism and Autonomy in Psychotherapy and Counselling (2nd Edn)*. Ross-on-Wye: PCCS.

Ingleby, D. (1985). Professionals as socializers: The 'psy complex'. In I. Parker (ed.) (2011) *Critical Psychology: Critical Concepts in Psychology, Volume 1, Dominant Understandings of Psychology and Their Limits* (pp. 279-307). London and New York: Routledge.

Ingleby, D. (Ed.) (1981). *Critical Psychiatry: The Politics of Mental Health*. Harmondsworth: Penguin.

Kovel, J. (2007). *The Enemy of Nature: The End of Capitalism or the End of the World? (2nd Revised Edn)*. London: Zed Books.

Lacan, J. (1961-1962). *The Seminar of Jacques Lacan, Book IX: Identification* (translated by C. Gallagher from unedited French manuscripts).

Lacan, J. (1981/1993). *The Psychoses: The Seminar of Jacques Lacan, Book III: 1955-1956*. London and New York: Routledge.

Lakeman, R., McGowan, P. & Walsh, J. (2007). Service users, authority, power and protest: A call for renewed activism. *Mental Health Practice*, 11(4), 12-16.

Layard, R. (2005). *Happiness: Lessons from a New Science*. Harmondsworth: Penguin.

Layard, R. (2006). *The Depression Report: A New Deal for Depression and Anxiety Disorders*. London: LSE Centre for Economic Performance, available at http://cep.lse.ac.uk/research/mentalhealth/default.asp (accessed 31 May 2012).

Leader, D. (2011). *What is Stress and distress?* London: Hamish Hamilton.

Loewenthal, D. and House, R. (Eds.). (2010). *Critically Engaging CBT in an Age of Happiness: Modality Perspectives*. Buckingham: Open University Press.

Maher, M. J. (2012). *Racism and cultural diversity: Cultivating racial harmony through counselling, Group Analysis, and psychotherapy*. London: Karnac.

Mandel, E. & Novack, G. (1970). *The Marxist Theory of Alienation*. New York: Pathfinder Press.

Marx, K. (1844). 'Economic and Philosophical Manuscripts', in New Left Review (Ed.) (1975). *Karl Marx: Early Writings* (pp. 279-400). Harmondsworth: Pelican.

McLaughlin, K. (2011). *Surviving Identity: Vulnerability and the Psychology of Recognition*. London and New York: Routledge.

McLaughlin, T. (1996). Coping with hearing voices: An empancipatory discourse analytic approach. In I. Parker (ed.) (2011). *Critical Psychology: Critical Concepts in Psychology, Volume 4, Alternatives and Visions for Change* (pp. 262-269). London and New York: Routledge.

McLaughlin, T. (2003). From the inside out: The view from democratic psychiatry. *European Journal of Counselling, Psychotherapy and Health*, 6(1), 63-66.

Moncrieff, J. (2009). *The Myth of the Chemical Cure: A Critique of Psychiatric Drug Treatment*. London: Palgrave.

Newnes, C., Holmes, G. & Dunn, C. (Eds.) (1999). *This is Stress and distress: A Critical Look at Psychiatry and the Future of Mental Health Services*. Ross-on-Wye: PCCS Books.

Newnes, C., Holmes, G. & Dunn, C. (Eds.) (2001). *This is Stress and distress Too: Critical Perspectives on Mental Health Services*. Ross-on-Wye: PCCS Books.

Parker, I. (Ed.) (1999). *Deconstructing Psychotherapy*. London: Sage.

Parker, I. (2007). *Revolution in Psychology: Alienation to Emancipation*. London: Pluto Press.

Parker, I. (2012). *Lacanian Psychoanalysis: Revolutions in Subjectivity*. London and New York: Routledge.

Parker, I. (2014). 'Psychology Politics Resistance: Theoretical Practice in Manchester', in B. Burstow, B. A. LeFrancois & S. Diamond (eds) *Psychiatry Disrupted: Theorizing Resistance and Crafting the (R)evolution*. Montreal, Quebec: McGill Queen's University Press.

Parker, I. (2020). *Psychology through Critical Auto-Ethnography: Academic Discipline, Professional Practice and Reflexive History*. London and New York: Routledge.

Parker, I., Georgaca, E., Harper, D., McLaughlin, T. & Stowell-Smith, M. (1995). *Deconstructing psychopathology*. London: Sage.

Parker, I. and Pavón-Cuéllar, D. (2021). *Psychoanalysis and Revolution: Critical Psychology for Liberation Movements*. London: 1968 Press

Parker, I. & Revelli, S. (Eds.). (2008). *Psychoanalytic Practice and State Regulation*. London: Karnac.

Pilgrim, D. (2008). Reading 'Happiness': CBT and the Layard thesis. *European Journal of Psychotherapy and Counselling*, 10(3), 247-260.

Pilgrim, D. & Rogers, A. (1993). *A Sociology of Mental Health and Illness*. Buckingham: Open University Press.

Ramon, S. (1988). *Psychiatry in transition: The British and Italian experiences*. London: Pluto Press.

Robinson, J. (1997). *The failure of psychiatry: a Marxist critique*. London: Index Books.

Romme, M. & Escher, S. (1993). *Accepting Voices*. London: MIND.

Selvini-Palazzoli, M., Boscolo, L. Cecchin, G. & Prata, G. (1980). Hypothesizing-circularity-neutrality: Three guidelines for the conductor of the session. *Family Process*, 19, 3-12.

Spandler, H. (2006). *Asylum to Action: Paddington Day Hospital, Therapeutic Communities and Beyond*. London and Philadelphia, PA: Jessica Kingsley.

Spiegel, A. (2005). The dictionary of disorder: How one man revolutionized psychiatry. *New Yorker*, 3 January, available at http://www.newyorker.com/fact/content/?050103fa_fact (accessed 14 June 2012).

Szasz, T. (1961). *The Myth of Mental Illness*. New York: Harper & Row.

Szasz, T. (1965). *The Ethics of Psychoanalysis: The Theory and Method of Autonomous Psychotherapy*. New York: Basic Books.

Szasz, T. (2009). *Antipsychiatry: Quackery squared*. New York: Syracuse University Press.

Vanheule, S. (2011). *The subject of psychosis: a Lacanian perspective*. London: Palgrave.

Vanheule, S. (2012). Diagnosis in the field of psychotherapy: a plea for an alternative to the DSM-5.x. *Psychology and Psychotherapy: Theory, Research and Practice*, 85, 128-142. doi: 10.1111/j.2044-8341.2012.02069.x

Verhaeghe, P. (2004). *On Being Normal and Other Disorders: A Manual for Clinical Psychodiagnostics*. New York: Other Press.

Walsh, J., Stevenson, C., Cutcliffe, J. & Zinck, K. (2008). Creating a space for recovery-focused psychiatric nursing care. *Nursing Inquiry*, 15(3), 251–259.

Warner, R. (1994). *Recovery from Schizophrenia: Psychiatry and Political Economy (2nd Edn)*. London and New York: Routledge.

White, M. (1989). The externalizing of the problem and the re-authoring of lives and relationships. In I. Parker (ed.) (2011). *Critical Psychology: Critical Concepts in Psychology, Volume 2, Contradictions in Psychology and Elements of Resistance* (pp. 169-201). London and New York: Routledge.

Wilkinson, R. & Pickett, K. (2010). *The Spirit Level: Why Equality is Better for Everyone*. Harmondsworth: Penguin.

Willoughby, C. J. (2012). Economics, the nurturance gap and social pain theory. *Journal of Critical Psychology, Counselling and Psychotherapy*, 12 (1), 14-25.

Young, R. M. (1994). *Mental Space*. London: Process Press.

Reconsidering the Diagnosis of Schizophrenia and Related Psychoses Through the Lens of the Integrative Model of Metacognition

Courtney N. Wiesepape, Aubrie R. Musselman, Sarah E. Queller, and Laura A. Faith

Abstract: *Although the recovery movement has gained traction over recent years, schizophrenia spectrum disorders remain some of the most stigmatized diagnoses in the general public and amongst mental health providers. Receiving the diagnosis of a schizophrenia spectrum disorder may have some benefits to the individual diagnosed but may also have adverse impacts on self-experience and narrative identity. In this chapter, we explore an existing framework that describes how deficits in metacognitive functioning lead to disturbances in self-experience and changes in narrative identity. We explore how traditional diagnostic labeling can further exacerbate these disruptions, potentially reinforcing stigma and hindering recovery. We introduce the integrated model of metacognition and Metacognitive Reflection and Insight Therapy (MERIT) as a way to reconceptualize the diagnosis of psychotic disorders and treat core changes in self-experience and narrative identity, respectively. This model provides a novel method of thinking about and describing "symptoms" observed in individuals who experience psychosis and related syndromes that utilizes their understanding of self, others, and community to further contextualize their lived experience.*

Introduction

Historically, recovery from psychosis has been considered a distant possibility; however, more contemporary models suggest that both personal (e.g., increased hope and connectedness) and functional (e.g., symptom remission) recovery from psychosis is not only possible, but the most likely outcome (Leonhardt et al., 2017). Despite the growing popularity of newer recovery models (e.g., CHIME framework; Leamy et al., 2011), schizophrenia and related disorders remain some of the most stigmatized diagnoses, both in the general population (Pescosolido et al., 2021) and among mental health providers (Valery & Prouteau, 2020). Further, receiving a diagnosis of a schizophrenia spectrum disorder and associated stigma may negatively impact lived experience.

In this chapter, we will begin to explore the connection between the diagnosis of a psychotic disorder and negative impacts to one's understanding of the self, others, and the wider world. We review some common critiques of diagnosis with an emphasis on schizophrenia spectrum disorders. Of note, we will refer to "psychotic disorders" and "individuals experiencing psychosis" throughout this chapter in an effort to avoid some of the downfalls of traditional, categorical diagnosis (e.g., schizophrenia); however, we acknowledge that our chosen terminology nevertheless reduces individual experience to a label.

We will briefly review existing frameworks of how deficits in metacognition impact self-experience, which is often expressed through disruptions in narrative identity. We will further explore the idea that diagnostic labeling may exacerbate core features of psychotic disorders, namely alterations in self-experience and narrative identity. Finally, we will discuss a metacognitive framework that begins to address some of these issues.

Impact of Diagnostic Labeling

Categorical labels, including psychiatric diagnoses, can be thought of as cognitive mechanisms that help manage perceptual complexity (Stolier & Freeman, 2016). Labeling helps to facilitate shared understanding and communication but can also lead to stereotyped thinking that precludes complexity and nuance. Ideally, diagnostic labels help guide treatment and self-understanding, but, unfortunately, labeling can reduce individuals who have been diagnosed with disorders along the psychosis spectrum to clusters of symptoms rather than complex individuals whose diagnosis explains one aspect of their lived experience.

Diagnostic labels can be beneficial to providers because these descriptors summarize commonly occurring symptom clusters, indicate potential etiological considerations, and facilitate communication about complex information (Jutel, 2009). Additionally, diagnoses may inform treatment selection (Reichenberg & Seligman, 2016) and provide access to reimbursement for services conferred by insurance agencies (Mayes & Horwitz, 2005).

From a service user perspective, the receipt of a diagnosis can provide a sense of understanding, control, relief, access to services, and a reduction of uncertainty (Craddock & Mynors-Wallis, 2014). Additionally, receiving a diagnosis can provide individuals with a sense of belonging and access to a community of relatable others (McNamara & Parsons, 2016).

Beyond the scope of the current chapter, critiques of our current psychiatric nosology are far-reaching (Stein et al., 2022). Receiving a diagnosis, because of potential overemphasis of the label itself, can result in the experience of disempowerment, hopelessness, stigma, discrimination, and disengagement from mental health services (Boysen et al., 2020; Dinos et al., 2004; Hagen & Nixon, 2011). Feelings of despair, demoralization, and grief may emerge, especially when the diagnosis is associated with poor perceptions of recovery and fewer options for treatment (Horn et al., 2007).

In addition, the receipt of a psychiatric diagnosis can result in the experience of stigmatization and resultant poor outcomes in multiple domains of life (Yanos, 2018). When individuals who have been diagnosed with a psychotic disorder experience societal stigma, it is possible that internalized stigma or self-stigma (i.e., the internalization of societal stigma into one's beliefs about oneself) will develop (Vrbova et al., 2016), which has also been connected to poor clinical and functional outcomes (Dubreucq et al., 2021).

Responses to the receipt of a psychiatric diagnosis are complex and varied. One recent review that focused on the consequences of both physical and psychiatric diagnoses found that 72% of studies reported negative psychosocial impacts of diagnostic labeling (e.g., confusion, bereavement) while 61% of studies reported positive impacts (e.g., validation, empowerment). This review also identified changes to self-identity and social identity as important themes after receiving a diagnostic label with both positive (e.g., transformation, empowerment) and negative (e.g., increased separation from others, viewing self as unwell or incompetent) impacts (Sims et al., 2021).

Although this study did not distinguish between physical and psychiatric diagnoses, we suggest it necessitates wider consideration of the impact of a diagnosis of a psychotic disorder on self-experience and identity, which can be understood through the framework of the integrated model of metacognition described below.

Metacognition in Psychosis

The integrated model of metacognition refers to the interplay between a spectrum of cognitive activities that supports one's understanding of self, others, and one's place in the world. The application of metacognition is an active process that utilizes information that is available in the moment and evolves over time. Importantly, metacognition is a measurable construct; researchers developed the Metacognition Assessment Scale-Abbreviated (MAS-A) to aid in research and monitoring progress in treatment (Lysaker, Minor et al., 2020; Lysaker & DiMaggio, 2014).

Metacognition is understood to be made up of four domains, each of which can be assessed using the MAS-A. The first domain, self-reflectivity, is the ability to think about oneself in increasingly complex and integrated ways. This capacity may range from being able to understand discrete experiences, such as thoughts or emotions, to having an integrative, complex, and nuanced understanding of the self both in the moment and over time (e.g., recognizing patterns in one's life narrative). Similarly, the second domain, understanding of the other's mind, is conceptualized as the ability to think about others in increasingly complex and integrated ways and may range from awareness of discrete experiences (e.g., specific thoughts or emotions) in others to a more holistic and complete understanding of others. Decentration, the third domain, is the capacity to understand that one is a part of a community made up of unique people with independent perspectives, cultures, and motives. The final domain, mastery, is the ability to use metacognitive information to respond to psychological challenges in increasingly complex and integrated ways.

Individuals with psychosis tend to have poorer metacognition compared with others, including healthy controls, individuals who have been diagnosed with bipolar disorder (Popolo et al., 2017) and individuals with other prolonged medical adversities (Lysaker et al., 2014). Metacognitive deficits are thought to originate from fragmentation in psychosis, originally conceptualized by Bleuler (1950) and characterized by a difficulty with integrating psychological information about oneself, others, and the world (Hamm, 2017).

When metacognitive functioning is intact, individuals can maintain a stable sense of self, pursue goals, and respond to psychological problems. In contrast, with metacognitive deficits as observed in those diagnosed with a psychotic disorder, individuals may have difficulty understanding themselves and others in complex ways, managing psychological problems, and engaging with the world. In other words, as a result of difficulty integrating complex information about the self, others, and the wider world, individuals with lower metacognitive capacity may lose a coherent sense of their identity, become isolated, and understand themselves in ways that appear incomprehensible to others (Lysaker, Minor et al., 2020).

In addition to the pitfalls of diagnostic labeling described above, assigning a psychiatric diagnosis to an individual with metacognitive deficits may result in further negative consequences as individuals struggle to make sense of and integrate complex information about the self, others, and wider world. For example, individuals with a diagnosis of psychosis and co-occurring metacognitive deficits may fail to reflect upon their unique experience of psychosis, experience difficulty understanding why others are reacting to them in discriminatory ways or have trouble developing masterful strategies to cope with difficult or distressing symptoms.

Taken together, metacognitive deficits and diagnostic labeling may also lead to other adverse effects in the way individuals experience themselves and share their life stories.

Disturbances in Self-Experience

The experience of psychosis involves changes in an individual's self-experience, intrinsically linked to metacognition, as documented by first person accounts and clinical observation (Conneely et al., 2021; Davidson, 2020). Disturbances in four interrelated dimensions of self-experience – purpose, possibility, positionality, and partiality – are theorized to characterize the phenomenological experience of psychosis and have a broader impact on personal identity (Lysaker & Lysaker, 2017). For individuals diagnosed with psychotic disorders, we suggest that disruptions in self-experience, as exacerbated by diagnostic labeling and metacognitive deficits, result in further disturbances in identity (see Figure 1 in Appendix A).

Purpose, the first of the dimensions of self-experience, refers to an individual's ongoing goals or what they are seeking in their life. Possibility, in turn, refers to an individual's sense of the means and barriers they may face moving towards their purpose. Together, an individual's purposes and possibilities inform the story of their pursuits and what results from these pursuits. The third dimension, positionality, can be understood as how an individual experiences the self contextually; that is, within their social roles, community, and historical context. Examples of one's positionality may include their role as a former student, current mentor, and longstanding friend. The final aspect of self-experience is partiality. The most complex of the four dimensions, partiality refers to the sense that the self is multidimensional, changes over time, and cannot be captured by one role or identity.

Discussed in detail elsewhere, these four dimensions of self-experience are impacted by deficits in metacognition (Lysaker et al., 2021). For example, decrements in the ability to understand the self in complex and integrated ways (self-reflectivity) may result in difficulty understanding one's purposes and possibilities in life. Difficulties grasping the idea that events in one's community result from emotional, cognitive, social, and environmental factors (decentration) may impede one's positionality, or ability to experience oneself contextually within their community.

We suggest that assigning a diagnostic label to an individual experiencing psychosis can further impede the development of self-experience. For example, if an individual is assigned a diagnostic label of schizophrenia, this label may become closely tied to their understanding of themselves. Partiality, or the sense that oneself is multidimensional and complex, might also be greatly impacted; for instance, the individual might overemphasize his identity as someone who is sick, disabled, and unable to live a normal life.

Ultimately, when these domains of self-experience are disrupted, we observe alterations to the stories individuals tell about their past, present, and future.

Disruptions in Narrative Identity

The construct of narrative identity is especially pertinent to understanding how diagnostic labeling and metacognitive deficits impact self-experience in individuals diagnosed with psychotic disorders. Narrative identity offers a method of studying difficult-to-measure changes in self-experience and has broader implications for treatment (Wiesepape et al., 2023). Stated differently, disruptions in self-experience are often expressed through alterations in one's narrative identity.

This aspect of identity is thought to be formed as individuals craft a life story or personal narrative made up of various experiences that have contributed to the person they are today (McAdams, 1996). This involves the ability to organize, make sense of, and incorporate events and experiences into a cohesive temporal narrative. Naturally, aspects of self-experience, including the consequences of disrupted self-experience, are subsumed within one's personal narrative identity. Importantly, personal narratives provide a sense of continuity with the past, purpose for the present, and direction for the future, and evolve as new experiences and information are incorporated (Lysaker et al., 2022).

The personal narratives of individuals who have been diagnosed with a psychotic disorder exhibit alterations in multiple domains, including their content, structure, and process (Cowan et al., 2021). The content of these narratives includes fewer themes of agency and communion and a more negative emotional valence or tone. For example, themes of isolation, adverse social interactions, and adverse life events have been observed in life narratives told by individuals diagnosed with a psychotic disorder (Chung-Zou et al., 2023).

Structurally, these narratives tend to lack temporal cohesion, rendering them disjointed or fragmented. Finally, these narratives often do not seem to respond to experience, leading to a narrative identity that fails to evolve and integrate information and events as they become available (Lysaker et al., 2022; Wiesepape et al., 2023).

Metacognitive deficits and diagnostic labeling can impact one's narrative identity in profound ways. For example, narrative themes, which already lack agency and communion, may become overwhelmed by experiences of societal stigma and thoughts of self-stigma (e.g., "I cannot recover" or "I am dangerous to myself and others"). The structure of personal narratives may lack a cohesive story of how one was diagnosed with a psychotic disorder and what has changed as a result.

A narrative that does not respond to experience may further concretize the idea that one's life is consumed by illness and lead to overidentifying with the "sick role." Importantly, these changes in narrative identity are driven by changes in self-experience such that deficits in understanding one's purpose, possibilities, positionality, and partiality contribute to the previously discussed changes in narrative.

The Metacognitive Framework as a Solution

Disturbances in self-experience and narrative identity, which we partly attribute to the impacts of metacognitive deficits and stigmatizing diagnostic labeling (Figure 1), can be understood and addressed through the integrated model of metacognition. We have suggested that deficits in metacognition and diagnostic labeling contribute to the changes in self-experience often seen in psychosis. These changes then impact the development of one's narrative identity.

The metacognitive model provides not only an alternative method of conceptualizing the experience of psychosis and related disorders without providing a traditional diagnostic label, but also offers a recovery-oriented treatment that can be utilized to address disturbances in self-experience and narrative identity.

Alternative Metacognitive Conceptualization

The integrated model of metacognition removes the emphasis of a diagnostic label by providing an alternative way to conceptualize individuals who experience psychosis that does not put a diagnosis at the center of treatment. Traditional models use diagnostic labels (e.g., "schizophrenia") and focus conceptualization and treatment on symptoms that align with said diagnosis (e.g., "hallucinations"). Because the metacognitive framework is transdiagnostic, a specific label is not necessary. Instead, a careful and individualized assessment of an individual's current metacognitive functioning is completed both at the start of treatment and during each psychotherapy session.

The assessment of metacognitive functioning is most often done utilizing the MAS-A described earlier in this chapter. Depending on the goals of the individual experiencing psychosis and various other factors, ideas and interventions surrounding metacognitive ability are often woven throughout treatment. By continuously assessing metacognition and focusing on individualized treatment that does not rely on targeting specific symptoms, traditional diagnostic labeling becomes increasingly extraneous.

In this approach, rather than categorizing an individual based on a specific label, there is movement toward understanding a person's experience in terms of how they understand themselves, others, and the world around them. Thus, understanding an individual's "symptoms" or experiences with psychosis is only part of the conceptualization.

With a metacognitively-oriented conceptualization, individuals with psychosis are seen as *whole people* with complex lives, challenges, and values that cannot be reduced to a diagnosis or discrete experiences such as psychiatric symptoms (e.g., hallucinations or delusions). As alluded to earlier, by avoiding focusing on a potentially stigmatizing diagnostic label, more opportunity arises to focus on and develop one's self-experience, including one's purpose, possibilities, positionality, and partiality. Of note, experiences of psychosis certainly impact one's self-experience, but using a metacognitive framework allows space for psychosis to occur within the context of one's life rather than the experience of psychosis becoming the primary or all-encompassing focus.

This shift allows for more purpose and possibilities, a diverse understanding of one's positionality, and the acknowledgment that the experience of psychosis is only one thread in the rich fabric of one's life story. This more nuanced experience of self then allows for the development of a narrative identity that may have, for example, more positive content themes, a more cohesive structure, and greater evolution in response to experience.

Metacognitive Psychotherapy

The integrated model of metacognition has led to the development of various metacognitively-oriented psychotherapies that directly target metacognition and are also likely to affects one's self-experience, narrative identity, and understanding of psychiatric diagnoses. For instance, Metacognitive Reflection and Insight Therapy (MERIT) is an integrative psychotherapy that utilizes six preconditions and eight treatment elements (see Table 1 in Appendix B) designed to promote metacognitive growth and treat the *whole person* rather than focusing on a diagnosis or specific symptoms (Lysaker & Klion, 2017; Lysaker, Gagen et al., 2020).

The elements of MERIT are thought to interact to produce meaningful change and promote recovery; in this chapter we will focus on the select few most pertinent to overcoming diagnostically-driven practice. Of the six preconditions, the beliefs that the experience of psychosis can be understood, and that stigma is present in everyone, seem to be the most relevant. Believing that the experience of psychosis can be understood negates the need for a specific diagnosis and instead encourages a more holistic understanding of the individual experiencing psychosis. The acknowledgement that stigma is present in everyone not only supports providers in confronting their own discriminatory ideas about psychosis, but also helps them become more thoughtful about the impact of psychiatric labeling.

Out of the eight treatment elements, eliciting narrative episodes and stimulating reflections about mastery seem especially important. In therapy, eliciting narrative episodes from the client's life helps them to know themselves as something more than a diagnosis or collection of symptoms. Similarly, stimulating mastery – using metacognitive information to manage distress – helps individuals experiencing psychosis to understand their problems as more than a diagnosis or specific symptom.

Finally, with the promotion of self-reflectivity, individuals may come to better understand themselves as protagonists in their own lives with complex thoughts and emotions, rich histories, and important connections to others. Broadly, this treatment approach improves the ability to understand the self, others, and the wider world. As one is better able to reflect upon and integrate information in these domains, self-experience improves and narrative identity becomes more integrated and complex.

Conclusion

Though the use of diagnostic labels provides practical benefits and a roadmap for treatment, we suggest that direct benefits to the individual diagnosed with said disorder come with fundamental limitations, most importantly, impeding recovery through promoting self-stigma and negatively impacting self-experience and narrative identity.

We posit that the integrative model of metacognition is a beneficial framework that allows for less emphasis on diagnostic labeling and more emphasis on the complexities of the lives of persons experiencing psychosis. This metacognitive model ultimately aims to offer a framework to improve conceptualization and treatments for individuals experiencing psychosis.

In Memoriam

This chapter is dedicated in memory of our mentor, Dr. Paul H. Lysaker, who died in July of 2023. Dr. Lysaker devoted countless hours and decades of his career to the metacognitive framework that informs this text and was foundational in developing Metacognitive Reflection and Insight Therapy (MERIT), the treatment we are proud to deliver to individuals who experience psychosis. He strongly believed that people are complex beings with unique goals, values, and motives, and that humanity cannot be reduced to a diagnostic label. We hope this chapter honors Dr. Lysaker's rich conceptualization of the metacognitive model of psychosis and invites readers to consider adapting elements of MERIT in their own work.

References

Bleuler, E. (1950). *Dementia praecox or the group of schizophrenias*. International Universities.

Boysen, G. A., Isaacs, R. A., Tretter, L., & Markowski, S. (2020). Evidence for blatant dehumanization of mental illness and its relation to stigma. *The Journal of Social Psychology, 160*(3), 346-356. https://doi.org/10.1080/00224545.2019.1671301

Chung-Zou, D. S., Faith, L. A., Wiesepape, C. N., Lysaker, P. H., & Kukla, M. (2023). Socialization, adversity, and growth in the life narratives of persons with serious mental illness: an exploratory qualitative study. *Psychosis*, 1-11. https://doi.org/10.1080/17522439.2023.2217709

Conneely, M., McNamee, P., Gupta, V., Richardson, J., Priebe, S., Jones, J. M., & Giacco, D. (2021). Understanding identity changes in psychosis: A systematic review and narrative synthesis. *Schizophrenia Bulletin, 47*(2), 309-322. https://doi.org/10.1093/schbul/sbaa124

Cowan, H. R., Mittal, V. A., & McAdams, D. P. (2021). Narrative identity in the psychosis spectrum: A systematic review and developmental model. *Clinical Psychology Review, 88*, 102067-102067. https://doi.org/10.1016/j.cpr.2021.102067

Craddock, N., & Mynors-Wallis, L. (2014). Psychiatric diagnosis: impersonal, imperfect and important. *The British Journal of Psychiatry, 204*(2), 93–95. http://doi.org/10.1192/bjp.bp.113.133090

Davidson, L. (2020). Recovering a sense of self in schizophrenia. *Journal of Personality, 88*(1), 122-132. https://doi.org/10.1111/jopy.12471

Dinos, S., Stevens, S., Serfaty, M., Weich, S., & King, M. (2004). Stigma: The feelings and experiences of 46 people with mental illness. Qualitative study. *The British Journal of Psychiatry, 184*, 176–181. https://doi.org/10.1192/bjp.184.2.176

Dubreucq, J., Plasse, J., & Franck, N. (2021). Self-stigma in serious mental illness: A systematic review of frequency, correlates, and consequences. *Schizophrenia Bulletin, 47*(5), 1261-1287. https://doi.org/10.1093/schbul/sbaa181

Hagen, B., & Nixon, G. (2011). Spider in a jar: Women who have recovered from psychosis and their experience of the mental health care system. *Ethical Human Psychology and Psychiatry, 13*(1), 47-63. https://doi.org/10.1891/1559-4343.13.1.47

Hamm, J. A., Buck, B., Leonhardt, B. L., Wasmuth, S., Lysaker, J. T., & Lysaker, P. H. (2017). Overcoming fragmentation in the treatment of persons with schizophrenia. *Journal of Theoretical and Philosophical Psychology, 37*(1), 21.

Horn, N., Johnstone, L., & Brooke, S. (2007). Some service user perspectives on the diagnosis of borderline personality disorder. *Journal of Mental Health, 16*(2), 255-269. https://doi.org/10.1080/09638230601056371

Jutel, A. (2009). Sociology of diagnosis: a preliminary review. *Sociology of Health & Illness, 31*(2), 278–299. https://doi.org/10.1111/j.1467-9566.2008.01152.x

Leamy, M., Bird, V., Boutillier, C. L., Williams, J., & Slade, M. (2011). Conceptual framework for personal recovery in mental health: Systematic review and narrative synthesis. *British Journal of Psychiatry, 199*(6), 445-452. https://doi.org/10.1192/bjp.bp.110.083733

Leonhardt, B. L., Huling, K., Hamm, J. A., Roe, D., Hasson-Ohayon, I., McLeod, H. J., & Lysaker, P. H. (2017). Recovery and serious mental illness: a review of current clinical and research paradigms and future directions. *Expert Review of Neurotherapeutics, 17*(11), 1117–1130. https://doi.org/10.1080/14737175.2017.1378099

Lysaker, P. H., & Dimaggio, G. (2014). Metacognitive capacities for reflection in schizophrenia: Implications for developing treatments. *Schizophrenia Bulletin, 40*(3), 487-491. https://doi.org/10.1093/schbul/sbu038

Lysaker, P. H., & Klion, R. E. (2017). *Recovery, meaning-making, and severe mental illness: A comprehensive guide to metacognitive reflection and insight therapy*. Routledge.

Lysaker, P. H., & Lysaker, J. T. (2017). Metacognition, self experience and the prospect of enhancing self management in schizophrenia spectrum disorders. *Philosophy, Psychiatry & Psychology, 24*(2), 169-178. https://doi.org/10.1353/ppp.2017.0021

Lysaker, P. H., Cheli, S., Dimaggio, G., Buck, B., Bonfils, K. A., Huling, K., Wiesepape, C., & Lysaker, J. T. (2021). Metacognition, social cognition, and mentalizing in psychosis: are these distinct constructs when it comes to subjective experience or are we just splitting hairs? *BMC Psychiatry, 21*(1), 329. https://doi.org/10.1186/s12888-021-03338-4

Lysaker, P. H., Gagen, E., Klion, R., Zalzala, A., Vohs, J., Faith, L. A., Leonhardt, B., Hamm, J., & Hasson-Ohayon, I. (2020). Metacognitive reflection and insight therapy: A recovery-oriented treatment approach for psychosis. *Psychology Research and Behavior Management, 13*, 331-341. https://doi.org/10.2147/PRBM.S198628

Lysaker, P. H., Holm, T., Kukla, M., Wiesepape, C. N., Faith, L. N., Musselman, A., & Lysaker, J. (2022). Psychosis and the challenges to narrative identity and the good life: Advances from research on the integrated model of metacognition. *Journal of Research in Personality, 100*, 104267. https://doi.org/10.1016/j.jrp.2022.104267.

Lysaker, P. H., Minor, K. S., Lysaker, J. T., Hasson-Ohayon, I., Bonfils, K., Hochheiser, J., & Vohs, J. L. (2020). Metacognitive function and fragmentation in schizophrenia: Relationship to cognition, self-experience and developing treatments. *Schizophrenia Research. Cognition, 19*, 100142-100142. https://doi.org/10.1016/j.scog.2019.100142

Lysaker, P. H., Vohs, J., Hamm, J. A., Kukla, M., Minor, K. S., de Jong, S., van Donkersgoed, R., Pijnenborg, M. H. M., Kent, J. S., Matthews, S. C., Ringer, J. M., Leonhardt, B. L., Francis, M. M., Buck, K. D., & Dimaggio, G. (2014).

Deficits in metacognitive capacity distinguish patients with schizophrenia from those with prolonged medical adversity. *Journal of Psychiatric Research, 55,* 126. https://doi.org/10.1016/j.jpsychires.2014.04.011

Mayes, R., & Horwitz, A. V. (2005). DSM-III and the revolution in the classification of mental illness. *Journal of the History of the Behavioral Sciences, 41*(3), 249-267. https://doi.org/10.1002/jhbs.20103

McAdams, D. P. (1996). Personality, modernity, and the storied self: A contemporary framework for studying persons. *Psychological Inquiry, 7*(4), 295-321. https://doi.org/10.1207/s15327965pli0704_1

McNamara, N., & Parsons, H. (2016). 'Everyone here wants everyone else to get better': The role of social identity in eating disorder recovery. *British Journal of Social Psychology, 55*(4), 662-680. https://doi.org/10.1111/bjso.12161

Pescosolido, B. A., Halpern-Manners, A., Luo, L., & Perry, B. (2021). Trends in public stigma of mental illness in the US, 1996-2018. *JAMA Network Open, 4*(12), e2140202. https://doi.org/10.1001/jamanetworkopen.2021.40202

Popolo, R., Smith, E., Lysaker, P. H., Lestingi, K., Cavallo, F., Melchiorre, L., Santone, C., & Dimaggio, G. (2017). Metacognitive profiles in schizophrenia and bipolar disorder: Comparisons with healthy controls and correlations with negative symptoms. *Psychiatry Research, 257,* 45. https://doi.org/10.1016/j.psychres.2017.07.022

Reichenberg, L. W., & Seligman, L. (2016). *Selecting effective treatments: A comprehensive, systematic guide to treating mental disorders* (5th ed.). Wiley.

Sims, R., Michaleff, Z. A., Glasziou, P., & Thomas, R. (2021). Consequences of a diagnostic label: A systematic scoping review and thematic framework. *Frontiers in Public Health, 9,* 725877. https://doi.org/10.3389/fpubh.2021.725877

Stein, D. J., Shoptaw, S. J., Vigo, D. V., Lund, C., Cuijpers, P., Bantjes, J., Sartorius, N., & Maj, M. (2022). Psychiatric diagnosis and treatment in the 21st century: Paradigm shifts versus incremental integration. *World Psychiatry, 21*(3), 393-414. https://doi.org/10.1002/wps.20998

Stolier, R. M., & Freeman, J. B. (2016). Chapter 7 - The neuroscience of social vision. *Neuroimaging Personality, Social Cognition, and Character* (pp. 139-157). Elsevier Inc. https://doi.org/10.1016/B978-0-12-800935-2.00007-5

Valery, K. M., & Prouteau, A. (2020). Schizophrenia stigma in mental health professionals and associated factors: A systematic review. *Psychiatry Research, 290,* 113068. https://doi.org/10.1016/j.psychres.2020.113068

Vrbova, K., Prasko, J., Holubova, M., Kamaradova, D., Ociskova, M., Marackova, M., Latalova, K., Grambal, A., Slepecky, M., & Zatkova, M. (2016). Self-stigma and schizophrenia: a cross-sectional study. *Neuropsychiatric Disease and Treatment, 12,* 3011–3020. https://doi.org/10.2147/NDT.S120298

Wiesepape, C. N., Lysaker, J. T., Queller, S. E., & Lysaker, P. H. (2023). Personal narratives and the pursuit of purpose and possibility in psychosis: Directions for developing recovery-oriented treatments. *Expert Review of Neurotherapeutics, 23*(6), 525. https://doi.org/10.1080/14737175.2023.2216384

Yanos, P. T. (2018). *Written off: Mental health stigma and the loss of human potential.* Cambridge University Press. https://doi.org/10.1017/9781108165006

Appendix A

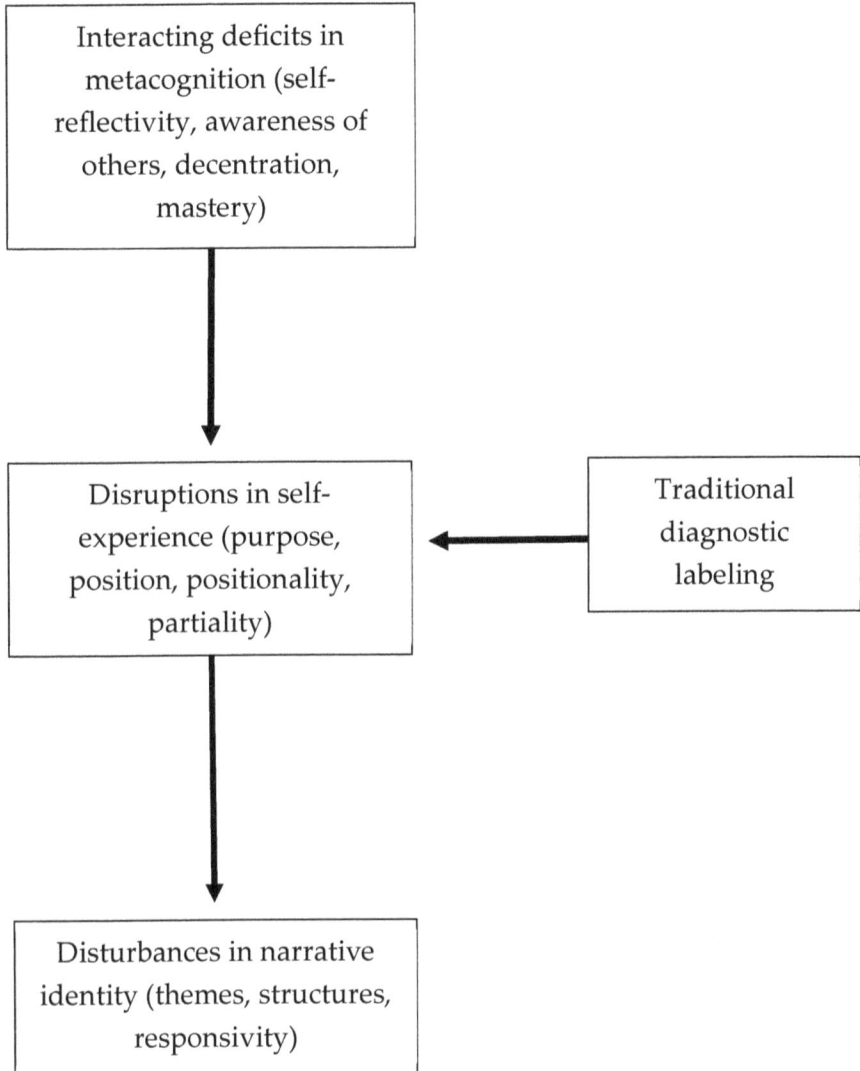

Figure 1: *Connections between metacognition, psychiatric diagnosis, self-experience and narrative identity*

Appendix B

Precondition
1. Recovery is possible
2. Patients are active agents in their recovery
3. The therapist is a consultant and equal participant
4. Psychosis can be understood
5. Greater awareness can lead to emotional distress
6. Social stigma can profoundly impact persons with psychosis

Element
1. Focus on the patient agenda
2. Insertion of therapist's mind
3. Eliciting narrative episodes
4. Eliciting the psychological problem
5. Reflection on the therapeutic relationship
6. Reflection upon progress
7. Stimulating reflections about self and others
8. Stimulating reflections about mastery

Table 1: *MERIT preconditions and elements*

Where Does Theory Take Us? Applying Systems Theory and Social Constructionism to the Process of a Psychiatric Paradigm Shift

Paul Blackburn and Gemma Dent

Abstract: *Written by advocates of the ERNI movement (Emotions aRe Not Illnesses), a critical group offering a challenge to the medicalisation of distress, the chapter considers social constructionism as a paradigm for understanding how meanings and truths are produced, and how changes to accepted truths and knowledges may be facilitated or, indeed, impeded. It borrows additional ideas from Systems Theory to discuss mechanisms for change in how we understand and have historically understood human distress and difference in the UK whilst being cognisant of the role of powerfully socially supported culturally specific narratives that exert force to pull back to the status quo. Recognising the complexity in the process of change, it considers how we might choose to position ourselves and invites a hopefulness for difference despite the challenges. It considers examples of current alternatives to the medical model and proposes that we might think of these as (1) Critical Philosophical Movements, (2) Alternative Conceptual Frameworks, and (3) Structured Systems of Implementation. Finally, it suggests some principles for thinking about how we position ourselves in relation to creating and being alongside ideas that resonate for each of us from an ethical, human rights lens.*

"All right then," said the Savage defiantly, "I'm claiming the right to be unhappy."
– Aldous Huxley, Brave New World (1932)

Systems theory (Von Bertalanffy, 1950) proposes that all interconnected organisms, including human systems through the homeostatic mechanism of negative feedback, resist change. How often do we hear that somebody "finds change difficult" and wonder privately about those who find no challenge in reorientation? How unsurprising is it to those of us working in the industry of distress that families more often seek help at times of family life cycle change (Carter and McGoldrick, 1988)? If we imagine this as a relatively generalisable soft reality, it should come as no revelation that it is much easier to grow an idea than to come up with an alternative.

But ideas do change. Eventually. Sometimes they evolve quickly, such as during periods of political instability or communal threat. Perhaps the ideas already exist but lack a good enough *purpose* for change or growth. Social Constructionist thinking would tell us that language and social action sit alongside each other in the process of shifting meanings. For example, whilst the Suffragette movement made women's rights visible and political, it was women's social action in the First World War efforts that resulted in legal change.

Sometimes the threat from "ideas as usual" is so significant that the pendulum swings so violently in opposition that new ideas blast those we once hailed as holy truths into the ether of space, never to be spoken or thought about again. It is hard to believe, for example, that Churchill—like many of his contemporary politicians, scientists and thinkers—was a proponent of the eugenic movement. Its association with Nazi ideology ensured an instant loss of momentum after the Second World War, though some would argue that the values base within it has not completely dissipated.

Often a new idea first finds an unlikely niche alongside the status quo, leading the same individual to have different understandings given different contexts without really noticing that this is the case. Suspending the risk of seeing this as hypocrisy, an example might be how a parent in 2023 may hold internally complex and not complimentary views of the education system as a byproduct of observing overnight change imposed by the global lockdown in 2020. They may hold both the typical 2019 view that all children have the right to be educated in school and a belief that rich education can be achieved at home.

We live in complex social worlds—and though change is hard, it is happening under our noses every day of our lives, in some places more than others. We all assimilate eventually, but what makes a strong idea overtake another is not individual preference or a contextless definition of morality or truth.

This chapter is to meander around the medical paradigm of distress with as much of a socially constructionist lens as is available. Vivien Burr (1995) referencing Gergen (1985) suggests that in order for a position or approach to be considered Social Constructionist in orientation, it needs to fulfil the following requirements:

1.   have a critical stance on take-for-granted knowledge
2.   understand meaning to have historical and cultural specificity
3.   assume knowledge to be sustained by social process and
4.   understand that knowledge and social action go together

Whilst it may be possible to focus wholly upon "theoretical alternatives to the psychiatric model of mental disorder labeling" without reference to the culture and beliefs in which the current dominant model exists, we are being disingenuous about the limits of our own creativity. Just as we need to recognise the chasm of ideas that exists for us as initiated community members, we also need to:

1.   make sure we overtly name the dominant ideas and stories that are around for us in 2023 Britain
2.   consider the processes through which ideas about "mental health" have and do change
3.   consider whether change is only possible and ethical when we have an off-the-shelf alternative

Mental Health in 2023: Some Stories of British Culture

In order to understand why we are consumed by ideas of "illness and health" in relation to our intra- and inter-psychic worlds, we perhaps need to note that science and scientific expertise have cultural status at this point in history, as they have done increasingly over the last two centuries. We don't have to be scientifically literate ourselves to know that "research" is synonymous with truth—and in a modernist world, scientific experts are the soothsayers.

Alongside the growth of secularism, and the move away from church leaders and the monarchy as sources of wisdom, we have seen the growth of modern medicine. Developments have led to greater life expectancy, prevention, and cures for ill remembered illnesses and the control of excruciating pain. Through careful and systematic means, doctors and scientists have changed all our lives. Few would argue that their power and status is incommensurate with their utility.

At this point in time, it is difficult to imagine a world where medical language doesn't dominate thought, feeling, and intention. It seems laughable to suggest that perhaps this is an arena where they were originally invited in to be kind doctors to the "hopeless and forgotten" (Reidbord, 2014, para. 12). Post First World War, at a time when one could not dispute the impact of devastating events on human functioning—and influenced by neurologist Freud to consider distress in the community to be indicative of disordered nerves—psychiatry was temporarily concerned with meanings and the unconscious, at least for those people who were not considered to need institutionalising.

However, with no strong evidence for psychotherapeutic approaches and with burgeoning opportunities for apparently less life-threatening drug treatments for the extremely distressed hospital population, it made sense for doctors to step away from the business of meaning-making and into what Scull (2016) describes as "Somatic Reductionism." Whereas after the Second World War the *DSM* (*Diagnostic and Statistical Manual of Mental Disorders*) and *ICD* (*International Classification of Diseases*) systems for categorising and classifying illness were influenced by knowledge of how what we now call "trauma" impacts behaviour, functioning and overt distress, the *DSM-III* (1980) marked a move away from the biopsychosocial model towards one with a somatic orientation (Kawa and Giordano, 2012).

No longer concerning itself with aetiology, using the language of medicine it provided clustered descriptions of how people present that lend themselves wholeheartedly to the discipline of drug studies. By 2013, the *DSM-V* had been published with its APA predecessor, Dr Allen Frances, outlining concerns that the descriptions were so inclusive as to shrink the range of normality still further.

Of course, what any brief analysis of social realities cannot do is detail the many non-dominant ideas that co-exist alongside the main model like croutons in a powerfully flavoured soup—adding little more than texture and temporary attention. In relation to what we now call "mental health," there is an accepted smudging of non-complimentary ideologies.

Whilst the language still nods back to a time in history when "health" was the opposite of maladaptation in early life (previously "hygiene") rather than illness, the everyman perspective is that poor "mental health" is some expertly understood medical problem applied to whatever we understand the mind to be. This poor mental health is perhaps "treatable" with drugs or maybe helped by packages of "talking therapies."

 Some of us may be described as "very unwell" and requiring doctors, nurses and hospitals—and others may be thought of as *having* some sort of disorder or condition. Most of us don't have time to trouble ourselves with Cartesian dualism and the epistemological problem of taking as scientific truths the self-reports of abnormality against which there is no valid or reliable comparison of normality. Campolonghi and Orrù (2023) suggest:

> [P]sychiatry emulates the medical approach by borrowing medical concepts such as symptom, disease, diagnosis, or syndrome, and using the health/disease axis as reference. (p. 3)

They point out that the "diagnosis" of Attention-Deficit/Hyperactivity Disorder, for instance, does not require any rationale or measure of normal attention. They suggest that the medical language seems to make sense on a "common sense level, but actually consist in purposively vague constructs, which mimic the medical outlook" (Campolonghi & Orrù, 2023, p. 4).

In 2022, psychology was the second-most popular A-Level subject within the UK (after mathematics) the curriculum of which includes what is described as "psychopathology" (AQA, 2021; CaSE, 2022). It reads like a mix of confused paradigms offering both a "cognitive" and "biological" approach to "treating" "OCD." In an era of "Mental Health Awareness," we are socialising and teaching our young people that, despite disorders and symptoms being the *same* thing and unrelated to any discernible medical aetiology, they still require "treatment" which may be drugs or talking. Clinical psychology does nothing but add the garnish to the medical soup.

If these ideas worked, then we would all be celebrating the advances in medical science that we have seen in every other area of the field. We would not be angry and sad that despite attempts to help those in extreme distress, our evolution as services has failed to produce anything other than poorer and poorer outcomes (Gottstein et al., 2023).

According to the charity, Young Minds (2023), over 1.2 million young people were referred to Child and Adolescent Mental Health Services (CAMHS) in 2022 with an increase in referral rates of 53% since 2019. In August 2023, the children's commissioner, Dame Rachel de Souza, outlined a hope to develop mental health support into every UK school in recognition of the "mental health crisis" (Whittaker, 2023). Newspapers and experts tell us that the only alternative to the horrifying failings of our professional care systems is to provide more of them in more places.

In 2023, British culture is saturated by the language of "mental health." The public knows that it is something that we need to be "aware" of and make "reasonable adjustments for." We know it includes things like "depression" and "anxiety," and we all know people who "suffer" with these or "have them." We may talk about the "genetics" of such and how it runs in our families—and is an inevitability for us.

As vigilant parents and teachers, we look for signs of it in our children. As caring friends and relatives, we make sure that the people around us know it is okay to talk to us about it. We also compassionately share that we know what it is like because we "have it" too.

The "it" that so many people "have" is more nebulous. Perhaps this is because after four generations, the languages of health and illness have merged in such a way that we are not sure what any of "it" actually is. Many believe that it is an "illness" with "symptoms" and turn to the professionals—the experts who say what "treatment" is needed.

We may feel that there is something "wrong" with us, but whether we know the "cause" or not only matters in relation to how we talk about it. Sometimes, it is just something that occurs spontaneously or in relation to a life event, but it is our genetics and biochemistry that predetermine whether or how we become "ill" as a result. Irrespective of the circular reasoning inherent in the descriptions of people having the thing because they have the symptoms and the symptoms "being" the thing, it all sounds pretty convincingly illness-y.

It is hard to believe, right now, that we will ever believe anything other than the dominant story of abnormality and illness, particularly if we think about the place of "power" in the privileging of ideas. When we hopefully skip in the opposite direction to the psychiatrists and psychologists, waving our new ideologies at them (and we are not suggesting we shouldn't), there is a naivety of process if we imagine that alternative narratives will magically transform or even chip away at the status quo rather than becoming subsumed or transformed by it.

Whilst social constructionist thought recognises that language creates meaning, it is also important to remember that it postulates that language and social action work together—and that for meaning to shift, there needs to be a perceived utility to those in power. A further premise is that we can only coherently relate to ideas that are within our own temporal and cultural repertoire and through our own experiential lens. It is, therefore, impossible, to consider as plausible those ideas that we haven't come across or that are unusual within our culture.

If we look at the current landscape in the UK from a constructionist position, we need to acknowledge that there are powerful institutions, people, processes, and social action that go together to legitimise the position outside of the clinic room (e.g., the NHS Trust or the commissioning contexts). James Davies, in his 2021 book, *Sedated*, discusses the mental health agenda in terms of it "thriving under the new style of capitalism" since the 1980s. He outlines the fit for the commoditisation of distress as part of a "pro-market agenda."

The bottom line is that these ideas and associated practices are not going anywhere fast—they are part of a huge profitable industry that has at the helm the pharmaceutical world. Capitalism has supercharged all of it, and often proponents of new ideas that are offered up as alternatives to the medical paradigm are blindly ignorant to the fact that they are also leaping into the marketing abyss with overreaching promises for exciting new therapies. Even if they were individually effective, and obviously people find many things helpful, they proliferate the idea that we need experts for our ever-expanding menu of "disorders." Capitalism and its focus upon the individual are the sea in which we all swim—so how would it make sense other than to sell packaged alternatives?

Arguably, in order for the incredible narrative that is the medical model to genuinely change, we perhaps need to understand that it can't without fundamental shifts in the socio-political regime and thought. At this point in time 2023, Britain holds holy ideas around the commercialisation of existence where everything has a problem and a marketable solution, whether it is the shame of a cracked heel, the lack-lustre of your social media posts, or the discomfort of living in what James Davies describes as "economic servitude." Every bit of our individual environment, body, identity and emotional worlds can be broken down and sold back to us.

Before seeming to contradict ourselves, we want to highlight that after years of working in this world, we have learned that whispers of new groups, services, approaches, and ways of talking have often made us feel that we are on the cusp of change. But the evidence seems to be that we are still waiting for that crisis that makes "the powerful" different. Systems theory would suggest that it will happen—"runaway" or "positive feedback" is the sister process to homeostasis.

As more development begets more development like an arms race, eventually some catastrophic process will kick in to stop it like an ever-expanding motorway in eventual gridlock. Whether this process involves war, political overthrowing, or some other horror or delight, it needs to knock the socks off the veneration of the next packaged thing.

At this point, there have to be alternatives available. We need to have the ideas ready and waiting, perhaps tried and tested. Crudely speaking, you can't make the "penny drop," but you can make sure it is there. But, perhaps sadly, those pennies can only be created in the context in which we currently exist.

There are many examples of cross-cultural ideas that have been helpful to those outside of Western understanding with much better outcomes than we could ever dream of, but it is unlikely that we would easily accommodate them without other change. Whilst this is clearly possible, we feel inclined to outline here some of the locally privileged ideas that are subjugated but understandable in the context of the here-and-now. In other words, they may be "oven ready," though a shame we haven't built the oven yet.

What Balloons Might We Select From?

Imagine that you are standing looking up at the sky. It is filled with balloons that are floating gently above your head, their strings dangling temptingly. Each balloon has within it a familiar idea or something you take to be real or true. You know that across the horizon is another person from another culture, and she has her own set of balloons. The balloons follow you around helpfully. They have been made by your country's leaders, the newspapers, your family, your books, the television, social media, your schoolteachers, and university lecturers.

When faced with a question, dilemma, life choice, creative project, or opportunity to speak, you can only select from those balloons that surround you. You look up and pull at the string. Your neighbour has her own strings to pull. When either of you does so, you proclaim, "Aha! That just makes sense."

The balloons about what the UK mostly calls "mental health" are familiar. You have seen that your neighbour has a balloon that is about the value of a shaman, but that sounds incomprehensible to you. She laughs at your balloon about the word "trauma." Some balloons may float between you both, but only if they are close. The balloons are not of equal size, and some have smaller ones attached to the strings. The bigger balloons are the philosophies, ideas and positions we connect with; the smaller, the means through which we act on them.

If we are to be ready for circumstances in which change can happen (either gradually or suddenly), we can only ever select from the balloons that are available to us now. Perhaps it is time to name some of those balloons? (See Appendix A) The illustration is a simple representation of some of the ideas that already have some status—and may implant deeper and blossom when there is a powerful context for great change. It is not necessarily a comment on what will be most helpful or ethical, though we have views on this.

Critical Philosophical Movements

The critical philosophical movements are a significant starting point for future social action. It has been said that there is no point in having ideas that, in essence, oppose the dominant one without also being able to say something clear about what would be a definitive, better alternative. We beg to differ.

Of course, we need to be able to take action and create new systems, but the starting point is to expose the deficits, risks, abuses, and illogicality of the current thinking. As psychologist activist Vikki Reynolds points out, "the fish in the bowl can't see the water." As more people become cognisant of that water, the opportunities to grow new languages, frameworks, understandings and, eventually, systems grow.

And if we as humans at this point in time see something to be doing harm, don't we have a duty (like Huxley's savage) to shout, "Stop!" In a future that has the capacity for radical change, those who have joined to say "this is a human rights issue" will be part of the think tank that is forced to create plausible alternatives in the void left behind. The movements highlighted influence others, collect like-minded allies, and gain strength together in what is otherwise a lonely invisible world.

Alternative Conceptual Frameworks

Some contemporary thinkers have gone on to offer alternative conceptual frameworks to those created by the medical model, but some alternatives are ideas that have been around for decades, though with very little status. Alternative conceptual frameworks are influenced by discourses that are familiar—ideas such as "attachment," "trauma," "behaviourism," and "occupational therapy."

Whilst many of us may be concerned about previous applications of behaviourism and even its current visibility in the Positive Behaviour Support world, it has gained popularity due to offering a simple, measurable, and generally understood way for people think of those at risk of distress, their immediate social contexts, and what they find rewarding. It is undeniably an alternative, though there is much to be critiqued in relation to consent, individualism, and powerful othering. A viable alternative does not, of course, make it more ethical.

The Power Threat Meaning Framework (2018) offers a philosophical alternative to the medical model, placing emphasis upon sense-making and the way in which power operates in an individual's life and experiences of difficulty. It may be considered constructionist in position whilst offering some purposefully tentative and open-ended ideas or patterns against which people may think about how they have responded to threat. The framework offers the idea that what the medical paradigm calls "symptoms" may be more helpfully thought of as "survival strategies," and places emphasis upon individual narratives rather than professionally imposed understandings. The language of the framework is sensitively informed by ideas relating to trauma, survivor movements, narrative approaches, and the notion of "formulation."

Of course, the relationship between critical philosophical movements, frameworks, and institutional structures is not linear. A Mutual Aid Network could be seen as a high context marker for all community functioning were the capitalist reign to collapse. Whilst not particular visible in the language of mental health, it offers a functional system for sharing, distribution of resource, and the rethinking of discourses of about the value and meaning of "work" and "employment" that could not help but influence the way in which we look at difference, need, and human distress.

Given the enormity of the place of medical model narratives in our culture, the processes required for slow or radical change, and our small place on the planet, it is easy to feel that "there is no point in trying" to talk, think and plan differently. We have spoken to people who share our concerns about human rights issues—the rise in distress and the ineffectiveness of the current regime—who feel that by trying to offer something different to an individual, that is as much as is possible.

We have no idea when things will be different and the "runaway" will crash, but as professionals working in the mental health system, we tend to hold a position that, in the meantime, we will try to connect with the following principles:

- The need to work at the highest context level available to *us*—we can't all be policymakers, writers, politicians, economists, et cetera. We can, however, have different conversations with families, employers, and teams. We can deconstruct the language used in our services and invite the possibility of change.
- The need to retain a curious stance in the face of taken-for-granted narratives or packaged ideas.
- The need to develop personal and professional lenses that are shaped by as broad of a landscape as is possible by engaging with those who have been subject to the power of the current systems and approaches; with those who have different ideas; and with those whose experiences are different from our own by virtue of age, culture, geography and belief systems.
- The need to find and create networks—and join allies who share concerns about the current paradigm but also offer alternative ways of thinking and doing.
- The need to be part of the group that remains open to change, and that plant seeds that may sprout in a desert but will flourish when the fishbowl cracks.

References and Suggested Resources

A Disorder 4 Everyone: Challenging the Culture of Psychiatric Diagnosis (2023). Website. https://www.adisorder4everyone.com

American Psychiatric Association. (1980). *Diagnostic and Statistical Manual of Mental Disorders* (3rd ed.).

AQA. (2021) *AS and A level Psychology Specification.* https://www.aqa.org.uk/subjects/psychology/as-and-a-level/psychology-7181-7182/specification-at-a-glance

Attachment Regulation and Competency Framework (2023). Website. www.arcframework.org

Berger, P. and Luckmann, T. (1966). *The Social Construction of Reality: A Treatise in the Sociology of Knowledge*, New York: Doubleday and Co.

Burr, V. (1995) *An introduction to social constructionism.* London: Routledge.

Campolonghi, S. & Orrù, L. (2023). Psychiatry as a Medical Discipline: Epistemological and Theoretical Issues. *Journal of Theoretical and Philosophical Psychology.* https://doi.org/10.1037/teo0000256.

Carr, E. G., & Horner, R. H. (2007). The Expanding Vision of Positive Behavior Support: Research Perspectives on Happiness, Helpfulness, Hopefulness. Journal of Positive Behavior Interventions, 9(1), 3–14. https://doi.org/10.1177/10983007070090010201

Carter, B., & McGoldrick, M. (Eds.). (1988). *The changing family life cycle: A framework for family therapy* (2nd ed.). Gardner Press.

CaSE: Campaign for Science and Engineering (2022). *A Level and GCSE results analysis 2022.* https://www.sciencecampaign.org.uk/analysis-and-publications/detail/a-level-and-gcse-results-analysis-2022/#:~:text=Five%20of%20the%20top%20ten,%25)%20and%20physics%20(4.7%25).

Council for Evidence Based Psychiatry (2023). Website. www.cepuk.org

Critical Psychiatry Network (2023). Website. https://www.criticalpsychiatry.co.uk

Davies, J. (2021). *Sedated: How Modern Capitalism Created our Mental Health Crisis.* Alantic Books.

Emotions aRe Not Illnesses (ERNI) (2023). Website. www.ernimovement.com

Föreningen Alternativ till Psykofarmaka (2023). Website.
https://www.alternativ-till-psykofarmaka.se

Frances, A. (2013). *Saving normal: An insider's revolt against out-of-control psychiatric diagnosis, DSM-5, Big Pharma, and the medicalization of ordinary life.* William Morrow & Co.

Gergen, K.J. (1985). 'The social constructionist movement in modern psychology', *American Psychologist* 40: 266-275

Gottstein, J.B, Gøtzsche, P.C., Cohen, D., Ruby, C., Myers, F. (2023). *Report on Improving Mental Health Outcomes,* Mad in America Website.

Hearing Voices Network. (2023). Website. https://www.hearing-voices.org

Huxley, A. (1932). *Brave New World.* New York: Harper Brothers.

Johnstone, L. & Boyle, M. with Cromby, J., Dillon, J., Harper, D., Kinderman, P., Longden, E., Pilgrim, D. & Read, J. (2018). *The Power Threat Meaning Framework: Towards the identification of patterns in emotional distress, unusual experiences and troubled or troubling behaviour, as an alternative to functional psychiatric diagnosis.* Leicester: British Psychological Society.

Kawa, S., Giordano, J. A brief historicity of the *Diagnostic and Statistical Manual of Mental Disorders*: Issues and implications for the future of psychiatric canon and practice. *Philos Ethics Humanit Med* 7, 2 (2012). https://doi.org/10.1186/1747-5341-7-2

Kesti, J. (2023). *Coalition to End Forced Psychiatric Drugging.* Website. https://www.youtube.com/playlist?list=PLxpCZsJvbOlEatOnUXkbhKsad MpKfcFw0

Mad in America. Science, Psychiatry and Social Justice website: https://www.madinamerica.com

Mutual Aid Networks: Website of the Humans Global Cooperative: https://mutualaidnetwork.org

Ostrow, L., & Hayes, S. L. (2015). Leadership and characteristics of nonprofit mental health Peer-Run organizations nationwide. *Psychiatric Services,* 66(4), 421–425. https://doi.org/10.1176/appi.ps.201400080

Reidbord, S. (2014). *A Brief History of Psychiatry. Biology and Psychology wrestle for the upper hand.* Psychology Today online.

https://www.psychologytoday.com/gb/blog/sacramento-street-psychiatry/201410/brief-history-psychiatry

Reynolds, V. (2023). Solidarity Talks. Youtube. Website. https://www.youtube.com/channel/UCUgoVQ_rPdHb-3MNyKZQNLQ

Sanderson, H., Thompson, J., & Kilbane, J. (2006). The Emergence of Person-Centred Planning as Evidence-Based Practice. *Journal of Integrated Care,* 14(2), 18–25.

Scull, A (2016). Madness in Historical Perspective. *Canadian Medical Association Journal.* 188(10) 756-758; https://doi.org/10.1503/cmaj.151418

Soteria Network (2023). Website. https://www.soterianetwork.org.uk/

Von Bertalanffy, L. (1950). An outline of general system theory. *British Journal for the Philosophy of Science, 1,* 134–165. https://doi.org/10.1093/bjps/I.2.134

Whittaker, F. (2023). Rise in Child Mental Health Demand Prompts call to Speed up School Support Reforms. Schoolsweek. Website. https://schoolsweek.co.uk/rise-in-child-mental-health-demand-prompts-call-to-speed-up-school-support-reforms/

Young Minds, (2023). Press Releases. *Yearly referrals to young people's mental health services have risen by 53% since 2019.* *https://www.youngminds.org.uk/about-us/media-centre/press-releases/yearly-referrals-to-young-people-s-mental-health-services-have-risen-by-53-since-2019/*

Appendix A

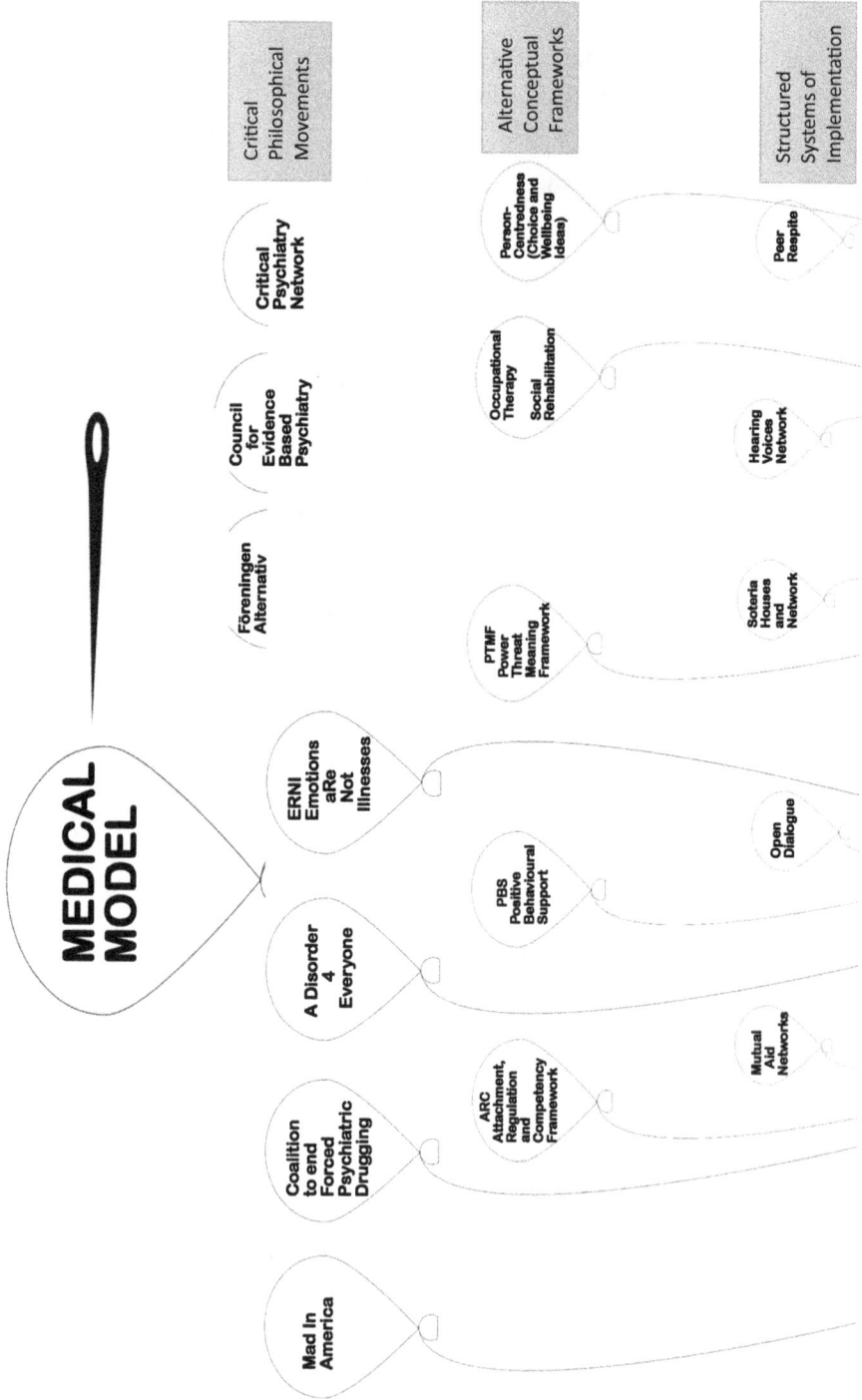

Critical Philosophical Movements

Alternative Conceptual Frameworks

Structured Systems of Implementation

MEDICAL MODEL

Föreningen Alternativ

Council for Evidence Based Psychiatry

Critical Psychiatry Network

ERNI Emotions aRe Not Illnesses

A Disorder 4 Everyone

Coalition to end Forced Psychiatric Drugging

Mad In America

Person-Centredness (Choice and Wellbeing Ideas)

Occupational Therapy Social Rehabilitation

PTMF Power Threat Meaning Framework

PBS Positive Behavioural Support

ARC Attachment, Regulation and Competency Framework

Peer Respite

Hearing Voices Network

Soteria Houses and Network

Open Dialogue

Mutual Aid Networks

Critiquing Contemporary Suicidology

Ian Marsh

Abstract: *In this chapter, the author outlines a number of key assumptions that underpin contemporary suicidology and calls into question the usefulness to practice each of these beliefs. He argues that by unsettling these taken-for-granted assumptions, we can create a space where new ideas and practices may emerge, allowing the field of suicidology to move away from its overreliance on expert notions of individual deficit and pathology and towards more genuinely inclusive, collaborative approaches that can draw on a wider range of knowledge and experiences in relation to suicide prevention.*

Acknowledgement: "Critiquing Contemporary Suicidology" was first published in the book *Critical Suicidology: Transforming Suicide Research and Prevention for the 21st Century* by UBC Press. It has been reprinted here with permission from UBC Press.

A picture held us captive. And we could not get outside it, for it lay in our language and language seemed to repeat it to us inexorably.
– Wittgenstein, Philosophical Investigations

How can we best understand what suicide and suicide prevention are now? By this I mean, how can we think about the ways we have come to conceptualize suicide, the assumptions we make about what it is, what should be done, and by whom? I do not think these are idle, abstract, academic questions, for the truths constructed in language about suicide (in defining what it is, and its causes and solutions, for example) produce many material effects in terms of national and international policies, research priorities and funding, and prevention practices. More subtly, a whole field of experience is formed in relation to authoritative knowledge of suicide – for suicidal people, attempt survivors, and their families and friends, as well as professionals involved in prevention and research.

One way of engaging with these questions is to map the discursive, practice, and institutional resources most commonly brought to bear in constructing "suicide" as a particular sort of issue that requires a certain set of responses in order to manage it. By attempting to map discourses[1] in relation to suicide, we can ask questions such as these:

- How is suicide most commonly talked about?
- What are constructed as the truths of suicide?

Similarly, if we look to map practices, we can ask:

- What is done in relation to suicide? By whom?

And if we look at the institutions most usually involved in conceptualizing and managing suicide as a problem, we can ask:

- Who gets to speak the truth of suicide?
- What happens to people identified as being at risk of suicide?

In attempting to explore the ways in which contemporary truths of suicide have come to be discursively formed, and the related "truth-effects," we are seeking to cast some light on the "kinds of familiar, unchallenged, unconsidered modes of thought [on which] the practices that we accept rest" (Foucault, 1988, p. 155). This form of inquiry has a critical and ethical dimension (Brookfield, 2011), for in looking to identify the assumptions that frame our thinking and determine our actions in relation to suicide, and in asking questions about the effects of so constituting the subject/field based on those assumptions, we can begin a discussion about whether the assumptions identified and examined could usefully be retained, modified, or discarded.

Again, these are not idle or abstract academic discussions, or mere questions of semantics, for how we frame the issue of suicide has material effects from the macro (e.g., in the formulation of national policies and the distribution of large-scale research funds) through to the micro (e.g., in the shaping of the conversational interaction between therapist and client). I would argue that such an inquiry is necessary today in suicidology, for what are in essence assumptions are too often unreflectively taken to be undeniable truths, and the effects of the continual production and reproduction of these truths have remained largely unexamined.

Suicidology Now

In a previous study (Marsh, 2010), I suggested that within contemporary suicidology, there are particular assumptions that dominate research and practice:

1. Suicide is pathological – ("People who kill themselves are mentally ill.")
2. Suicidology is science – ("We will come to the best understanding of suicide through studying it objectively, using the tools of Western medical science.")
3. Suicide is individual – ("Suicidality arises from, and is located within, the 'interiority' of a separate, singular, individual subject.")

These three assumptions could usefully be critiqued in terms of their value and utility. Each is outlined in more detail below. I show how they enter into and guide research and practice by reference to a chapter in *The International Handbook of Suicide Prevention* (Silverman, 2011). I then discuss the limitations unnecessarily placed on our understanding of suicide by the insistence on the truth and necessity of these assumptions, alongside a brief consideration of other possibilities for thought and action that are opened up once one breaks free from such constraints.

Suicide Is Pathological ("People who kill themselves are mentally ill")

This is, I think, the most commonly held (and defended) assumption in suicidology. In many ways it is the dominant assumption that drives research, policy, and practice. Modern suicidology is founded on this claim (Marsh, 2010). It seems to have been implicitly accepted as a truth of the field, albeit sometimes expressed overtly:

In all the major investigations to date, 90 to 95 percent of people who committed suicide had a diagnosable psychiatric illness. (Jamison, 1999, p. 100)

Approximately 95 percent of people who die by suicide experienced a mental disorder at the time of death. (Joiner, 2005, p. 191)

A review of 31 studies involving 15,629 cases of suicide reported that 98% had ICD- or DSM-defined mental disorder. (Kapur and Gask, 2006, p. 260)

The presence of a psychiatric disorder is among the most consistently reported risk factors for suicidal behavior. Psychological autopsy studies reveal that 90–95 percent of the people who die by suicide had a diagnosable psychiatric disorder at the time of the suicide. (Nock et al., 2008, p. 139)

Such a position (that people who kill themselves are mentally ill) tends not to be offered up as one possible reading among many (White and Morris, 2010), but rather as the most important factor, one that should not be overlooked. Kay Redfield Jamison (1999, p. 255), for instance, writes that to ignore "the biological and psychopathological causes and treatments of suicidal behavior is clinically and ethically indefensible."

These claims are often framed as unassailable truths, and they have come to dominate thinking on suicide to such an extent that it is now hard to think otherwise about the issue, or to imagine suicide prevention practices not in some way diagrammed in relation to mental illness and its detection and treatment. Margaret Pabst Battin (2005, p. 173) writes of the "uniform assumption that suicide is the causal product of mental illness, the normatively monolithic assumption seemingly so prevalent in contemporary times," and argues that "the only substantive discussions about suicide in current Western culture have concerned whether access to psychotherapy, or improved suicide-prevention programs, or more effective antidepressant medications should form the principal lines of defense" (p. 164).

Of course it hasn't always been thus. Prior to its modern "medicalization," suicide in Europe had for a long time been thought of and managed predominantly as a sin and a crime (MacDonald and Murphy, 1990; Watt, 2004). With the emergence of a recognizable "psychiatric" profession in England and France from the late eighteenth century, alongside the rise of the asylum as a site of containment and study of the "mentally ill," patient suicide came to be formed as a distinct type of problem (see Esquirol, 1821, for example), and responsibility for the care and management of the suicidal increasingly fell to (or was claimed by) asylum physicians, alienists, "mad doctors," and attendants (Hacking, 1990; Marsh, 2010).

Without doubt this reformulation of suicide as a question of pathology opened up many possibilities for thought and action (as is evidenced by the vast psychiatric, psychological, and psychotherapeutic literature on the subject), but it is perhaps worth noting here the somewhat arbitrary nature of the early-nineteenth-century claiming of suicide for medicine – for there was no discovery of pathological anatomy (Esquirol, 1821; Forbes, 1840), or of diseased instincts or impulses (Prichard, 1840), to support medical claims of expertise. An aetiological link between underlying pathology and signs and symptoms of "suicidality" has been theorized in many different forms since, but empirical support has proved to be elusive.[2]

What *has* been established, though, is a self-authenticating style of reasoning that, in Ian Hacking's terms (1992, p. 132), "generates its own standard of objectivity and its own ideology." Such a "regime of truth" (Foucault, 2002, p. 131), formed around a "compulsory ontology of pathology" (Marsh, 2010), has been productive, but, perhaps due to the unresolved uncertainties associated with the main disciplines involved in suicidology (psychiatry and psychology) with regard to the truth-status and utility of the knowledge it generates, it is a field that has remained somewhat defensive, unreflective, and uncritical in relation to the assumptions under which it operates.

Although there remains a lack of convincing empirical findings of a link between underlying (physical or mental) pathology and suicidal acts (Hjelmeland, Dieserud, Dyregrov, Knizek, and Leenaars, 2012), there is still an obvious strategic logic to the idea that mental illness causes suicide and that we should therefore work to identify and treat those unwell but currently un- or under-treated in order to reduce deaths.[3] It is perhaps the limitations of such an approach that need to be acknowledged more openly, and the assumptions that underpin it more thoroughly held up to critical inquiry.

At the very least, even if operating from within a predominantly health or medical paradigm in relation to suicide, we should question the often-assumed aetiological link between mental illness and suicide, acknowledge that the identification of those at risk remains highly problematic in the absence of observable clinical signs or objective tests (Law, Wong, and Yip, 2010), and admit that the evidence for the effectiveness of interventions once "suicidality" has been identified is sparse (van Praag, 2005; Johannessen, Dieserud, Claussen, and Zahl, 2011; Nock et al., 2013). Such a critical stance can help us cast light on the utility of allowing the assumption that suicide is best understood (or should only be understood) in terms of individual mental illness to dominate suicide theory, research and prevention practices to the extent that it does.

Suicidology Is Science ("We will come to the best understanding of suicide through studying it objectively, using the tools of Western science")

That suicide should be studied "scientifically" has become another truth within suicidology. The opening sentence of the *International Handbook of Suicide Prevention* (2011) has it that "suicidology *is* the science of suicide and suicide prevention" (O'Connor, Platt, and Gordon, 2011, p. 1; emphasis added). In theory, such a stance is unproblematic – if science is taken to be "the intellectual and practical activity encompassing the systematic study of the structure and behaviour of the physical and natural world through observation and experiment" that leads to "a systematically organized body of know- ledge on a particular subject" (Oxford Dictionaries).

In practice, however, what constitutes a "scientific" approach within suicidology has come to be defined in a very narrow way. The editor of one of the main suicide journals, *Suicide and Life-Threatening Behavior*, wrote of the "values, priorities, and procedures" (Joiner, 2011, p. 471) in place at the journal, concluding that it was only by means of "hypothesis testing with fair tests using valid and quantifiable metrics" (Joiner, 2011) that the field of suicidology would advance. Thus, the "accurate translation of complex phenomena into numbers, numbers then amenable to inferential statistical analysis, or, at the very least, descriptive statistical analysis," is taken to be the most desirable approach to studying the subject. In terms of papers that would be considered for publication in the journal, a hierarchy is established whereby

> the fully experimental design is advantaged over the quasi-experimental and the quasi-experimental over the nonexperimental. All other things being equal, the multistudy paper will compete for journal space more successfully than the single study (because of, among other factors, the emphasis on reproducibility), as will the longitudinal more than the cross-sectional, and the quantitative more than the qualitative (Joiner, 2011, p. 471)

This positioning of suicidology as a particular sort of (positivist) scientific venture produces many effects, not the least of which concerns the sorts of research that are deemed legitimate, fundable, and publishable. Hjelmeland and Knizek (2010, p. 74) report that

> in the period 2005–2007, less than 3% of the studies (research articles) published in the three main international suicidological journals had used qualitative methods. In Archives of Suicide Research 1.9% (n = 2), in Crisis 6.6% (n = 4), and in Suicide and Life-Threatening Behavior 2.1% (n = 4) of the studies published had used a qualitative approach, most often in addition to a quantitative one.

Such figures reflect the dominance of quantitative approaches and the search for objective, empirically grounded facts of suicide, and the marginalization of approaches to research that do not promise such certainties. However, whereas the current editor of *Suicide and Life-Threatening Behavior* sees "an insistence on the rigorously and quantitatively scientific ... as a natural next phase for a maturing field of knowledge ... without which genuine progress is distinctly unlikely" (Joiner, 2011, pp.

471–72), for others this retreat into numbers, measuring, and counting is highly problematic.

Jennifer White (2012, p. 48) points to the tendency of suicidology to favour "narrowly defined conceptualizations of 'scientific rigor'" and argues that such an approach "may not give us a deep appreciation or sufficient understanding of the fluctuating, historically contingent, and relationally constructed nature of youth or suicide. Nor do they make room for multiple, emergent and contextually specific possibilities for doing prevention work." Similarly, Heidi Hjelmeland and Birthe Knizek (2011, p. 604) argue that suicidology needs to move away from "simply explaining suicidal behaviour to understanding it" and needs to embrace "pluralistic methodologies to develop new suicidological knowledge." This favouring of "explaining" over "understanding" is, again, not just a purely academic or research issue, but one that has "real world" effects. David Webb (2010, p. 40), from an attempt-survivor perspective, expresses it thus:

> The academic and professional discipline of suicidology strives hard to be an objective science, but in doing so renders itself virtually blind to what are in fact the most "substantial" and important issues being faced by the suicidal person. To me, as someone who has lived with and recovered from persistent suicidal feelings, when I look at the academic discipline of suicidology, it feels as if the expert "suicidologists" are looking at us through the wrong end of their telescope. Their remote, long-distance (objective, empirical) view of suicide transforms the subjective reality and meaning of the suicidal crisis of the self – that is, the actual suicidal person – into almost invisible pinpricks in the far distance.

The knowledge gained through quantitative studies can be important in the attempt to establish an "evidence base" in suicidology, but it is also limited (Hjelmeland, 2011; Hjelmeland and Knizek, 2011). Other forms of knowledge and knowledge production are needed, ones perhaps founded on a different set of assumptions from those currently favoured within suicidology about the nature of suicide and how best to understand and respond to its prevalence and persistence.

Suicide Is Individual ("Suicidality arises from, and is located within, the 'interiority' of a separate, singular, individual subject")

The final assumption that I think underlies most suicide research and strongly informs practice is the belief that suicidality (suicidal thoughts, feelings, and behaviours) arises from, and is located within, the "interiority" of a (separate, singular) individual subject. Michael Kral (1998, p. 229) has talked of the "great origin myth" in suicidology – the implicit notion that "the ultimate origin of suicide, whatever the stressful precursors, lies within the person." Kral (1998, pp. 229–30) argues that:

> Whether examining biological, psychological, or social factors related to suicide, the received explanation has been that the idea of suicide ultimately originates within the person. That is, the conscious decision to end one's life is believed to be some product of an aggregate of personal factors for a given individual ... We believe that if we identify enough of the right individual factors, we might one day be able to predict or prevent suicide. This belief in an individual-centered style of explanation in suicidology holds us powerfully within its frame.

Others have noted the strongly "individualized" way we have come to conceptualize suicide in the West. For Katrina Jaworski (2010, p. 51), the very definition of suicide as "the act of deliberately taking one's own life" already establishes it as something individual in nature: "The definition summons an individual as the author of the act, solely responsible for the act. There is an agent behind the act, recognised as being the one who decides on the act. As such, the deliberate choice decided by the agent appears to be determined largely by the activities of a disembodied mind."

When suicide is defined and explained in this way, such deaths come to be understood as private, individual events largely divorced from issues of social justice, practices of exclusion and oppression, politics, stigma, relations of power, and hate. Suicidality is taken to originate either from an internal mental/psychic space (as in the literature that constitutes suicide as primarily a result of individual psychological or psychiatric disturbance), or from some form of internal bodily pathology (as in, for example, in [neuro]biological accounts), or from a combination of the two. Such "interiorities" are taken to require expert reading by mental health professionals, who look to find and treat ahistorical and acultural signs and symptoms of illness in the individual (Marsh, 2010).

The historical and cultural formation of suicidal subjects cannot be read within such a scheme, and, just as importantly, the historical and cultural resources potentially able to counteract or resist suicide come to be viewed as only marginally salient relative to the identification and treatment of individual mental disorders, abnormalities, or disturbances. Yet as Heidi Hjelmeland (2010, p. 34) makes clear, "suicidal behaviour always occurs and is embedded within a cultural context and no suicidal act is conducted without reference to the prevailing normative standards and attitudes of a cultural community." Later in the chapter I say more about approaches that endeavour to more broadly contextualize the issue of suicide (by drawing on a range of ethical, political, and community-oriented frames of thought), but first I wish to look at an example of how the assumptions discussed above can enter into and guide research and practice.

An Illustration

It's not too hard to see these three assumptions at work in the field of suicidology – in research papers presented at conferences, and in journal articles and textbooks, but also in policy documents (e.g., national suicide prevention strategies) and, most importantly, in practice, where suicide is almost always read as pathological and individual in nature, with medical-scientific language and practices taken to be the best (and, it is often implied, the only) way of conceptualizing and managing the problem.

By way of illustration, I want to look in more detail at one article that, I think, exemplifies the way the assumptions discussed above are embedded in suicidology discourse, and how they are presented as natural and necessary truths.

For the multi-authored *International Handbook of Suicide Prevention* (O'Connor, Platt, and Gordon, 2011), Morton M. Silverman has provided the opening chapter – "Challenges to Classifying Suicidal Ideations, Communications, and Behaviours." That chapter argues that there is a problem in the lack of uniformity in the "terms, definitions and classifications for the range of thoughts, communications, and behaviours that are related to self-injurious behaviours, with or without the intent to die" (Silverman, 2011, p. 9). It reviews these issues from a historical perspective and sets out "current efforts to improve our ability to communicate clearly, consistently, and confidently about suicidal individuals" (p. 9). Finally, "recommendations are made as to the next steps in the process of developing and implementing a standardized nomenclature and classification system for the field of suicidology" (p. 9).

Assumptions about suicide being individual and pathological and about the study of it needing to proceed along scientific/positivist lines are encountered throughout the chapter. For example, Silverman (2011, p. 10) writes that "suicidal behaviour is often undiagnosed, under-treated, or mistreated in clinical settings because it is misunderstood" and that "one of the major difficulties in communicating about suicidal phenomena with our patients and within our discipline (as well as across disciplines) is that we do not speak the same scientific language."

Silverman argues that there is a need for uniformity in language use and in the ways phenomena and behaviours are categorized, and that a lack of standardization is holding back research and prevention efforts. The effects of this drive to uniformity within suicidology strike me as problematic. It seems that what is being worked towards (and Silverman's chapter is not an isolated example of this style of thought) is a narrowing down of the linguistic and practical resources available to us to make sense of, and to engage with, issues around suicide.

This would appear to be driven by a belief that suicide is somehow a singular and stable "thing" or phenomenon and thus readily amenable to singular description. (Silverman [2011, p. 11] writes that the "ongoing debate concerning nomenclature" is perpetuating "the use of multiple terms to refer to the same behaviour.") Alongside this drive towards linguistic uniformity is a desire to seek out "objective" elements of suicide that can be accurately measured, compared, and categorized:

Consensus is required with regard to the development, implementation, and evaluation of clinical and preventive interventions [Silverman, 2006, p. 21]. All the components of the suicidal process then must be identified, labelled, and classified if we are ever to reach the point where we all can share information and observations to help identify and treat truly suicidal individuals and develop interventions to prevent the onset, maintenance, duration, intensity, frequency, and recurrence of suicidal thoughts and behaviours. Classifying individuals on the basis of the intent of their self- injury is a useful scientific and clinical endeavor.

Silverman (2011, p. 14) argues that for this to happen, it is necessary to move away from "our almost total reliance on self-report for understanding and recording such important components of the suicidal process as suicidal thoughts, intent, motivation, planning, accurately remembering and reporting prior life events, assigning significance to life events, appraisal of current stressors, history of prior self-destructive behaviours, etc."

In the conclusions to his chapter, Silverman (2011, p. 22) sets out what he sees as an ideal destination or goal of this endeavour:

An ideal goal is to develop, for example, a classification system similar to that used in oncology, where first a tumour is classified by type of cancer, and then by staging (e.g., based on size, location, degree of invasiveness, extent of metastasis, etc.), which not only informs diagnosis, but also treatment, management, monitoring, and prognosis. In a similar fashion, "staging" criteria for suicidal behaviours might be degree of intent, lethality of method used, likelihood of rescue, degree of planning (impulsivity), and presence and status of psychiatric or medical illness. Scales or ranking systems can be developed to measure these elements and provide clinicians and researchers with a richly nuanced approach to classifying the full range of suicidal thoughts, communications, and behaviours.

Uniformity of language use, it is argued, could potentially (and usefully) lead to the development of scales and ranking systems to objectively classify types and stages of suicidal thoughts, communications, and behaviours. Suicidal behaviour could thus be read as a form of individual pathology amenable to the sort of categorization found in "mainstream" medicine, which would then inform "treatment, management, monitoring, and prognosis" (p. 22). Such a goal has obvious appeal, but for me, it also raises certain questions.

Imagine for a moment being told you had a "type 2, stage 4 suicidal state" that came with a "30% chance of survival over 2 years" or some such like. What would you do with that information? What effects would that information have on you? And at a more general level, how amenable are "suicide," "suicidal behaviours," and "the suicidal process" to singular, objective descriptions and categorizations? Is suicidal behaviour analogous to cancer? Is suicide prevention that similar to oncology?

The medical analogy Silverman is drawing on in his chapter is certainly a powerful one. The suggestion is that "suicidal behaviours" could be (with a sufficiently uniform use of language) objectively measured and categorized as if they were tumours, and thus not only "diagnosis" "but also treatment, management, monitoring, and prognosis" (2011, p. 22) of a suicidal individual could proceed along similar lines to those of a cancer patient. For the comparison to work, however, we have to take the "degree of intent, lethality of method used, likelihood of rescue, degree of planning (impulsivity), and presence and status of psychiatric or medical illness" as analogous to the "size, location, degree of invasiveness, extent of metastasis" of a tumour.

But most tumours present as visible and measurable "things" that can (with the right equipment) be observed, measured, and categorized in a way that intentions, likelihood of rescue, impulsivity, and the presence or absence of psychiatric illnesses cannot, and I don't think that is simply a problem of uniformity of language use. The elements that constitute the stages of a tumour, being observable and measurable, offer a degree of certainty and predictability of outcome that does not map well against the mutable and contingent elements of the "suicidal process."

For example, the changeable social, cultural, and relational elements of a person's life surely have effects on the "suicidal process" far in excess of what they would have on the progress and outcome of a tumour (e.g., reconciliation with spouse, finding a new job). It is the same with the meanings given to events and situations by the clients themselves. It is suggested that because such elements cannot be "objectively" observed and measured, they should be set aside in favour of factors that can be. The danger is that if we exclude such elements from any conceptualizing and categorizing of the "suicidal process," we will lose sight of the importance of these contextual, relational, or "subjective" factors, and this can have effects beyond research.

It is often those more subjective, contextual, and relational factors, by dint of their transience and contingency or changeableness, that allow for hope to be part of any intervention with a suicidal person, and our language should remain open and flexible enough to allow for those to be part of the conversation. By excluding from our vocabulary terms that fall outside the medical-scientific, we would be reducing the possibilities for thought and action available to the field of prevention. By insisting that suicide be read as an issue primarily (or even exclusively) of individual pathology, as something analogous to oncology, we would be limiting the field to an unnecessarily impoverished and decontextualized set of discursive resources.

Conclusion

This chapter has suggested that three assumptions dominate suicidology now: that suicide is pathological, that suicidology is (or should be) science, and that suicide is individual. These assumptions, to paraphrase Wittgenstein (1953), lie in our language, and the medical-scientific language of individual pathology and deficit is repeated inexorably. As Judith Butler (2004, p. 309) notes, "certain kinds of practices which are designed to handle certain kinds of problems produce, over time, a settled domain of ontology as their consequence, and this ontological domain, in turn, constrains our understanding of what is possible." This is the case with suicidology, where the (somewhat arbitrary) early-nineteenth-century claiming of suicide for medicine, and the introduction of "medical"/

psychiatric practices (identification, diagnosis, and treatment of "cases" within a medical setting), theorizing (relationship between various, and contingent, categories of pathology and suicide), and forms of inquiry (epidemiological studies, case studies) have led to a "settled domain of ontology," but one that is highly problematic.

Medical-scientific discourse has undoubtedly been productive in terms of generating theories, monographs, conferences, journals, academic careers, and so on, but it also limits and restricts, to a troublesome degree, what can be authoritatively said and done in relation to the issue of suicide. Silverman's proposals (analyzed above), while undoubtedly well-meant and thoughtfully considered, exemplify what suicidology has become and where it is heading (unless checked). As the field becomes further enmeshed in practices of categorizing, measuring, and counting, it risks losing the means to understand and engage with the complex and changing contexts in which suicidal individuals are formed and suicides occur.

However, the assumptions, beliefs, and formulations that underlie thought and practice in relation to suicide are such that redescription is always possible and that we can draw on alternative vocabularies and constructs, setting aside assumptions not taken to be useful and formulating issues in ways not bound by them. In seeking to develop "a nomenclature that is free of bias – philosophical, theoretical, biological, sociological, political, religious, cultural, etc." (2011, p. 13) – Silverman frames the plurality of language resources available for constituting our understanding of suicide as problematic in that they somehow compromise objective scientific description.

By drawing on these diverse and multiple discourses in thoughtful and creative ways, we might begin to construct understandings of, and responses to, suicide that are culturally congruent and meaningful and that are able to deal with the fluidity and contingency of the cultural production of suicide. We might move beyond the idea that the language we employ is somehow representative of reality, ideologically neutral, and without constituting effects.

We might begin to reflect on the ways our language practices work in productive and ideological ways, sensitive to how language produces effects. As an example of this, in her paper "Wasted Lives: The Social Dynamics of Shame and Youth Suicide," Simone Fullagar (2003, p. 301) points to the ways in which "authoritative" accounts of suicide, based on assumptions of individual pathology, can have unintended negative consequences, both in terms of "privatizing" such acts (i.e., denying the social contexts in which they are created) and in terms of constituting subjects in ways that can exacerbate rather than relieve suffering:

> Discourses of mental health and illness within suicide policy and prevention programmes actually work to invisiblize the effects of culture on the embodied self. The emphasis on diagnosis and treatment of suicidal ideation, depression and self-harm as mental health problems may actually participate in the process of subjectification whereby the subject "sees" their own self as pathological and hence shameful.

Today, many researchers and clinicians are attempting to redirect the field of suicidology away from its reliance on individualized, pathology-based ways of constructing and responding to the issue (e.g., Kral and Idlout, 2009; White and Morris, 2010; White, 2012). They accept and embrace a multiplicity of descriptions, they strive to be inclusive in their research designs and interventions, they value conversational approaches over expert monologue, and they look to build solutions from the ground up rather than impose them from above.

These approaches are noticeably community (rather than service) owned and led; the experts (including "at risk" groups, such as youth, mental health service users, and prisoners, as well as "front line" practitioners) are taken to be in the community and are looking to build collaborative, relationally focused solutions founded on strengths-based (rather than deficit) models.

How we think and act in relation to suicide is necessarily grounded in the assumptions we make about what it is and how it should be studied, understood, and responded to. By critically engaging with these assumptions, paying close attention to the context in which they have come to be formed, and analyzing the effects of constituting the issue in those ways, we can ask questions about the value and utility of current, dominant ways of constructing the subject (Brookfield, 2011).

From here we can begin to imagine and explore possibilities other than those the present seems to impose on us. We have come to think about suicide almost solely in terms of individual mental illness and risk, and as a consequence "an individualised, 'internalised,' pathologised, depoliticised and ultimately tragic form of suicide has come to be produced, with alternative interpretations of acts of self-accomplished death marginalised or foreclosed" (Marsh, 2010, p. 219). But if suicide is a problem, it is as much a social, ethical, and political issue as a mental health one, and we need to be able to draw upon a wide range of discursive resources in order to adequately frame and respond to its possibility or actuality.

Notes

[1] Sets of "meanings, metaphors, representations, images, stories, statements and so on that in some way together produce a particular version of events" (Burr, 1995, p. 48).

[2] It is a field, however, that draws much on anticipatory or proleptic discourse – the sense that we are on the cusp of a medical/scientific breakthrough in relation to the etiology of suicide has been a feature of psychiatric writings on the subject for nearly two centuries.

[3] As an example of this style of thought, Isacsson, Rich, and De Leo (2003, p. 457) argue that "depression is a necessary cause of most suicides. Based on this proposition, it has been suggested that effective suicide prevention must focus on improving identification and treatment of depression in the population."

References

Battin, M.P. (2005). *Ending life: Ethics and the way we die*. Oxford: Oxford University Press.

Brookfield, S. (2011). *Teaching for critical thinking: Tools and techniques to help students question their assumptions*. San Francisco: Jossey-Bass.

Burr, V. (1995). *An introduction to social constructionism*. London: Routledge. http://dx.doi.org/10.4324/9780203299968

Butler, J. (2004). What is critique? In S. Salih (Ed.), *The Judith Butler reader* (302–22). Oxford: Blackwell.

Esquirol, J.-E.D. (1821) Suicide, in *Dictionaire des sciences médicales: Par une société de médecins et de chirurgiens* (53rd ed.). Paris: Panckoucke.

Foucault, M. (1988). "Practicing criticism, or Is it really important to think?" May 30–31, 1981. Didier Eribon interview. In L. Kritzman, *Foucault, politics, philosophy, culture*. New York and London: Routledge.

–. (2002). *Essential works of Foucault (1954–1984): Vol. 3, Power*. J.D. Faubion (Ed.). London: Penguin.

Fullagar, S. (2003). Wasted lives: The social dynamics of shame and youth suicide. *Journal of Sociology (Melbourne, Vic.), 39*(3), 291–307. http://dx.doi.org/ 10.1177/0004869003035076

Hacking, I. (1990). *The taming of chance*. Cambridge: Cambridge University Press.

Hjelmeland, H. (2010). Cultural research in suicidology: Challenges and opportunities. *Suicidology Online*, 1, 34–52.

–. (2011). Cultural context is critical in suicide research and prevention. *Crisis, 32*(2), 61–64. http://dx.doi.org/10.1027/0227-5910/a000097

Hjelmeland, H., Dieserud, G., Dyregrov, K., Knizek, B.L., and Leenaars, A.A. (2012). Psychological autopsy studies as diagnostic tools: Are they methodologically flawed? *Death Studies, 36*(7), 605–26. http://dx.doi.org/10.1080/07481187.2011.584015

Hjelmeland, H., and Knizek, B.L. (2010). Why we need qualitative research in suicidology. *Suicide and Life-Threatening Behavior, 40*(1), 74–80. http://dx.doi. org/10.1521/suli.2010.40.1.74

–. (2011). What kind of research do we need in suicidology today? In R.C. O'Connor, S. Platt, and J. Gordon (Eds.), *International handbook of suicide prevention: Research, policy, and practice* (591–608). Chichester, England: John Wiley. http://dx.doi.org/10.1002/9781119998556.ch34

Isacsson, G., Rich, C.L., and De Leo, D. (2003). Getting closer to suicide prevention. *British Journal of Psychiatry, 182*(5), 457–58. http://dx.doi.org/10.1192/ bjp.182.5.4547

Jamison, K.R. (1999). *Night falls fast: Understanding suicide*. New York: Vintage Books.

Jaworski, K. (2010). The gender-ing of suicide. *Australian Feminist Studies, 25*(63), 47–61. http://dx.doi.org/10.1080/08164640903499752

Johannessen, H.A., Dieserud, G., Claussen, B., and Zahl, P.-H. (2011). Changes in mental health services and suicide mortality in Norway: An ecological study. *BMC Health Services Research, 11*(1), 68. http://dx.doi.org/10.1186/ 1472-6963-11-68

Joiner, T. (2005). *Why people die by suicide*. Cambridge, MA: Harvard University Press.

Joiner, T., Jr. (2011). Editorial: Scientific rigor as the guiding heuristic for SLTB's editorial stance. *Suicide and Life-Threatening Behavior, 41*(5), 471–73. http://dx.doi.org/10.1111/j.1943-278X.2011.00056.x

Kapur, N., and Gask, L. (2006). Introduction to suicide and self-harm. *Psychiatry, 5*(8), 259–62. http://dx.doi.org/10.1053/j.mppsy.2006.05.004

Kral, M.J. (1998). Suicide and the internalization of culture: Three questions. *Transcultural Psychiatry, 35*(2), 221–33.

Kral, M.J., and Idlout, L. (2009). Community wellness and social action in the Canadian Arctic: Collective agency as subjective well-being. In L.J. Kirmayer and G. Valaskakis (Eds.), *Healing traditions: The mental health of Aboriginal peoples in Canada* (315–34). Vancouver, BC: University of British Columbia Press.

Law, Y., Wong, P.W.C., and Yip, P.S.F. (2010). Suicide with psychiatric diagnosis and without utilization of psychiatric service. *BMC Public Health, 10*(1), 431. http://dx.doi.org/10.1186/1471-2458-10-431

MacDonald, M., and Murphy, T.R. (1990). *Sleepless souls: Suicide in early modern England*. Oxford: Oxford University Press.

Marsh, I. (2010). *Suicide: Foucault, history, and truth*. Cambridge: Cambridge University Press.

Nock, M.K., Borges, G., Bromet, E.J., Cha, C.B., Kessler, R.C., and Lee, S. (2008). Suicide and suicidal behavior. *Epidemiologic Reviews, 30*(1), 133–54. http:// dx.doi.org/10.1093/epirev/mxn002

Nock, M.K., Green, J.G., Hwang, I., McLaughlin, K.A., Sampson, N.A., Zaslavsky, A.M., and Kessler, R.C. (2013). Prevalence, correlates, and treatment of life- time suicidal behavior among adolescents. *JAMA Psychiatry, 70*(3), 300–10.

O'Connor, R.C., Platt, S., and Gordon, J. (Eds.). (2011). *International handbook of suicide prevention: Research, policy, and practice*. Chichester, UK: John Wiley and Sons. http://dx.doi.org/10.1002/9781119998556

Prichard, J.C. (1840). Suicide. In A. Tweedie (Ed.), *A system of practical medicine, comprised in a series of original dissertations* (120–23). London: Whittaker and Co.

Silverman, M.M. (2006). The language of suicidology. *Suicide and Life- Threatening Behavior, 36*(5), 519–32.

–. (2011). Challenges to classifying suicidal ideations, communications, and behaviors. In R.C.

O'Connor, S. Platt, and J. Gordon (Eds.), *International handbook of suicide prevention: Research, policy, and practice* (9–25). Chichester, UK: Wiley/Blackwell.

van Praag, H. (2005). The resistance of suicide: Why have antidepressants not reduced suicide rates? In K. Hawton (Ed.), *Prevention and treatment of suicidal behaviour: From science to practice* (239–60). Oxford: Oxford University Press. http://dx.doi.org/10.1093/med/9780198529767.003.0014

Watt, J. (Ed.). (2004). *From sin to insanity: Suicide in early modern Europe*. Ithaca, NY: Cornell University Press.

Webb, D. (2010). *Thinking about suicide: Contemplating and comprehending the urge to die*. Ross-on-Wye, UK: PCCS Books Ltd.

White, J. (2012). Youth suicide as a "wild problem": Implications for prevention practice. *Suicidology Online, 3*, 42–50. http://www.suicidology-online.com/pdf/ SOL-2012-3-42-50.pdf

White, J., and Morris, J. (2010). Precarious spaces: Risk, responsibility, and uncertainty in school-based suicide prevention programs. *Social Science and Medicine, 71*(12), 2187–94. http://dx.doi.org/10.1016/j.socscimed.2010.09.046

Winslow, Forbes. (1840). *The anatomy of suicide*. London: Henry Renshaw. Wittgenstein, L. (1953). *Philosophical investigations* (G.E.M. Anscombe, Trans.). Oxford: Blackwell.

The Power Threat Meaning Framework and Eating Distress

Jo Watson

Abstract: *In this chapter, I argue that The Power Threat Meaning Framework could offer an infinitely more hopeful and respectful way of responding to eating distress than the traditional illness narrative imposed by psychiatry. In the words of Lucy Johnstone and Mary Boyle, lead authors of the PTMF: "The Power Threat Meaning Framework can be used as a way of helping people to create more hopeful narratives or stories about their lives and the difficulties they have faced or are still facing, instead of seeing themselves as blameworthy, weak, deficient or 'mentally ill'."*

Acknowledgement: The chapter below is updated from a piece written by me and the late great Paula J. Caplan, PhD titled "Why Must People Pathologize Eating Problems?". It was originally published on madinamerica.com and republished on madintheuk.com in February 2020.

What is the Power Threat Meaning Framework?

The Power Threat Meaning Framework, published by the British Psychological Society[1,2] in 2018 and co-produced with survivors of the psychiatric system, is a new perspective on why people sometimes experience a whole range of forms of distress, confusion, fear, despair, and troubled or troubling behaviour. It is an alternative to the more traditional models based on psychiatric diagnosis. It applies not just to people who

---

[1] Johnstone, L. & Boyle, M. with Cromby, J., Dillon, J., Harper, D., Kinderman, P., Longden, E., Pilgrim, D. & Read, J. (2018). *The Power Threat Meaning Framework: Overview*. Leicester: British Psychological Society

[2] https://www.pccs-books.co.uk/products/a-straight-talking-introduction-to-the-power-threat-meaning-framework-an-alternative-to-psychiatric-diagnosis

have been in contact with the mental health or criminal justice systems, but to all of us.

The Framework summarises and integrates a great deal of evidence about the role of various kinds of power in people's lives; the kinds of threat that misuses of power pose to us; and the ways we have learned as human beings to respond to threat. In traditional mental health practice, these threat responses are sometimes called 'symptoms'. The Framework also looks at how we make sense of these difficult experiences, and how messages from wider society can increase our feelings of shame, self-blame, isolation, fear, and guilt.

The main aspects of the Framework are summarised in these questions, which can apply to individuals, families, or social groups:

- 'What has happened to you?' (How is **Power** operating in your life?)
- 'How did it affect you?' (What kind of **Threats** does this pose?)
- 'What sense did you make of it?' (What is the **Meaning** of these situations and experiences to you?)
- 'What did you have to do to survive?' (What kinds of **Threat Responses** are you using?)

In addition, the two questions below help us think about what skills and resources people might have, and how we might pull all these ideas and responses together into a personal narrative or story:

- 'What are your strengths?' (What access to **Power resources** do you have?)
- 'What is your story?' (How does all this fit together?)

The Framework describes the many different strategies people use, from automatic bodily reactions to deliberately-chosen ways of coping with overwhelming emotions, in order to survive and protect themselves and meet their core needs. It suggests a wide range of ways that may help people move forward. For some people, this may be therapy or other standard interventions including (if they help someone to cope) psychiatric drugs.

For others, the main needs will be for practical help and resources, perhaps along with peer support, art, music, exercise, nutrition, community activism and so on. Underpinning all this, the Framework offers a new perspective on distress which takes us beyond the individual and shows that we are all part of a wider struggle for a fairer society.

In addition, the Framework offers a way of thinking about culturally-specific understandings of distress without seeing them through a Western diagnostic model. It encourages respect for the many creative and non-medical ways of supporting people around the world, and the varied forms of narrative and healing practices that are used across cultures.

Current understandings of eating distress

A recent issue of the Sunday *New York Times* (February 7, 2020) had a full-page essay[3] in its "Modern Love" series in which the writer Lauren Covalucci, an intelligent and self-aware woman, describes having been shamed since age three in her ballet class because her tights dug into her waist. At age 13, she writes, "my body had stretched and thinned" and her teacher said to her, "You finally look like a dancer."

You might think that would be enough to convince her that such intolerable pressures – which pervade not only the ballet studio but the wider societies of many countries across the globe – are unconscionable and that something is wrong with the perpetrators of those pressures, not with those who are made to feel horribly inadequate and even to hate themselves.

Sadly, Covalucci reports that after she began feeling better about her body thanks to being in a relationship with a man who treated her well – "Another person's comfort with you can make you forget your discomfort with yourself," she says – her therapist announced that she had an "eating disorder." The result of that diagnosis was despair: "That's when I really plummeted…. I spent mornings on the floor in a corner…wailing because I couldn't speak in complete sentences anymore and my brain, my beautiful, Harvard-trained brain wouldn't work right." As psychologist

---

[3] https://www.nytimes.com/2020/02/07/style/the-unhealthy-math-of-skinny-pretty-good.html

Michael Cornwall has written[4], assigning someone a psychiatric diagnosis is the "infliction of what amounts to a medical curse."

Covalucci writes that, eventually, she got better. And although she started taking psychiatric drugs that she says helped, it was the ongoing love and respect of her partner that made a huge difference. (She later mentions Prozac, which often causes weight gain, and reports that she has become "fat" and is trying to have a positive attitude about that.) Even when at one point her partner mentions that she has gained weight because of his loving attitude toward her, "The words lost their venom coming from him."

What would have helped, she says, is if her therapist had not told her she had an eating *disorder*, thus making it seem like she was "mentally ill," that there was some kind of internal, individual difficulty she had rather than that she was responding to terrible pressures from her ballet teacher and society in general.

Given that the societal factors leading girls and women to panic about their weight are crystal clear, why didn't her therapist address that with her instead of doing the most harmful thing, classifying her as mentally ill? That, too, would have been helpful, as the work of Prof. Carla Rice,[5] former director of the Body Image Project at Women's College Hospital in Toronto showed decades ago.

Once girls and women come to understand that they have been acting out impossibly strict societal standards with regard to eating and that their often-distorted images of how they look have resulted from those standards, it is easier for them to begin to challenge them, keeping them in acutely conscious view, and to find other ways to feel good about themselves.

Indeed, why is it that so many people, even some astute critics of the traditional mental health system who are happy to challenge the pathologizing of emotional distress generally, cling uncritically to the term

---

[4] https://www.madinamerica.com/2017/09/psychiatric-diagnosis-impact-medical-curse/
[5] https://family.uoguelph.ca/people/carla-rice

and concept of "eating disorders"? We come across it all the time and are genuinely confused and frustrated.

A critical omission

Those who challenge psychiatric diagnoses overall usually do so because, on the whole, they lack scientific foundation, certainly lack scientific validity, and are, in fact, constructs invented by committees of people with vested interests![6] Unlike physical illnesses such as diabetes and cancer, there are not, never have been, and are never likely to be objective tests for the so-called psychiatric illnesses.

Critics of psychiatric diagnoses generally readily acknowledge that, for instance, "Borderline Personality Disorder," "Schizophrenia," and "Attention-Deficit/Hyperactivity Disorder" are constructs without biological basis, and have been invented and promoted by a collective of powerful people with questionable objectives that are mainly concerned with increasing their profits, power, and territory.

It is alarming that, too often, "eating disorders" diagnoses have been left out of the critical dialogue, leading to a bizarre situation in which almost every class of psychiatric "disorder" is challenged except this one. Why is it alarming? Why, indeed, would the pathologizing of emotional distress that involves food, eating, and body image be any more acceptable than the pathologizing of emotional distress that gives rise to obsessive thinking, dissociative experiences, or suicidal thoughts and actions?

The concept of "eating disorders" is just as dubious as all of the other so-called "disorders." It is just as much a construct, and it is no more justified to call it "pathological" than, for instance, "PTSD."

Traditional mental health professionals have capitalized in many ways on pathologizing socially created problems, and the "eating disorders" concept does this especially blatantly given the well-documented ways that patriarchal society puts intolerable pressure on girls and women to believe

[6] Caplan, P. J. (1995). *They Say You're Crazy: How the World's Most Powerful Psychiatrists Decide Who's Normal.* Da Capo Press.

they can never be too thin; persuading them that if they weigh "too much," they will be unattractive and devalued by men, specifically, and by society, generally. In the process, it has become unusual for girls and women to be comfortable with their bodies *even when they become dangerously thin.*

So why do some people who otherwise challenge "mental disorders" claim that the label "eating disorders" is legitimate and must be retained? One argument is, "It's a biological problem, fundamentally physiological!" But the fact that depriving oneself of or bingeing on food has physical *consequences* no more justifies calling such behavior psychiatrically disordered than it would justify creating the concept "sprained ankle disorder."

Like most people who take comfort in being psychiatrically labeled, some women and men may suppose that the therapist gave them a label because he or she believes they are suffering. But that validation could just as easily be achieved by the statement, "I believe you are suffering," which would not add to their burden by conveying the notion that they are also "sick."

Besides masking the powerful social factors causing eating problems, to diagnose someone with an eating "disorder" is to make it extremely likely that they will be told something is wrong with their brain and that they need psychiatric drugs. Also, because severe restriction of food can have, at worst, fatal effects, caring family members may understandably agree to have the diagnosed person hospitalized and will sometimes even ask for this. But once hospitalized, in far too many cases the person is increasingly medicated and stripped of their sense of agency.

Case study

Consider the not unusual case of a teenage girl who had starved herself in reaction to her parents' ignoring her pleas that they should get a divorce because she could not bear their constant fighting and her father's demeaning of her mother. Her parents resisted, though both longed to be out of the marriage instead of staying together "for the daughter's sake." Talk about turning her reality upside down!

When she was hospitalized in a psychiatric ward, her therapist advised her parents to forbid her to participate in the extracurricular activities she adored, the very activities where her immersion in the arts and her warm friendships were important in giving her strength to endure her difficult home life. Allowing her to go home on a brief visit, the therapist also told the parents, "If you put 15 grapes on her plate, you have to make her eat all 15 grapes."

Thus, she was deprived of her sources of emotional sanctuary and infantilized, just as her parents' and the doctor's pathologizing of *her* as the source of the problem involved a stunning lack of respect and regard for the suffering caused by her home situation. And all the while, no one addressed the forces that led to her using starvation as a coping mechanism: her father's demeaning views of real women and society's message that the route to happiness and regard is through weight loss. Many unhappy women go on strict diets when they feel that important parts of their lives are beyond their control, but dieting is something they *can* control.

What would likely have helped that young woman would have been if, first, her parents and therapists had really listened to the pain that her parents' awful relationship and her father's demeaning view of women were causing her—and then had worked with her to find ways to reduce that pain. Both parents could have considered her needs rather than the abstract principle that even a terrible marriage should continue because it is better for the child than a divorce.

The psychiatrist could also have helped the daughter spend more time and energy in rewarding activities like her choir practice rather than forbidding them unless she ate what the therapist considered to be "enough." He could also have helped her find ways to gain a sense of agency given how helpless she was feeling, living with parents who were miserable and a father who demeaned women. And he could have helped her find ways to earn friendship, love, and respect other than by trying to become impossibly thin.

The Power Threat Meaning Framework could offer an infinitely more hopeful and respectful way of responding to eating distress than the traditional illness narrative imposed by psychiatry. It shows that "what may be called psychiatric symptoms are understandable responses to often very adverse environments and that these responses, both evolved and socially influenced, serve protective functions and demonstrate the human capacity for meaning-making and agency." In relation to eating problems, it would suggest that these can be seen as a reaction to difficult experiences—as a threat response, a way of surviving the intolerable, that is understandable in the context of someone's life.

The Framework is ultimately about the process of that sense being made, and surely few would disagree that there are always reasons, always stories behind every type of eating problem. The adverse environments of the woman and the girl described above were clear, and starving themselves was in both cases a way to try to take some control over how people evaluated and treated them. As such, helping them understand that the adverse factors in their environment were unreasonable, inhumane, and harmful; to consider other ways to think about themselves; and to find different, life-enhancing, life-enriching, self-respecting, safe ways to feel a sense of belonging, being loved, and caring for themselves would have been natural consequences of a Power Threat Meaning approach to so-called eating disorders.

The PTMF has attracted widespread interest not just in the UK but across the world—and has been translated into several languages, with more planned. Perhaps the narrative is beginning to change? I remember too many reasons and stories, just as I remember too many women who I've come across over the years who had internalized the belief that they had/have an "eating disorder." Just like any other psychiatric diagnosis, it has all too often robbed them of their power, taken away their agency, and stolen their hope. The diagnosis of "eating disorder" in all its forms is as much a curse of psychiatry as any of its numerous others. Isn't it time we called it that?

In Memoriam

Some words about Paula. Paula Joan Caplan, PhD—a prolific writer, playwright, and social activist—was one of the most prominent critics of psychiatry and its diagnoses. She was also my friend. Many years before the day I met her in a Downtown Manhattan café, I loved her through her courageous change-making work that had so massively influenced my life—but meeting her, feeling her support, encouragement and love was a pure blessing.

Paula's work in terms of publications, contribution to academia and her tireless activism was simply extraordinary. The publication of *They Say You're Crazy: How the World's Most Powerful Psychiatrists Decide Who's Normal* is a truth-telling game-changer in the thinking around how we understand psychiatry that came directly from her experience as a consultant to DSM committees and her bravery in speaking out about what she discovered. No one else has exposed the deceit and corruption in quite the same way. And her masterpiece of the play Call Me Crazy brought these ideas to new audiences again and again.

In July 2021, we lost a true warrior. Her legacy is immense and the example that she left to always challenge psychiatry's lies and injustice inspires me every day.

Expanding Suicidological Training and Practice: A Critical Place for Clinical Social Work

Josh Bylotas[1] and Arnoldo Cantú

Abstract: *Suicide is one of the leading causes of death across demographics in the United States. Despite significant efforts and resources invested to address this issue, the overall suicide rate for some populations continues to increase. The academic discipline of suicidology is said to be multidisciplinary, yet social work contributes comparatively less than other fields to the cumulative body of suicide research. This is despite social work's significant presence in the provision of mental health and suicide prevention services. In addition, contemporary practices addressing acute suicidality framed by the biomedical model of mental health typically support coercive practices - such as involuntary hospitalization for individuals at risk of attempting suicide - with questionable effectiveness. This chapter advocates for the expansion of social work research and practice within the field of suicidology so that it may align more consistently with social work values. Additionally, it briefly reviews critical perspectives and alternative intervention strategies consistent with the principles and ethics of the social work profession. It concludes with a call to action for the field to contribute more to the suicidological body of research and practice in innovative ways, adding to the non-pathologizing interventions and frameworks already developed.*

Author's Note[1]: The views expressed in this article are those of the author and do not reflect the official policy or position of the United States Air Force, Department of Defense, or the U.S. Government.

Introduction

Suicide is a leading cause of death in the United States and a public health crisis of escalating proportions (Hedegaard et al., 2021). In 2021, suicide occurred at an age-adjusted rate of 14.4 per 100,000 people, with an estimated 132 suicide deaths occurring daily (American Foundation for Suicide Prevention [AFSP], 2023). To stem the tide of rising suicide rates, serious financial, programmatic, and clinical efforts have been poured into preventing and treating these deaths of despair over the course of the past fifty years (Barnhorst et al., 2021).

Yet, despite these efforts, appreciable change has yet to occur, with the overall rate of suicide increasing for many populations (Curtin et al., 2016). Our collective ability to predict who will die by suicide, and when, remains poor. As former director of the National Institute of Mental Health (NIMH), Thomas Insel (Rogers, 2017), pointedly stated while summarizing his career there:

> I spent 13 years at NIMH really pushing on the neuroscience and genetics of mental disorders, and when I look back on that I realize that while I think I succeeded at getting lots of really cool papers published by cool scientists at fairly large costs---I think $20 billion---I don't think we moved the needle in reducing suicide, reducing hospitalizations, improving recovery for the tens of millions of people who have mental illness. (para. 6)

Why has progress in preventing suicide death stalled, despite notable advances in understanding and attention? The field of suicidology is both broad and multidisciplinary, ranging from public health to psychiatry to name a few of the disciplines engaged in this work. Among those engaged in suicide prevention, social workers stand on the front lines of prevention work as they represent the largest percentage of clinical mental health providers in the United States (Heisler, 2018). Given their substantial role in the delivery of mental health services, social workers have the potential to create meaningful change across the spectrum of suicide prevention.

Surprisingly, however, social work has been underrepresented in the production of research (Maple, 2016). Additionally, social work education programs have (largely) failed to adequately train students in suicide prevention (Feldman & Freedenthal, 2006), leading to junior professionals feeling ill-equipped to implement social work methods in suicide prevention practice (Ruth et al., 2012). To advance social work's potential contribution to suicide prevention, it is necessary to acknowledge the various ways in which social work has been complicit in the stagnation of prevention efforts and highlight opportunities to move the field forward.

We assert the multifaceted central problem: social work has co-opted and embraced as a handmaiden a psychiatric model that 1) portrays suicidality as resulting from mental illness, which contributes to a 2) medicalized response that favors psychiatric interventions like medication and hospitalization, further perpetuating shame, stigma, and perceived hopelessness. This adoption of the biomedical model runs counter to existing suicidological research, generally accepted prevention practice, and social work values.

A contextual approach to understanding and preventing suicide is needed, incorporating such frameworks are already broadly recognized in concepts such as social determinants of health and ecological systems theory (Bronfenbrenner, 1979; Cramer & Kapusta, 2017; World Health Organization, 2008) or public health concerns like homelessness, poverty, and cycles of violence. Additionally, alternative non-medicalized and non-coercive responses to suicidality that prioritize harm reduction over prediction provide promising signposts for future practice.

To that end, the purpose of this chapter is to identify challenges embedded within contemporary suicide prevention and intervention as practiced by social workers, highlight ways in which these approaches may contribute to persistent stigma and perpetuate stagnant prevention efforts running contrary to the field's self-proclaimed designation of being "anti-oppressive," and offer varying perspectives and methods as alternatives to current practice.

In the context of this writing, the psychiatric model of care and the biomedical model are used interchangeably. A central tool employed by the biomedical model is the *Diagnostic and Statistical Manual of Mental Disorders,* or *DSM,* purported to be an "authoritative volume that defines and classifies mental disorders to improve diagnoses, treatment, and research" by the American Psychiatric Association (APA) (APA, n.d., para. 2). When applied within the field of mental health, the biomedical model and *DSM* posit that human suffering stems primarily from biological factors gone awry *within* the individual which are, subsequently, conceptualized as mental disorders (Fritscher, 2020), effectively pathologizing the individual. However, a consequence of this model is the discounting of contextual and environmental factors that influence suicidality.

Together, these approaches and perspectives comprise a contemporary approach to suicide prevention that often supports the involuntary hospitalization of individuals who are perceived as being an imminent risk of harm to themselves (VA/DoD, 2019). However, despite the normalization of these treatment practices as a trusted intervention for the suicidal person, the efficacy of inpatient hospitalization remains in question at best and harmful at worst (Gomory et al., 2011; Jordan & McNiel, 2020; Kirk et al., 2013; Zalsman et al., 2016). Standards for hospitalization are often inconsistent; individuals may leave restrictive, higher level-of-care settings at increased risk for suicide (Ward-Ciesielski & Rizvi, 2021); and an overall ability to reliably predict suicidal behavior is questionable (Franklin et al., 2017).

In short, the biomedical model of mental health – including psychiatric hospitalization – has not produced the kinds of clinical outcomes needed to reduce suicide risk and improve overall mental health outcomes. Consequently, we argue that clinical social workers must contribute to a system that reprioritizes clinical training, expertise, client preference, and consideration of contextual factors that contribute to suicidality on equal footing with the psychiatric model – both in practice and research. Several promising alternative intervention strategies and frameworks have emerged that comprise an underrepresented portion of suicidological prevention practice and, more accurately, reflect the guiding principles and values of social work practice (National Association of Social Workers [NASW], 2021).

Clinical Social Work and the Genesis of Contemporary Suicide Prevention

Clinical social workers represent the single largest professional category of mental health service providers (Heisler, 2018). Yet, despite social work's significant role in the provision of mental health and suicide prevention services, the profession contributes comparatively little to the cumulative body of suicide research (Maple et al., 2016). Applying clinical evidence rooted in the professional goals and mandates of the biomedical model limits the voice of social work and deprioritizes the implementation of social work values.

Suicidology is generally recognized as being inherently multidisciplinary (Fitzpatrick et al., 2015). However, social work's narrow contribution to the field (compared to other disciplines) restricts the presence of its key professional values within suicide prevention practice. Social work's adoption of the psychiatric model has been facilitated by the profession's sparse contribution to the body of research and limited training offered in schools of social work. As a result, biomedically focused perspectives of the suicidal person permeate suicide intervention and prevention efforts enacted by social work professionals.

The uptake of these practices by social workers serves to pathologize the individual through the guise of the biomedical model. That is, the lens applied insufficiently acknowledges the importance of social, cultural, circumstantial, and environmental factors that contribute to suicidality (Manning, 2020). People experiencing suicidal ideation are categorized as experiencing medical abnormalities and individual psychopathology. These views (i.e., suffering from "mental illnesses/disorders") are inextricably linked with the biomedical model of mental health which reinforces the notion that biomedical practices are needed to protect the impacted individual (East et al., 2021). As United Nations Special Rapporteur, Dainius Pūras, stated, once a psychiatric label is applied, "everything that then happens is seen through that prism, and then only biomedical decisions and treatments will be applied" (as quoted in Davies, 2021, p. 323).

As such, suicide prevention and treatment frequently involve the application of risk management practices in which a client's civil liberties, autonomy, and decision-making are removed to reduce the anxieties and liability of clinical providers (Blocker & Miller, 2013). These practices typically include requiring psychiatric hospitalization for individuals at high risk of suicide to maintain the individual's safety (Department of Veterans Affairs [VA] & Department of Defense [DoD], 2019). Presumably, this is to allow one to "aggressively target modifiable factors," including "acute mental illness" (p. 11) such as "depression" (VA/DoD, 2019, p. 13).

Social work's tacit endorsement of the biomedical model has narrowed the lens through which suicide is interpreted. This has been to the exclusion of person-in-environment and biopsychosocial perspectives central to social work practice (Karls et al., 1997). This limits the tools available to clinical social workers in addressing suicidality. The result has been the emergence of a perception that hospitalization is the safest and most efficacious means of supporting individuals in crisis. This process reaffirms the misdirected notion that through the application of a biomedical framework, suicide may be reliably predicted and prevented. This is not the case. For example, among young adults, the rate of suicide has continued to grow over the past decade increasing by 57% from 2007 to 2018 (Curtin, 2020). A meta-analysis of 50 years of risk factors research further reiterates the failure of this strategy to reliably predict lethal or near-lethal suicidal behavior (Franklin et al., 2017).

Paradoxically, psychiatric hospitalization has been shown to lead to increased suicide rates following the client's discharge from the hospital (Chung et al., 2017; Olfson et al., 2016) in addition to recurring psychiatric re-admissions known as the "revolving door syndrome" (Centers for Disease Control and Prevention, 2020; Garrido & Saraiva, 2012). Regardless, coercive interventions for suicide are increasingly used within contemporary clinical practice (Sashidharan & Saraceno, 2017) with the social work profession complicit in perpetuating the practice.

Further limitations perpetuated by a biomedical model

Related to the approach that psychiatrically hospitalizing an individual allows one to "target modifiable factors" such as a "mental illness" (VA & DoD, 2019, p. 11), there is also the oft-referenced statistic that up to 90% of suicide deaths have evidence of a diagnosable mental illness/disorder (Bertolote & Fleischmann, 2002; Conwell et al., 1996; Lyubov & Zotov, 2022) which, arguably, attempts to bolster the utility of the biomedical model and use of psychiatric diagnoses within suicide prevention efforts.

However, following enduring issues related to psychiatric diagnoses' decreasing rates of reliability (Carney, 2013; Regier et al., 2013) and, perhaps more concerningly, their lack of validity as putative medical conditions (Lynch, 2018; Johnstone, 2022), one should caution against their use as an explanatory system or cause of suicide. Some suggest it is improbable for mental illness and psychiatric diagnoses to approximate reality (Kendler, 2021; Plakun, 2015). This is perhaps due to the supposed existence of psychiatric diagnoses *a priori* – that is, *presumed independent* of empirical support (Internet Encyclopedia of Philosophy, n.d.) – without "evidence of ontological reality" (Kirk et al., 2013, p. 128).

Conversely, others argue psychiatric diagnoses are social and cultural constructs brought into existence by voting, not science (Council for Evidence-based Psychiatry, 2015). They are "pseudo-diagnoses" that primarily *describe* – not explain the causes of – varying emotional, behavioral, and psychological difficulties (Timimi, 2021). Therefore, statistics proclaiming that up to 90% of deaths by suicide had a mental illness are merely purporting the obvious reality that those individuals suffered from extreme distress, although to the exclusion of considering if or which environmental and circumstantial factors (e.g., poverty, abuse, loneliness, etc.) played a role.

It can also be argued that the biomedical model of mental health is antithetical to foundational social work principles. Clinical social workers are trained to utilize a contextual *strengths-based* approach, one in which a client's sense of agency is honored and supported *collaboratively* while, instead of emphasizing their "pathologies", their resources and strengths are highlighted (Saleebey, 2012). Conversely, what is often perceived by clinical social workers as best practices, such as psychiatrically hospitalizing someone to treat a "mental illness" despite questionable efficacy of the practice (Gomory et al., 2011), typically promote a *deficits-based* lens by attempting to define pathology, abnormality, and illness by affixing psychiatric diagnoses onto a designated "patient" embedded in a medical milieu. The result can be psychiatric diagnoses that brand people with labels that can stick like glue—defining the entire person while creating a pernicious expectation of hardship (Duncan et al., 2004). As one example in a study by Kemp and colleagues (2014), when a biomedical explanation of their difficulties was given to participants, it worsened self-blame, self-efficacy, and prognostic pessimism.

The use of mental disorders and psychiatric labeling can also negatively influence practitioners in a client-clinician encounter. When a client is said to be suffering from a mental illness, the professional may maintain lessened expectations for that individual (Hodge, 2016). The practitioner may also presume the client to be negatively predestined after generalizing from others who have received similar labels (Haslam & Kvaale, 2015; Satel & Lilienfeld, 2015). Lebowitz and Ahn (2014) have also shown that biological explanations can evoke significantly less empathy in clinicians— a crucial ingredient in psychotherapy encounters. As such, the clinician who adheres to this restrictive biomedical ideology of an inappropriately implemented practice is presumed to be applying the best evidence in intervention; however, they may not see how they are being guided to see problems in a *certain* way – that is, to treat *the average* instead of *the individual* – consequently degrading clinical practice (Fava, 2017).

Additionally, wholesale adoption of the biomedical model in relation to suicide prevention can also blur political, cultural, environmental, and social factors contributing to human suffering. Contemporary practice of using psychiatric diagnoses places the problem within the person. This act relabels social problems (e.g., poverty) as medical (e.g., an "anxiety disorder" or "mental illness" [in response to experiencing stress amid poverty]) and relocates intractable areas of social policy (e.g., addressing social inequalities, neighborhood violence, etc.) into the hands of the healthcare professional community (Moncrieff, 2010). This runs against social work's approach of appreciating the broader context of one's experience, contradicting an Ethical Principle emphasizing the importance of helping maintain the dignity and holistic worth of the person (NASW, 2021).

The speciousness of social work professional organizations

A recent update to the Council on Social Work Education's (CSWE) Educational Policy and Accreditation Standards (EPAS) states that "social workers understand and critique the history and current structures of social policies and services and the role of policy in service delivery through rights-based, *anti-oppressive*...lenses [emphasis added]" (Council on Social Work Education [CSWE], 2022, p. 10). (The CSWE is the sole accrediting agency for social work education in the United States.)

Similarly, the NASW's Code of Ethics comprises the field's values, of which one is social justice. Its associated ethical principle delineates that social workers "pursue social change, particularly with and on behalf of vulnerable and oppressed individuals and groups of people...Social workers strive to ensure access to needed information, services, and resources; equality of opportunity; and meaningful participation in decision making for all people" (NASW, 2021).

Despite the discipline's immense presence in the field of mental health, unavoidable entanglement with the psychiatric model and explicit commitment to engaging in anti-oppressive practices, its response to the harms inflicted by a biomedical model of mental health and desires for reform have been virtually nonexistent except for a handful of outspoken and fiercely critical social workers (e.g., Carney, 2014). For example, in anticipation of the controversial *DSM-5*'s publication in 2013, a petition challenging the *DSM* and expressing concern was widely circulated online (see Robbins, n.d.). In addition to thousands of signatories, the petition contains a list of professional organizations who signed up as sponsors for the petition. However, an organization notably absent from that list is the National Association of Social Workers (NASW).

Irrespective of the NASW's Code of Ethics emphasis of social justice as one of its values and description of social workers being those who "pursue social change, particularly with and on behalf of vulnerable and oppressed individuals and groups of people" (NASW, 2021), anything pertaining to mental health and challenging oppressive characteristics of the psychiatric model are absent from its list of Social Justice Priorities (NASW, n.d.-a). Instead, its description of clinical social work practice continues to subscribe to the questionable notion of mental illness as it explicates that clinical social work is "a specialty practice area of social work which focuses on the assessment, diagnosis, treatment, and prevention of mental illness, emotional, and other behavioral disturbances" (NASW, n.d.-b).

Notably, the same webpage states that the NASW "advocates for clinical social workers through the legislative and regulatory process," a statement for which it would be opportune to convey a commitment to reforming the mental health system—a commitment worth mentioning, to be sure, if only one existed. Additionally, the Grand Challenges for Social Work launched in 2016 by the American Academy of Social Work & Social Welfare (AASWSW) makes no mention of challenging the psychiatric model as part of any of their challenges put forth (*Grand Challenges for Social Work*, n.d.). To be clear, we assert as others have that suicide prevention is a social justice issue (e.g., Button & Marsh, 2020).

As previously noted, social workers represent the largest segment of clinical mental health providers in the United States (Heisler, 2018). With this context established, it is worth critiquing the profession's key stakeholders and pointing out the posturing that abounds among influential social work organizations. Their lack of promoting critical and alternative perspectives to suicide prevention as part of their training or pedagogical standards, in effect, allow for the field to be complicit in perpetuating a questionable, unscientific, and harmful model of mental health while voicing a supposed commitment to engaging in anti-oppressive practices and research.

Returning to the CSWE as the sole accrediting agency for social work education in the United States, it is possible that part of the lack of a field-wide response to challenging the psychiatric model can be tied to what the CSWE requires (or does not require) in their "explicit curriculum" educational policies delineated in the recently revised EPAS (CSWE, 2022). Although dated, if Lacasse and Gomory's 2003 study still holds true, it could be that most social work education continues to lack critical and alternative perspectives pertaining to psychiatry, the *DSM*, and the field of mental health. In reviewing a sample of 71 psychopathology course syllabi from 58 different graduate schools of social work across the United States, their study demonstrated little evidence that graduate school psychopathology courses review critical perspectives in addition to the traditional and predominant biomedical psychiatry views (Lacasse & Gomory, 2003).

Taken together, these kinds of critiques have led others to deem the field of social work to be simply a "handmaiden to psychiatry" (Gomory et al., 2011). Others argued nearly three decades ago that the discipline had already lost its traditional mission of promoting social justice in favor of pursuing professional status on par with psychiatry (Specht & Courtney, 1995). Lacasse and Gomory (2003) have added that social work becoming a handmaiden to psychiatry has much to do with "the profession's inability to set itself apart ideologically from psychiatry" (p. 398). However, if the field of social work wants to truly embrace and implement anti-oppressive practices, push for social change, and advocate for social justice on behalf of a vulnerable and oppressed segment of the population in a field in which they maintain a significant presence, challenging the psychiatric model and advocating for humanistic alternatives more aligned with the field's values and ethics is ripe for the picking.

Towards a Contextual Understanding of Suicide

The biomedical model's focus on defining internal psychopathology pivots away from social work's general concern with family, culture, and contexts in assessment and support (Kirk et al., 1989). Regardless of the number of those labeled with a reified mental disorder, this practice can influence public opinion, policymakers, clinicians, and researchers alike into thinking that mental health treatment is the *only* solution to the problem of suicide; however, approaches to preventing suicide must be multifaceted and contextual (Reed, 2013).

Epidemiologist Richard Wilkinson has stated how "we rarely ask why a society living with such unprecedented levels of physical comfort suffers such an appalling burden of mental and emotional difficulties…there are structural explanations for this, and that's the central problem" (as quoted in Davies, 2021, p. 332). A contextual and multifaceted approach – that is, placing environmental and psychosocial factors on equal footing with individual biomedical characteristics– can more effectively fall under the wheelhouse of clinical social workers if a pivot away from the *DSM* and the biomedical model occurs. The understanding of human beings and their suffering *must be contextual* as people cannot be understood separate from their environments (Witkin & Iversen, 2012). The human organism does not operate in a vacuum—the external environment can have a powerful influence.

The biomedical model of mental health -- in practice -- does not sufficiently consider if an individual is experiencing psychosocial stressors. It excludes, for example, adequate consideration of social determinants of health (SDH) identified by the World Health Organization (World Health Organization, 2008); these comprise of (but are not limited to) poverty, unemployment and job insecurity, working life conditions and dissatisfaction, low educational attainment, sexism, housing and basic amenities, social exclusion and discrimination, and access to affordable health services (Black Dog Institute, 2020) that can shape and influence suicidality.

Social inequality (i.e., increasing income gaps) is also associated with increased levels of emotional, behavioral, and psychological problems accompanied by rises in reported rates of distress and suicide (Wilkinson & Pickett, 2009), though it is not captured by the current biomedical model. Research has also found that adults who have experienced trauma and adverse childhood experiences (ACEs) (e.g., psychological, physical, and sexual abuse; emotional and physical neglect; witnessing violence; disruption within the family, etc.) are more likely to attempt suicide in their lifetime than those who have not experienced ACEs (Choi et al., 2017).

The utilization of alternative frameworks to the biomedical model and its accompanying *DSM* is also imperative. A notable example is the Power Threat Meaning Framework (PTMF) (Johnstone & Boyle, 2018; Boyle & Johnstone, 2020). PTMF attempts to integrate the role of power in people's lives to understand what has happened to the individual; elucidate how power has affected the individual through "threats"; and identify ways people have learned to respond to said threats in order to survive — responses, such as suicidal ideation and acts, usually labeled as "symptoms" of a "mental illness/disorder" within the biomedical model. The PTMF also examines how people make sense of their difficult experiences in conjunction with how messages from the greater society can influence people's feelings of shame, self-blame, isolation, and guilt.

The *Indicative Trauma Impact Manual (ITIM)* (VictimFocus, 2023) was recently published as a trauma-informed, non-diagnostic alternative to the DSM. The manual provides a multitude of emotional, behavioral, and psychological responses to trauma that the authors argue have been typically labeled as symptoms of a mental disorder. Similarly, Kousteni (2018) suggests that the three traditional factors comprising evidenced-based practices in psychotherapy (i.e., research, client characteristics, and therapist attributes) should be augmented by a fourth factor; that is, the context of therapy. In this framework, consideration of the context of therapy allows one to acknowledge how the "outcome of therapy is shaped by socioeconomic, political, and cultural factors that can have an impact on clients and therapists" (Kousteni, 2018, p. 37).

Alternative Non-pathologizing Suicide Prevention Practices

Despite the prevalence of coercive and restrictive biomedical practices within contemporary suicide prevention (Sashidharan & Saraceno, 2017), multiple efforts to move beyond the highly entrenched epistemology and methodologies of these practices are currently being undertaken. Lived experience support groups of varying formats have sought to build upon the peer-based group model that has been effective for individuals experiencing mental health difficulties (Bellamy et al., 2017). These peer support models provide a space for individuals with lived experience to seek connection and belonging outside of a biomedical model that has misunderstood them (Stratford et al., 2017).

Yet, despite some initial evidence indicating the utility of this model when applied to individuals with histories of engagement with the medical system and suicidality, few research studies have explored these efforts. As a result, limited data regarding effectiveness is available with concrete conclusions remaining elusive (Schlichthorst et al., 2020). These interventions leave ample room for further exploration regarding how peer connection may support individuals experiencing thoughts of suicide over traditional interventions.

Community-based treatment

Additional community-based treatment alternatives have emerged which demonstrate the potential utility of moving beyond treatment-as-usual approaches. Acute day facilities, crisis resolution teams, and residential crisis houses all represent promising alternatives with positive preliminary results (Lloyd-Evans & Johnson, 2019). These peer respite programs, which provide voluntary residential services to persons with self-reporting mental health crises, are an alternative to restrictive and coercive treatment options (Croft & İsvan, 2015).

Despite relatively few peer respite programs in the United States, findings from the limited research available suggest individuals using these programs for support are less likely to need emergency services after discharge, and treatment care costs are lower than patients receiving treatment as usual options (Bouchery et al., 2018; Croft & İsvan, 2015; National Empowerment Center, 2023). Although there is a growing body of research indicating the viability of alternative treatments – and compounding evidence revealing concerns regarding modern suicide intervention as restrictive – meaningful change has yet to be realized (Callaghan et al., 2013; Sashidharan & Saraceno, 2017).

Examples of emerging prevention resources that expand beyond the psychiatric model of care and incorporate person-centered, harm reduction approaches include The Yarrow Collective and Wildflower Alliance. The Yarrow Collective offers several peer support groups, notably including an Alternatives to Suicide Peer Support group, in which "we do not assume you have an illness, do not assess for risk or involuntary intervention, and do not call the police." (The Yarrow Collective, 2023). Such an approach moves beyond the implicit assumptions by the psychiatric model that persons experiencing suicidal thoughts and behaviors are experiencing mental illness and must be protected from themselves at the expense of individual autonomy and dignity.

The Wildflower Alliance approaches these public health challenges from a similar perspective, focusing on peer support, training, and advocacy. These services are grounded in a validation of individual experience and focus on the role of community in establishing an ecology of resilience (Wildflower Alliance, 2023). Similarly, initiatives such as the Humane Clinic offer a variety of services that sidestep the use of pathologizing labels as they work to support people experiencing extreme states such as suicidality and hearing voices (Humane Clinic, n.d.).

The living room model

Yet another promising prevention resource for individuals experiencing mental health crises is the Living Room Model. Although this approach has received very little research attention relative to its utility in supporting individuals experiencing suicidal thoughts and behaviors, it has notable potential to meet the highly contextualized demands of prevention practice. The Living Room Model "is a community crisis center that offers people experiencing a mental health crisis an alternative to hospitalization" (St. Margarets Health Center, 2023). That is, this model provides a critical middle-ground service option for those who may be deciding whether to navigate a crisis on their own or seek hospital admission.

Among the limited research findings that explore the efficacy of the Living Room Model, themes of safe-harbor and judgment-free intervention emerge (Shattell et al., 2014). Considering the concerns presented here regarding the limitations of the biomedical model and its contribution to the perpetuation of suicide stigma, alternative treatment options such as The Living Room Model offer person-centered, harm reduction approaches that align with the priorities of the social work profession.

Conclusion

In response to the limitations of the psychiatric model and social work's adoption of a biomedical model of practice, the profession must reprioritize suicide prevention efforts to a system that values clinical expertise and client preference on equal footing with the prerogatives of psychiatric interventions. Similarly, this must include a fundamental rethinking of how the individual experiencing suicidal ideation is perceived.

Rather than portray suicidality in the light of the biomedical model in which suicidality is nearly always the result of "mental illness" reflecting a person incapable of fully making decisions to support themselves, applying greater contextual understanding – for example, recognizing psychosocial, political, and economic factors that influence a person's experience of the world around them – is needed. This includes the implementation of alternative noncoercive supportive options. Several alternative and innovative approaches already exist, though they require continued research and support.

Suicide prevention stands at a long overdue crossroads. The arguments presented here raise concern regarding how social work's attachment to the biomedical conceptualization of suicide stymies prevention and has run astray of its professional values. We are not the first authors to argue such (e.g., Hightower et al., 2023). Yet we add our voices to these calls for change in order to further advance suicide prevention and treatment in social work.

Social work's significant presence within the mental health community represents an opportunity to affect change. These changes do not necessitate scrapping systems entirely; rather, they require social workers to assert professional values and apply them despite the competing interests of a psychiatric model. The social work perspective has much to offer prevention science and suicidology. However, this requires social workers to lead change, challenge the status quo when necessary, and present practical, useful alternatives to meet these needs.

References

American Psychiatric Association. (n.d.). *About DSM-5-TR.* https://www.psychiatry.org/psychiatrists/practice/dsm/about-dsm

American Foundation for Suicide Prevention. (2023, September 1). https://afsp.org/

Barnhorst, A., Gonzales, H., & Asif-Sattar, R. (2021). Suicide prevention efforts in the United States and their effectiveness. *Current opinion in psychiatry,* *34*(3), 299.

Bellamy, C., Schmutte, T., & Davidson, L. (2017). An update on the growing evidence base for peer support. *Mental Health and Social Inclusion, 21.* https://www.emerald.com/insight/content/doi/10.1108/MHSI-03-2017-0014/full/html

Bertolote, J. M., & Fleischmann, A. (2002). Suicide and psychiatric diagnosis: A worldwide perspective. *World Psychiatry, 1*(3), 181–185. https://www.ncbi.nlm.nih.gov/pmc/articles/PMC1489848/

Black Dog Institute. (2020, October). *What can be done to decrease suicidal behaviour in Australia?* https://www.blackdoginstitute.org.au/suicide-prevention-white-paper/

Blocker, G. M., & Miller, J. A. (2013). Unintended Consequences: Stigma and Suicide Prevention Efforts. *Military Medicine, 178*(5), 473–473. https://doi.org/10.7205/MILMED-D-13-00056

Bouchery, E. E., Barna, M., Babalola, E., Friend, D., Brown, J. D., Blyler, C., & Ireys, H. T. (2018). The Effectiveness of a Peer-Staffed Crisis Respite Program as an Alternative to Hospitalization. *Psychiatric Services, 69*(10), 1069–1074.

Boyle, M., & Johnstone, L. (2020). *A straight talking introduction to the power threat meaning framework: An alternative to psychiatric diagnosis.* PCCS Books.

Bronfenbrenner, U. (1979). *The ecology of human development: Experiments by nature and design.* Harvard University Press.

Button, M. E., & Marsh, I. (Eds.). (2020). *Suicide and social justice: New perspectives on the politics of suicide and suicide prevention.* Routledge.

Callaghan, S., Ryan, C., & Kerridge, I. (2013). Risk of suicide is insufficient warrant for coercive treatment for mental illness. *International Journal of Law and Psychiatry, 36*(5), 374–385. https://doi.org/10.1016/j.ijlp.2013.06.021

Carney, J. (2013, May 3). The DSM-5 field trials: Inter-Rater reliability ratings take a nose dive. *Mad In America.* https://www.madinamerica.com/2013/03/the-dsm-5-field-trials-inter-rater-reliability-ratings-take-a-nose-dive/

Carney, J. (2014). Where are the social workers? One social worker's road to active opposition to the new *DSM. Ethical Human Psychology and Psychiatry, 16*(1), 63–79. https://doi.org/10.1891/1559-4343.16.1.63

Centers for Disease Control and Prevention. (2020, February 7). *"Revolving door" syndrome.* Retrieved from https://wwwn.cdc.gov/WPVHC/Nurses/Course/Slide/Unit3_11

Choi, N. G., DiNitto, D. M., Marti, C. N., & Segal, S. P. (2017). Adverse childhood experiences and suicide attempts among those with mental and substance use disorders. *Child Abuse & Neglect, 69,* 252–262. https://doi.org/10.1016/j.chiabu.2017.04.024

Chung, D. T., Ryan, C. J., Hadzi-Pavlovic, D., Singh, S. P., Stanton, C., & Large, M. M. (2017). Suicide rates after discharge from psychiatric facilities. *JAMA Psychiatry, 74*(7), 694. https://doi.org/10.1001/jamapsychiatry.2017.1044

Conwell, Y., Duberstein, P. R., Cox, C., Herrmann, J. H., Forbes, N. T., & Caine, E. D. (1996). Relationships of age and axis I diagnoses in victims of completed suicide: a psychological autopsy study. *American Journal of Psychiatry, 153*(8), 1001–1008. https://doi.org/10.1176/ajp.153.8.1001

Council for Evidence-based Psychiatry. (2015, September 30). *Dr James Davies: The origins of the DSM* [Video]. YouTube. https://www.youtube.com/watch?v=6JPgpasgueQ

Council on Social Work Education. (2022). *2022 educational policy and accreditation standards.* CSWE. https://www.cswe.org/accreditation/standards/2022-epas/

Cramer, R. J., & Kapusta, N. D. (2017). A social-ecological framework of theory, assessment, and prevention of suicide. *Frontiers in psychology, 8,* 1756. https://doi.org/10.3389/fpsyg.2017.01756

Croft, B., & İsvan, N. (2015). Impact of the 2nd Story Peer Respite Program on Use of Inpatient and Emergency Services. *Psychiatric Services, 66*(6), 632–637. https://doi.org/10.1176/appi.ps.201400266

Curtin, S. C. (2020). State suicide rates among adolescents and young adults aged 10–24: United States, 2000–2018.

Curtin, S. C., Warner, M., & Hedegaard, H. (2016). *Increase in suicide in the United States, 1999-2014* (No. 241). US Department of Health and Human Services, Centers for Disease Control and Prevention, National Center for Health Statistics.

Davies, J. (2021). *Sedated: How modern capitalism created our mental health crisis.* Atlantic Books.

Department of Veterans Affairs & Department of Defense. (2019). *The assessment and management of patients at risk for suicide - provider summary.* https://www.healthquality.va.gov/guidelines/MH/srb/VADoDSuicideRisk CPGProviderSummaryFinal5088212019.pdf

Duncan, B. L., Miller, S. D., & Sparks, J. A. (2004). *The heroic client: A revolutionary way to improve effectiveness through client-directed, outcome-Informed therapy.* Jossey-Bass.

East, L., Dorozenko, K. P., & Martin, R. (2021). The construction of people in suicide prevention documents. *Death Studies, 45*(3), 182–190. https://doi.org/10.1080/07481187.2019.1626938

Fava, G. A. (2017). Evidence-based medicine was bound to fail: A report to Alvan Feinstein. *Journal of Clinical Epidemiology, 84*, 3–7. https://doi.org/10.1016/j.jclinepi.2017.01.012

Feldman, B. N., & Freedenthal, S. (2006). Social work education in suicide intervention and prevention: An unmet need? *Suicide and Life-Threatening Behavior, 36*(4), 467–480. https://doi.org/10.1521/suli.2006.36.4.467

Fitzpatrick, S. J., Hooker, C., & Kerridge, I. (2015). Suicidology as a Social Practice. *Social Epistemology, 29*(3), 303–322. https://doi.org/10.1080/02691728.2014.895448

Franklin, J. C., Ribeiro, J. D., Fox, K. R., Bentley, K. H., Kleiman, E. M., Huang, X., Musacchio, K. M., Jaroszewski, A. C., Chang, B. P., & Nock, M. K. (2017). Risk factors for suicidal thoughts and behaviors: A meta-analysis of

50 years of research. *Psychological Bulletin, 143*(2), 187–232. https://doi.org/10.1037/bul0000084

Fritscher, L. (2020, March 10). *How the medical model for mental disorders works in psychology.* Verywell Mind. Retrieved from https://www.verywellmind.com/medical-model-2671617

Gomory, T., Wong, S. E., Cohen, D., & Lacasse, J. R. (2011). Clinical social work and the biomedical industrial complex. *The Journal of Sociology & Social Welfare, 38*(4), 135–165. https://scholarworks.wmich.edu/jssw/vol38/iss4/8

Garrido, P., & Saraiva, C. (2012). P-601 - understanding the revolving door syndrome. *European Psychiatry, 27*, 1. https://doi.org/10.1016/s0924-9338(12)74768-5

Grand challenges for social work. (n.d.). Grand Challenges for Social Work. Retrieved from https://grandchallengesforsocialwork.org/#the-challenges

Hightower, H., Almeida, J., & Anderson, J. (2023). Reimagining Suicide Prevention as a Social Justice Issue: Getting Back to Social Work's Roots. *Social work, 68*(2), 167-169.

Haslam, N., & Kvaale, E. P. (2015). Biogenetic explanations of mental disorder. *Current Directions in Psychological Science, 24*(5), 399–404. https://doi.org/10.1177/0963721415588082

Hedegaard, H., Curtin, S. C., & Warner, M. (2021). *Suicide mortality in the United States, 1999-2019.* https://doi.org/10.15620/cdc:101761

Heisler, E. J. (2018). The Mental Health Workforce: A Primer. 18. *Congressional Research Service.* CRS R43255. Retrieved from https://sgp.fas.org/crs/misc/R43255.pdf

Hodge, N. (2016). Schools without labels. In K. Runswick-Cole, R. Mallett, & S. Timimi (Eds.), *Re-Thinking Autism: Diagnosis, Identity and Equality* (pp. 156–172). Jessica Kingsley Publishers.

Humane Clinic. (n.d.). *Our story.* https://www.humaneclinic.com.au/about-4

Internet Encyclopedia of Philosophy. (n.d.). *A priori and a posteriori.* Retrieved from https://iep.utm.edu/apriori/

Johnstone, L. (2022). *A straight talking introduction to psychiatric diagnosis* (2nd ed.). PCCS Books.

Johnstone, L., & Boyle, M. (2018). The power threat meaning framework: An alternative nondiagnostic conceptual system. *Journal of Humanistic Psychology*. https://doi.org/10.1177/0022167818793289

Jordan, J. T., & McNiel, D. E. (2020). Perceived Coercion During Admission Into Psychiatric Hospitalization Increases Risk of Suicide Attempts After Discharge. *Suicide and Life-Threatening Behavior, 50*(1), 180–188. https://doi.org/10.1111/sltb.12560

Karls, J. M., Lowery, C. T., Mattaini, M. A., & Wandrei, K. E. (1997). The use of the PIE (person-in-environment) system in social work education. *Journal of Social Work Education, 33*(1), 48-58.

Kemp, J. J., Lickel, J. J., & Deacon, B. J. (2014). Effects of a chemical imbalance causal explanation on individuals' perceptions of their depressive symptoms. *Behaviour Research and Therapy, 56*, 47–52. https://doi.org/10.1016/j.brat.2014.02.009

Kendler, K. S. (2021). Potential lessons for DSM from contemporary philosophy of science. *JAMA Psychiatry*. https://doi.org/10.1001/jamapsychiatry.2021.3559

Kirk, S. A., Gomory, T., & Cohen, D. (2013). *Mad science: Psychiatric coercion, diagnosis, and drugs*. Routledge.

Kirk, S. A., Siporin, M., & Kutchins, H. (1989). The prognosis for social work diagnosis. *Social Casework, 70*(5), 295–304. https://doi.org/10.1177/104438948907000505

Kousteni, I. D. (2018). Toward an extended view of Evidence-Based psychotherapy: Diversity and societal factors. *Journal of Humanistic Psychology*. https://doi.org/10.1177/0022167818762651

Lacasse, J. R., & Gomory, T. (2003). Is graduate social work education promoting a critical approach to mental health practice? *Journal of Social Work Education, 39*(3), 383–408. https://doi.org/10.1080/10437797.2003.10779145

Lebowitz, M. S., & Ahn, W. K. (2014). Effects of biological explanations for mental disorders on clinicians' empathy. *Proceedings of the National Academy of Sciences, 111*(50), 17786–17790. https://doi.org/10.1073/pnas.1414058111

Lloyd-Evans, B., & Johnson, S. (2019). Community alternatives to inpatient admissions in psychiatry. *World Psychiatry, 18*(1), 31–32. https://doi.org/10.1002/wps.20587

Lynch, T. (2018). The validity of the DSM: An overview. *The Irish Journal of Counselling and Psychotherapy, 18*(2), 5–10.

Lyubov, E. B., & Zotov, P. B. (2022). "Suicidal disease" as psychiatric diagnosis: Scientific and practical rationale. *Suicidology, 13*(04(49)). https://doi.org/10.32878/suiciderus.22-13-04(49)-91-112

Manning, J. (2020). *Suicide: The social causes of self-destruction.* University of Virginia Press.

Maple, M., Pearce, T., Sanford, R., & Cerel, J. (2016). The Role of Social Work in Suicide Prevention, Intervention, and Postvention: A Scoping Review. *Australian Social Work, 70,* 1–13. https://doi.org/10.1080/0312407X.2016.1213871

Moncrieff, J. (2010). Psychiatric diagnosis as a political device. *Social Theory & Health, 8*(4), 370–382. https://doi.org/10.1057/sth.2009.11

National Association of Social Workers. (n.d.-a). *Social justice priorities.* NASW. Retrieved from https://www.socialworkers.org/Advocacy/Social-Justice/Social-Justice-Priorities

National Association of Social Workers. (n.d.-b). *Clinical social work.* NASW. Retrieved from https://www.socialworkers.org/Practice/Clinical-Social-Work

National Association of Social Workers. (2021). *Code of ethics of the National Association of Social Workers.* https://www.socialworkers.org/About/Ethics/Code-of-Ethics/Code-of-Ethics-English

National Empowerment Center. (2023). *Directory of peer respites.* Retrieved from https://power2u.org/directory-of-peer-respites/

Olfson, M., Wall, M., Wang, S., Crystal, S., Liu, S. M., Gerhard, T., & Blanco, C. (2016). Short-term suicide risk after psychiatric hospital discharge. *JAMA Psychiatry, 73*(11), 1119. https://doi.org/10.1001/jamapsychiatry.2016.2035

Plakun, E. M. (2015). Correcting psychiatry's false assumptions and implementing parity. *Psychiatric Times.* Retrieved from https://www.psychiatrictimes.com/view/correcting-psychiatrys-false-assumptions-and-implementing-parity

Reed, J. (2013, November 7). *90 percent*. Suicide Prevention Resource Center. Retrieved from https://www.sprc.org/news/90-percent

Regier, D. A., Narrow, W. E., Clarke, D. E., Kraemer, H. C., Kuramoto, S. J., Kuhl, E. A., & Kupfer, D. J. (2013). DSM-5 field trials in the United States and Canada, part II: Test-Retest reliability of selected categorical diagnoses. *American Journal of Psychiatry, 170*(1), 59–70. https://doi.org/10.1176/appi.ajp.2012.12070999

Rogers, A. (2017, May 11). Star neuroscientist Tom Insel leaves the Google-Spawned verily for . . . A startup? *WIRED*. Retrieved from https://www.wired.com/2017/05/star-neuroscientist-tom-insel-leaves-google-spawned-verily-startup/

Ruth, B. J., Gianino, M., Muroff, J., McLaughlin, D., & Feldman, B. N. (2012). You Can't Recover From Suicide: Perspectives on Suicide Education in MSW Programs. *Journal of Social Work Education, 48*(3), 501–516. https://doi.org/10.5175/JSWE.2012.201000095

Robbins, B. (n.d.). *Open letter to the DSM-5*. iPetitions. Retrieved from https://www.ipetitions.com/petition/dsm5

Saleebey, D. (2012). *The strengths perspective in social work practice* (6th ed.). Pearson.

Sashidharan, S. P., & Saraceno, B. (2017). Is psychiatry becoming more coercive? *BMJ*, j2904. https://doi.org/10.1136/bmj.j2904

Satel, S., & Lilienfeld, S. O. (2015). *Brainwashed: The seductive appeal of mindless neuroscience*. Basic Books.

Schlichthorst, M., Ozols, I., Reifels, L., & Morgan, A. (2020). Lived experience peer support programs for suicide prevention: A systematic scoping review. *International Journal of Mental Health Systems, 14*(1), 65. https://doi.org/10.1186/s13033-020-00396-1

Shattell, M. M., Harris, B., Beavers, J., Tomlinson, S. K., Prasek, L., Geevarghese, S., Emery, C. L., &

Heyland, M. (2014). A Recovery-Oriented Alternative to Hospital Emergency Departments for Persons in Emotional Distress: "The Living Room." *Issues*

in Mental Health Nursing, 35(1), 4–12.
https://doi.org/10.3109/01612840.2013.835012

Specht, H., & Courtney, M. E. (1995). *Unfaithful angels: How social work has abandoned its mission.* Free Press.

St. Margarets Health Center (n.d.). *The Living Room Model.* St. Margarets Health Center for Holistic Health and Wellness. Retrieved from https://smhchhw.org/the-living-room-model/

Stratford, A., Halpin, M., Phillips, K., Skerritt, F., Beales, A., Cheng, V., Hammond, M., O'Hagan, M., Loreto, C., Tiengtom, K., Kobe, B., Harrington, S., Fisher, D., & Davidson, L. (2017). The growth of peer support: An international charter. *Journal of Mental Health, 28,* 1–6. https://doi.org/10.1080/09638237.2017.1340593

The Yarrow Collective (n.d.). *Peer Support Groups.* Retrieved from https://www.yarrowcollective.org/peer-support-groups

Timimi, S. (2021). *Insane medicine: How the mental health industry creates damaging treatment traps and how you can escape them.* Independently published.

VictimFocus. (2023). Indicative trauma impact manual: ITIM for professionals. Independently published.

Ward-Ciesielski, E. F., & Rizvi, S. L. (2021). The potential iatrogenic effects of psychiatric hospitalization for suicidal behavior: A critical review and recommendations for research. *Clinical Psychology: Science and Practice, 28*(1), 60–71. https://doi.org/10.1111/cpsp.12332

Wildflower Alliance (2023). *Peer to Peer Supports.* The Wildflower Alliance. Retrieved from https://wildfloweralliance.org/peer-to-peer-supports/

Wilkinson, R. D., & Pickett, K. (2009). *The spirit level: Why greater equality makes societies stronger.* Bloomsbury Publishing.

Witkin, S. L., & Iversen, R. R. (2012). Contemporary issues in social work. In C. N. Dulmus & K. M. Sowers (Eds.), *The Profession of Social Work: Guided by History, Led by Evidence* (1st ed., pp. 225–261). Wiley.

World Health Organization. (2008). *Closing the gap in a generation: Health equity through action on the social determinants of health.* World Health Organization. https://www.ncbi.nlm.nih.gov/nlmcatalog/101488674

Zalsman, G., Hawton, K., Wasserman, D., van Heeringen, K., Arensman, E., Sarchiapone, M., Carli, V., Höschl, C., Barzilay, R., Balazs, J., Purebl, G., Kahn, J. P., Sáiz, P. A., Lipsicas,Bobes, C.B., Cozman, J., Hegerl, D., & Zohar, J. (2016). Suicide prevention strategies revisited: 10-year systematic review. *The Lancet Psychiatry*, *3*(7), 646–659. https://doi.org/10.1016/S2215-0366(16)30030-X

Madness-as-Strategy as an Alternative to Psychiatry's Dysfunction-Centered Model

Justin Garson

Abstract: *A broad base of agreement among the contributors to this volume is that there is a distinctive paradigm called "psychiatry's medical model," "medical psychiatry," or "the medical view of psychiatry." Because of a complex array of institutional, economic, social, and political factors, this model has become so deeply entrenched in our collective thinking about madness that it can be hard to see a way out of it. In the following, I present, on the basis of extensive historical research, one particular alternative. I call it madness-as-strategy and oppose it to the now-dominant view, which I call madness-as-dysfunction. My goal here is to clarify the meaning of madness-as-strategy, to show how it surfaces repeatedly throughout the history of madness in different forms and guises, to gesture toward some contemporary research projects that exemplify this framework, and to describe its continuing relevance.*

Some Working Assumptions

These reflections stem from a basic set of assumptions that I believe I share with all of the volume's contributors. These are a set of postulates that won't be defended here, but that will be adopted as working assumptions—as the intellectual soil for new growth. I will enumerate seven of those postulates.

First, there is *something*—a set of beliefs, a way of seeing, an intellectual paradigm—called "medical psychiatry" or the "medicalized view of psychiatry." Though this vision has been with us for millennia, it has in the last few decades managed to become so deeply entrenched in the public conversation—about mental health in the West—that it can be hard to even see it as a distinctive paradigm, much less to envision alternatives. I have documented this extensively in my book, *Madness: A Philosophical Exploration* (Garson 2022), and the following represents a distillation of the core points.

Second, this medical vision manifests itself through empirically observable facts: for example, that at least 15% of the population of the UK are on antidepressant drugs[1]; that one in five American college students are on psychiatric drugs[2]; that there is a $30 billion plus industry that seeks to promote disease-centered framings of mental health problems and thrives on this basis; and the conceptual foundation of which is the belief that mental distress represents a medical problem akin to diabetes or cancer.[3]

Third, there's likely no one person or small group of people to blame for the entrenchment of the medical vision. It probably represents the outcome of the confluence of various psychological, sociological, historical, and institutional forces—in addition to powerful personalities such as Robert Spitzer (Wakefield in prep) or Solomon Snyder (Garson in prep); that is, forces that are appropriate subjects for historical and sociological analysis (e.g., Moncrieff 2013; Harrington 2019).

Fourth, a core intellectual mission of medical psychiatry's critics is not merely to expose how deeply entrenched it has become, but to explore alternative, more empowering framings for making sense of and coping with the distressing, disturbing, extreme or unusual experiences (modes of cognition, forms of interpersonal interaction, etc.) that currently fall under the rubric of "mental disorder."

Fifth, this medical vision, though not without benefits for some suffering people, has extensive and well-documented harms; that is, both harms associated with overmedication and subsequent withdrawal symptoms as well as relational and emotional harms from framing one's experiences or choices as the byproduct of an inner dysfunction or disorder (e.g., Kvaale et al. 2013; Lebowitz and Ahn 2014; Haslam and Kvaale 2015; Pescolido et al. 2021; Schomerus et al. 2022; Schroder et al. 2022). Other harms include the fact that, by seeking to explain distress in terms of a breakdown in the individual, it often draws attention away from relevant social and political

---

[1] https://www.bbc.com/news/uk-scotland-66430817.amp
[2] https://www.statista.com/statistics/1126744/percentage-of-college-students-using-psychotropic-medications-us/
[3] https://www.globaldata.com/media/pharma/global-sales-of-psychiatric-drugs-could-reach-more-than-40bn-by-2025-due-to-coronavirus-says-globaldata/

causes of suffering and thereby neutralizes attempts to address those causes directly (e.g., Davies 2021).

Sixth, psychiatry has not, contrary to some of its proponents, abandoned this medical model; rather, it tends to reaffirm it under various guises. For example, what is sometimes called the bio-psycho-social model is, often enough, just one guise under which this medical vision asserts itself (Read 2005). That is because, on at least one natural way of understanding what the bio-psycho-social model is, it is simply a way of seeing one's mental health problems as the result of an inner dysfunction that is precipitated by psychological and social factors.

Seventh, this model additionally manifests itself through the proliferation of disease language; that is, the disease-related terminology that has permeated the way we talk about mental health: "disorder," "dysfunction," "intervention," "diagnosis," "prescription," "medication," and so on (Johnstone 2022). In Eleanor Longden and John Read's (2017) memorable words, this vision is unable to see "people with problems" but only "patients with illnesses."

That said, how can a philosopher and historian of ideas intervene into this medical vision?

In my academic work, I study the history of madness with special attention to the ideas and intellectual frameworks that coexist or succeed one another in various eras. This work has not only helped me appreciate the historical contingency and fragility of our current medical framework—it has also led me to identify a handful of recurring motifs that, historically, permeate our thinking and theorizing on the topic of madness.

(Note that I generally prefer using the term "madness" to terms like "mental disorder" or "mental illness" as I want to move away from these quasi-medical framings. I realize that "madness" is not a perfect term because it alludes primarily to psychosis; it doesn't typically incorporate experiences like sinking into a deep depression, experiencing overwhelming panic, having difficulties understanding the expectations of the social world or adjusting one's behavior to meet them, and so on. But I will use the term "madness" anyway with the qualification that I mean it to include a broader range of experiences than the term usually connotes.)

It is tempting to think about the history of madness as an unmanageable plurality of different viewpoints that arrange themselves chronologically ("in the West, the mad were first thought to be shamans; then they were thought demon-possessed; then they were thought lazy; then they were thought infantile; now they are thought diseased…"). Even historians as perceptive as Foucault (2006/1961) or Scull (2015) sometimes suggest such a picture.

I found, rather, that there were two main viewpoints that seemed to crop up again and again but in such diverse guises that it was sometimes difficult to see them as variations on a theme. Moreover, I found that, rather than chronologically alternating with one another, they seemed to exist everywhere simultaneously with one or the other enjoying a slight dominance in the public and professional imagination at any given time. I've called these two paradigms madness-as-strategy and madness-as-dysfunction.

My goal here is simple. I begin by articulating what I mean by this distinction, and how my distinction differs from the traditional distinction between "biogenic" and "psychogenic" perspectives. Then I illustrate how these two paradigms (framings, perspectives, ways of seeing) have alternated and sometimes moved hand-in-hand throughout the history of madness. Finally, I will show how madness-as-strategy represents a powerful alternative to psychiatry's medical vision—and indicate some of the current research that exemplifies it and that will continue to make this paradigm relevant far into the future.

Madness-as-Dysfunction

The first point of view that we can use for thinking about madness is what I call madness-as-dysfunction. The basic idea is that when somebody is mad, something inside of them isn't working the way that it's supposed to; something isn't working as it ought or as nature intended. If we think of the sane mind as a well-functioning machine, the mad mind represents a machine with one of its cogs loose, misplaced, or its parts disarranged.

From the standpoint of madness-as-dysfunction, the doctor's job is, at least in theory, quite simple: to figure out what exactly went wrong within the mad person and fix it.

A crucial point about madness-as-dysfunction, and what makes my approach differ from the approach many historians have adopted, is that madness-as-dysfunction isn't wedded to a *biological* vision of the mind. It is not the same thing as the view that sees mental disorders in terms of brain dysfunctions. Rather, the operative idea is the more abstract notion of something not "working right." Something is broken.

The "something" that is broken could be a biological sort of thing. It could be that one's brain is broken (dysfunctional, defective) in that it is producing too much dopamine or too little serotonin, and this chemical imbalance somehow distorts our ability to gate sensory perceptions accurately, which in turn leads to hallucinations, delusions, or mood fluctuations.

It is possible, however, to think that this inner "something" is broken in a purely psychological way. For example, cognitive behavioral therapists often describe panic disorder in terms of a dysfunctional and self-perpetuating pattern of thoughts, feelings, and actions (e.g., Clark 1997). This is a way of seeing something broken or dysfunctional inside the patient—but it is not a biological something. It's a psychological something. I count this, too, as an instance of madness-as-dysfunction.

Madness-as-dysfunction is by no means a new paradigm. It goes back thousands of years, at least in the West. The Hippocratic author of *On the Sacred Disease*, probably penned around 400 BC, tells us that all the different varieties of madness involve a disruption of the flow of air to different parts of the brain. As I have argued in my book (Garson 2022, Chapter 1), the real originality of the Hippocratic vision is not that it frames madness as natural (rather than supernatural), but as the byproduct of an inner brokenness.

Madness-as-dysfunction resurfaces again in Late Renaissance Europe in the duels between the physicians and the exorcists about specific forms of distress. For example, suppose a group of investigators are presented with a young woman with symptoms such as *"suffocation* in the throate...crowing of Cockes, barking of Dogges, garring of Crowes, frenzies, convulsions, hickcockes, laughing, singing, weeping, crying, &c."* (Jorden 1603, 2), and the exorcist diagnoses demonic possession. Physicians like Edward Jordan, in contrast, argued that it resulted from a natural organic pathology: "suffocation of the mother," also known as hysteria. According to Jorden, hysteria takes place when the womb detaches from its ordinary position in the body and begins to press into and disrupt various organ systems.

This dysfunction-centered orientation became standardized in nineteenth-century psychiatric textbooks, such as those written by Cox (1806), Rush (1835), and Spurzheim (1836). It also formed the intellectual backbone of the period in late nineteenth century Germany, which historians sometimes describe as "German imperial psychiatry" (Engstrom 2003). This dysfunction-centered view reaches a zenith in the writings of the great nosologist, Emil Kraepelin. I think, for various social, political, and economic reasons that are impossible to delve into here, madness-as-dysfunction had, by the 1980s, managed to practically eliminate alternative frameworks.

Madness-as-Strategy

In contrast to madness-as-dysfunction, the point of view that I call madness-as-strategy holds that when somebody is mad, everything inside of them is working exactly the way it is supposed to. Everything is working exactly as it ought. Perhaps madness has a function or a purpose, and if we could just unlock that purpose or reason, we would have the key to healing and wholeness.

Again, the goal is not to divide up the history of madness into biological and psychological points of view where "madness-as-dysfunction" is synonymous with the biological perspective and "madness-as-strategy" with the psychological perspective. It is to divide it into those thinkers who primarily see madness in terms of its intrinsic purposiveness, and those who see it as a breakdown or violation of this purposiveness. Put as simply as possible, the proponent of madness-as-dysfunction is inclined to make sense of madness as the result of a broken mechanism, and that of madness-as-strategy as a well-functioning mechanism. Like madness-as-dysfunction, madness-as-strategy resurfaces in different times and in different eras.

I don't want to be overly simplistic. We cannot classify specific thinkers in a very sharp way. We often see some intermingling of both themes in any particular thinker or theorist. In this respect, describing theorists as falling into two camps is sort of like describing Americans in terms of whether they are politically "liberal" or "conservative." Distinguishing people in that way does not imply that conservatives have no liberal beliefs, liberals have no conservative beliefs, or that there are some people who fall somewhere in the middle. It's meant to capture an unmistakable trend of thought—a firm disposition to view social problems in certain ways and to pursue certain types of solutions.

One thinker that exemplifies the madness-as-strategy viewpoint in a fairly strict form is the early seventeenth century theologian and scholar Robert Burton (1577-1640) who penned *The Anatomy of Melancholy*. He often describes melancholy and other forms of madness as having a *divine* purposiveness. At the time, one of the core theoretical problems of madness was: why would God allow madness? Why would God allow such terrible suffering to befall his beloved children?

The answer that Burton gave is that madness acts both as a punishment for sin and as a rod of correction—as God's wakeup call to the sinful individual: "He is desirous of our salvation...and for that cause pulls us by the ear many times, to put us in mind of our duties" (2001/1621, I. 132-3). Understanding the divine purpose of madness, he thought, might provide the tool for healing.

Madness-as-strategy also finds expression in the French physician Philippe Pinel (1745-1826), who is famously depicted as breaking off the chains of the mad patients at the Salpêtrière women's asylum in Paris and is known for promoting the "moral treatment of the insane." But Pinel had other radical ideas, too. One of his ideas was that certain kinds of psychotic episodes, which he called *accès de Manie*, are actually cathartic and healing.

They're purposeful, not pathological. He likened them to fever, the body's natural mechanism for fighting infection. In general—and like fever, he thought—they should typically be allowed to run their course in a safe environment with medical intervention (drugging, vomiting, etc.) used only as a last resort. Given time, he thought, they would be healed by the "salutary efforts of nature [*efforts salutaires de la nature*]" (1800, 267).

Another with similar views was the German Johann Christian August Heinroth (1773-1843) whose massive *Textbook of Mental Disturbances* was published in 1818. There, he describes one particular form of madness which Schmorak translates as "insanity with dementia and rage" [*Wahnsinn mit Verrücktheit und Tollheit*]. This takes place when the patient slips from reality into a kind of dream world—a world of hallucinations and delusions. But this slippage, he thought, was a coping mechanism for trauma: *nature itself*, he insisted, heals the patient by allowing them to escape, temporarily, from their troubles. This is not a disease but the manifestation of the mind's intrinsic design. In the best scenario, he thought, such cases would run their course and remit spontaneously.

I see Freud, likewise, as primarily a proponent of madness-as-strategy. Despite the fact that he occasionally used more dysfunction-centered terminology, he thought of many mental health problems, such as hysteria, phobias, obsessive thoughts, or delusions, as *strategies* rather than defects. They were *unconscious* strategies that the mind deploys to release the pent-up energy (libido) associated with forbidden ideas or desires. For example, consider his 1911 paper on Judge Schreber, "Psycho-analytic notes on an autobiographical account of a case of paranoia (dementia paranoides)":

> And the paranoic builds [his world] up again, not more splendid, it is true, but at least so that he can once more live in it. He builds it up by the work of his delusions. *The delusional formation, which we take to be the pathological product, is in reality an attempt at recovery, a process of reconstruction.*[4]

---

[4] SE (12: 70-1). All citations to Freud refer to the volume and page number of *The Standard Edition of the Complete Psychological Works of Sigmund Freud*.

This basic vision, madness-as-strategy, was woven into the first edition of the American *Diagnostic and Statistical Manual of Mental Disorders* (DSM) of 1952. DSM divides all of the "non-organic" mental disorders into three main classes: the psychotic, the neurotic, and the personality disorders. Intriguingly, each class is defined as a *different sort of coping mechanism* that the mind uses to deal with stressors. For example, the psychotic patient is described as coping with stressors by withdrawing from reality:

> ...a psychotic reaction may be defined as one in which the personality, in its struggle for adjustment to internal and external stresses, utilizes severe affective disturbance, profound autism and withdrawal from reality, and/or formation of delusions or hallucinations. (APA 1952, 12)

Viewed in this light, one of the core intellectual transformations of the famous third edition of the *Diagnostic and Statistical Manual of Mental Disorders*, DSM-III, of 1980, was not to implement a *biological* vision of madness—it was to implement a *dysfunction-centered* vision of madness. Right at the outset, the DSM-III Task Force insists, rather sharply, that *all* mental disorders involve "behavioral, psychological, or biological dysfunction[s]" rather than merely "[disturbances] in the relationship between the individual and society" (APA 1980, 6). (This passage has a somewhat long and complex history that I cannot go into here [see Garson 2022, Chapter 14]).

The reemergence, or entrenchment, of this dysfunction-centered vision of madness in the 1980s went hand-in-hand with the promotion, on the part of influential psychiatrists such as Solomon Snyder, of the idea that most mental disorders, such as schizophrenia, depression, ADHD, and bipolar disorder, resulted from neurotransmitter abnormalities that could, in theory, be reversed or supplemented by using the right medication (e.g., Snyder 1986). Snyder (1976) himself formulated the "dopamine hypothesis of schizophrenia" and spent many years tirelessly promoting it and similar theories. As psychiatrist and historian Joanna Moncrieff (2013) has documented, such theories helped to solidify, in the public consciousness, the idea that mental disorders were brain diseases that could be cured, or at least managed, by pills. This is an era that I believe we are still waking up from.

There are signs, however, of an emerging paradigm shift. One reason that I sought to develop this terminology and this historical analysis—that is, viewing the history of madness as a clash or confrontation between madness-as-dysfunction and madness-as-strategy rather than a clash between psychogenic and biogenic perspectives—was to give us a conceptual *lever* to help lift us out of the dysfunction-centered vision.

It seems to me quite impossible to move away from madness-as-dysfunction until we can see it clearly for what it is and, thereby, begin constructing alternatives. Only then can we treat it for what it is: as a contingent historical formation—one that could, and quite possibly should, be changed.

I don't mean to suggest that madness-as-dysfunction is *never* an appropriate stance to adopt toward a specific mental disorder. To my knowledge, the mental confusion associated with Lewy body dementia stems from a buildup of misfolded proteins in the brain. I do think, however, that it's deeply morally problematic for psychiatrists, psychologists, and other mental health professionals to promote a dysfunction-centered vision as if it is the only scientifically credible framework.

Rather, as I will argue shortly, I believe that as a rule, people have the right to be exposed to different frameworks for making sense of their suffering so long as those frameworks are scientifically credible.

Current research projects

Before wrapping up, I want to describe four current research projects that exemplify madness-as-strategy, and that provide a welcome counterpoint to the entrenched madness-as-dysfunction perspective. These concern the way we think about depression, borderline personality disorder, delusions, and dyslexia, respectively. I think it's important to grasp the way all four of these projects manage to see purpose, rather than pathology, in various mental health problems—and to that extent they share a similar spirit despite their outward differences.

I've been fortunate to be able to write about these in more detail in a blog for PsychologyToday.com where one can find more information and citations to follow up on.[5] The point of this section is to summarize a large amount of evidence without attempting to document it extensively as that documentation has been provided elsewhere.

My first example is depression. By the late 1980s, it became very common to think of depression as a byproduct of a chemical imbalance in the brain, a notion that was reinforced by the commercial success of Prozac and other antidepressant medications.[6] The theory that supported that notion—the idea that depression stems from low serotonin—has been all but refuted (Moncrieff et al. 2023a; Moncrieff et al. 2023b). At the very least, the evidence for that idea turned out to be far weaker than many of us were led to believe at the time.

In contrast, some evolutionary psychiatrists, such as Randolph Nesse (2000), have been promoting a very different point of view (for a recent overview of evolutionary psychiatry, see Abed and St John-Smith 2022). In this view, depression, far from being a brain dysfunction, has an evolved purpose.[7] Put differently, it doesn't represent a broken mechanism, but a mechanism that is serving its purpose exactly as "designed." Specifically, it represents the brain's evolved mechanism for showing a person that something in their life is going wrong and needs more attention.

Although the details of these evolutionary theories differ somewhat, they share a common presumption that depression represents an evolved feature of the human brain rather than a broken mechanism. If this view is

---

[5] https://www.psychologytoday.com/us/blog/the-biology-human-nature
[6] Whittaker provides a journalistic overview of the emergence of the chemical imbalance metaphor and the interaction of psychiatrists, journalists, and pharmaceutical companies in promoting it: see
https://www.madinamerica.com/2022/08/psychiatry-fraud-and-the-case-for-a-class-action-lawsuit/
[7] https://www.psychologytoday.com/us/blog/the-biology-human-nature/202208/what-depression-may-be-trying-tell-us

correct, it would have profound therapeutic significance. It would suggest that, in many cases, the right approach to treating depression is not to bombard it with medication, but to listen to what it's trying to say. Intriguingly, recent evidence even shows that framing a person's depression as an evolved signal, rather than a chemical imbalance, may actually promote superior treatment outcomes (Schroder et al., 2022).[8]

A second example comes from the realm of (so-called) personality disorders, particularly borderline personality disorder (BPD). BPD describes a cluster of traits associated with deep mistrust of other people, volatile interpersonal relationships, impulsiveness, and sometimes self-harm. Until recently, it was common for psychiatrists to think of BPD as the result of a frontal lobe defect or as a failure of executive functioning.

But an emerging point of view holds that some BPD traits, such as mistrust, are survival strategies and not brain defects.[9] Some evidence suggests that up to 80% of people who've received a diagnosis of BPD have a history of trauma, abuse, or neglect. From that point of view, it becomes far more plausible to construe mistrust as a perfectly coherent strategy for navigating a hostile social environment.

Suppose we choose to see BPD traits as survival strategies rather than brain defects. Two things, I think, immediately follow. First, we should discard the language of disease, disorder, and dysfunction—terms which, as the evidence is starting to show, only foment stigma rather than alleviate it. Second and more importantly, it suggests an important approach to treatment where treatment is deemed desirable. It would indicate that the best path forward is not to search for a hypothetical brain dysfunction, but to ask whether and how those strategies—strategies that might have been sensible enough at one point in life—may have outlived their usefulness. It would prompt us to consider which alternative strategies might be more beneficial.

---

[8] https://www.psychologytoday.com/us/blog/the-biology-of-human-nature/202306/how-seeing-depression-as-purposeful-may-promote-healing
[9] https://www.psychologytoday.com/us/blog/the-biology-human-nature/202208/is-borderline-personality-disorder-actually-adaptation

A third example comes from the study of delusions. Although the very idea of a delusion is hard to define precisely (see Bortolotti 2023 for discussion), we can think of them as bizarre beliefs that have no social sanction: that I'm the second coming of Christ; that God has given me a special mission; that a famous actress is communicating with me telepathically. Surely, delusions must represent some sort of brain dysfunction? An alternative point of view holds that some delusions actually serve a protective function. They are designed to buffer the mind from a reality that is just too difficult to confront—a view that harks back to earlier views such as Heinroth or Freud.

Recently, Ritunnano et al. (2022) described a whole class of delusions that are almost impossible to understand without recognizing them as an attempt to give the sufferer a sense of meaning, purpose, and significance in life.[10] Additionally, Isham et al. (2022) recently showed that there is a correlation between the grandiosity of one's delusions and having a sense of purpose or significance in life. If this is right, it has deep therapeutic implications, for it suggests that the point of treatment is not always to bombard delusions with antipsychotic medications. The point, rather, is to try to figure out what the purpose of these delusions are and to devise healthier strategies for achieving the same end.

My last example is dyslexia, though I suspect that similar points might be made about ADHD and, perhaps, some forms of autism.[11] Dyslexia is often described as a neurodevelopmental disorder that disrupts the ability to read or write well. Emerging evidence, however—evidence drawn from a variety of sources—suggests that dyslexia might actually represent an evolved cognitive style. In other words, it might be a unique style of processing information, one with its own strengths and trade-offs.

---

[10] https://www.psychologytoday.com/us/blog/the-biology-human-nature/202209/grandiose-delusions-and-the-meaning-life
[11] On dyslexia, see https://www.psychologytoday.com/us/blog/the-biology-human-nature/202207/seeing-dyslexia-unique-cognitive-strength-rather-disorder. On ADHD, see https://www.psychologytoday.com/us/blog/the-biology-of-human-nature/202211/did-adhd-evolve-to-help-us

People with dyslexia tend to excel at what one might call "big picture thinking." For example, there's evidence that they are quicker to notice when a painting depicts an impossible figure (such as M. C. Escher's *Waterfall*). They also excel at divergent thinking, the ability to devise multiple solutions to the same problem. In fact, some surveys suggest that up to one third of American entrepreneurs have dyslexia.

This evidence points to the same conclusion that dyslexia is not a dysfunction but a distinctive cognitive style. It is quite possible that framing dyslexia as a distinct cognitive style could be extremely useful for young people who suffer from it for it would help to imbue them with the sense that dyslexia gives them unique cognitive strengths rather than merely limitations (Taylor and Vestergaard 2022).

I suspect that for nearly any alleged mental disorder we care to name, there are at least two contrasting ways of understanding it, researching it, and framing it. We can frame it as the breakdown of a designed mechanism in the brain or, alternatively, we can frame it as a designed mechanism in its own right. But it is important to appreciate that the fact that these two quite distinctive perspectives are *available* to us does not mean that there's no "fact of the matter" as to which one is correct in any given case.

I've given reasons for thinking that, in many cases, depression, BPD, delusions, and dyslexia are in fact designed mechanisms, not dysfunctions. Continuing to promote a dysfunction-centered perspective on mental illness is, in my view, not only scientifically dubious but morally problematic.

Conclusion

I feel quite optimistic about the future of mental health framings. It seems to me that society is not only waking up to the fact that our language and conceptualization of mental health is mired in an entrenched dysfunction-centered framing, but we are also waking up to how harmful these framings can be and to the extent of alternatives to them.

To be clear, I do not hold that we should simply *replace* dysfunction framings with function framings, or that madness-as-strategy should be the new intellectual norm that governs mental health research for the next few decades until people find problems with it in turn. I'm quite aware, moreover, that there are mental health service users and ex-patients who have found some comfort in dysfunction framings of their distressing experiences, and I have no wish to rob them of this tool.

What I want to insist upon rather sharply, however, is that people who have distressing, disturbing, or otherwise extreme experiences have a right to be exposed to *multiple, scientifically-credible* frameworks for making sense of and navigating those experiences. If someone comes to accept a dysfunction-centered framing, it should be because they have been exposed to diverse ways of making sense of their problems and they have selected that framework as the best path forward for them.

References

Abed, R., and St John-Smith, P. (Eds.) 2022. *Evolutionary Psychiatry: Current Perspectives on Evolution and Mental Health.* Cambridge: Cambridge University Press.

American Psychiatric Association. 1952. *Diagnostic and Statistical Manual of Mental Disorders.* Washington, D. C.: American Psychiatric Association.

American Psychiatric Association. 1980. *Diagnostic and Statistical Manual of Mental Disorders: DSM-III.* Washington, DC: American Psychiatric Association.

Bortolotti, L. 2023. *Why Delusions Matter.* London: Bloomsbury.

Burton, R. 2001/1621. *The Anatomy of Melancholy.* New York: New York Review of Books.

Clark, D. M. 1997. Panic disorder and social phobia. In *Science and Practice of Cognitive Behaviour Therapy,* edited by D. M. Clark, and C. G. Fairburn, 119-153. Oxford: Oxford University Press.

Cox, J. M. 1806. *Practical Observations on Insanity. 2nd edition.* London: J. Murray.

Davies, J. 2021. *Sedated: How Modern Capitalism Created our Mental Health Crisis.* London: Atlantic.

Engstrom, E. J. 2003. *Clinical Psychiatry in Imperial Germany: A History of Psychiatric Practice.* Ithaca, NY: Cornell University Press.

Foucault, M. 2006/1961. *History of Madness.* New York: Routledge.

Freud, S., Strachey, J., Freud, A., and Rothgeb, C. L. 1953. *The Standard Edition of the Complete Psychological Works of Sigmund Freud.* London: Hogarth Press and the Institute of Psycho-Analysis.

Garson, J. 2022. *Madness: A Philosophical Exploration.* New York: Oxford University Press.

Garson, J. in prep. *The Madness Pill: The Quest to Create Insanity and One Doctor's Discovery that Transformed Psychiatry.* New York: St. Martin's Press.

Harrington, A. 2019. *Mind Fixers: Psychiatry's Troubled Search for the Biology of Mental Illness.* New York: W. W. Norton and Co.

Haslam, N., and Kvaale, E. P. 2015. Biogenetic explanations of mental disorder: The mixed-blessings model. *Current Directions in Psychological Science* 24(5): 399-404. doi.org/10.1177/0963721415588082

Isham, L., et al. 2022. The meaning in grandiose delusions: measure development and cohort studies in clinical psychosis and non-clinical general population groups in the UK and Ireland. *The Lancet Psychiatry* 9(10): 792-803.

Johnstone, L. 2022. *A Straight Talking Introduction to Psychiatric Diagnosis.* Monmouth: PCCS Books.

Jorden, E. 1603. *A Briefe Discourse of a Disease Called the Suffocation of the Mother.* London: John Windet.

Kvaale, E. P., Gottdiener, W. H., and Haslam, N. 2013. Biogenic explanations and stigma: A meta-analytic review of associations among lay people. *Social Science and Medicine* 96:95-103. doi: 10.1016/j.socscimed.2013.07.017

Lebowitz, M., and Ahn, W. 2014. Effects of biological explanations for mental disorders on clinicians' empathy. *PNAS* 111(50): 17786-17790. doi: 10.1073/pnas.1414058111

Longden, E., and Read, J. 2017. 'People with problems, not patients with illnesses': Using psychosocial frameworks to reduce the stigma of psychosis. *The Israel Journal of Psychiatry and Related Sciences* 54(1): 24-28.

Moncrieff, J. 2013. *The Bitterest Pills: The Troubling Story of Antipsychotic Drugs*. New York: Palgrave MacMillan.

Moncrieff, J. 2023a. The serotonin theory of depression: a systematic umbrella review of the evidence. *Molecular Psychiatry* 28: 3243-3256. https://doi.org/10.1038/s41380-022-01661-0

Moncrieff, J. 2023b. The serotonin theory of depression: both long discarded and still supported? *Molecular Psychiatry* 28: 3160-3163. https://www.nature.com/articles/s41380-023-02094-z

Nesse, R. M. 2000. Is depression an adaptation? *Archives of General Psychiatry* 57: 14-20.

Pescolido, B. A., Halpern-Manners, A, Luo, L., et al. 2021. Trends in public stigma of mental illness in the US, 1996-2018. *Jama Network Open* 4(12): e2140202. doi:10.1001/jamanetworkopen.2021.40202

Pinel, P. 1800. *Traité Médico-Philosophique sur L'Aliénation Mentale, ou La Manie*. Paris: Richard, Caille, et Ravier Libraires.

Read, J. 2005. The *bio-bio-bio* model of madness. *The Psychologist*, 18(10), 596–597.

Ritunnano, R., et al. 2022. Subjective experience and meaning of delusions in psychosis: a systematic review and qualitative evidence synthesis. *The Lancet Psychiatry* 9(6): 458-476.

Rush, B. 1835. *Medical Inquiries and Observations Upon the Diseases of the Mind. 5th edition*. Philadelphia: Grigg and Elliot.

Schomerus, G., Schindler, S., Sander, C., Baumann, E., and Angermeyer, M. 2022. Changes in mental illness stigma over 30 years – Improvement, persistence, or deterioration? *European Psychiatry*, 65(1): E78. doi:10.1192/j.eurpsy.2022.2337

Schroder, H. S. Devendorf, A, and Zikmund-Fisher, B. J. 2022. Framing depression as a functional signal, not a disease: Rationale and initial randomized control trial. *Social Science and Medicine* 328, 115995. doi.org/10.1016/j.socscimed.2023.115995

Scull, A. 2015. *Madness in Civilization*. Princeton: Princeton University Press.

Snyder, S. H. 1976. The dopamine hypothesis of schizophrenia: Focus on the dopamine receptor. *American Journal of Psychiatry* 133(2): 197-202.

Snyder, S. H. 1986. *Drugs and the Brain*. New York: W. H. Freeman and Co.

Spurzheim, J. G. 1836. *Observations on the Deranged Manifestations of the Mind; or, Insanity*. Boston: Marsh, Capen, and Lyon.

Taylor, H., and Vestergaard, M. D. 2022. Developmental dyslexia: Disorder or specialization of exploration? *Frontiers in Psychology* 13: 889245. https://doi.org/10.3389/fpsyg.2022.889245

Wakefield, J. in prep. *Psychiatrist as Philosopher: Robert Spitzer's Quest for a Definition of Mental Disorder*. Oxford: Oxford University Press.

Traumatic Immobility: Depression as a Stress Response

Sarah Knutson

Abstract: *This chapter challenges the claim of mainstream psychiatry that "major depressive disorder" is necessarily the result of genetic defects or abnormal brain functioning. It posits that evolutionary survival responses wired into human physiology can produce essentially the same phenomena. The author points out similarities between the Defense Cascade proposed by trauma researchers to explain involuntary immobility responses in the face of overwhelming stress, and the DSM criteria for depression and its subtypes. The criteria for depression are analyzed and explained through a survival lens—in particular, the Fright, Flag and Faint responses of the Defense Cascade—demonstrating that the clinical (and, allegedly, pathological) criteria are virtually indistinguishable from responses that would be predicted by normal human survival activation. In addition to explaining its incapacitating features, the author argues that the trauma model accounts for the subjective experience of depression in ways the DSM has yet failed to capture. Given the added value, not to mention the profound overlap, the author suggests that the survival paradigm offers individuals and supporters new options for working with physically and mentally immobilizing phenomena—with or without clinical or pharmacological aid. The author additionally proposes reconceptualizing depression as a human vulnerability at the species level, rather than an illness or defect at the individual level.*

Acknowledgement: A version of this chapter was first published by Mad in America on January 27, 2019.

I don't know about you, but for me the lines between trauma, stress, and suicidal depression can get pretty blurred. Whatever you call it, I feel like I'm being attacked from all sides. The universe is out to get me. Nothing I do can make any difference. My mind and body have betrayed me. *Family and friends become suspects or spies. Help degrades to force or manipulation.*

Reassurance mutates into lies. Neuronal connections to happy, hopeful memories drop like flies.

I once spent four years of my life like this—the lion's share of it, I was praying to die. Life was a prison camp with no future. Just torture or death in a hold so deep and dark no sunlight made it to the walls. The last fight left was with myself. Conscience in chains, I watched my integrity slither away and disappear through a gap in the bars.

I tried to describe what was happening to my doctor: *Are you sure this is depression? Because it feels like abject terror to me. It's as if some portentous wraith showed up, hijacked my body, and opened a refuge for underworld drifters. Now, they're all hanging out, making themselves at home, feeding on my energy and laughing at what a goner I am. It's no use trying to kick them out. The next day they're back in force with a new pack of goons, mocking me for trying and tormenting me all the more.*

Doctor: *You're depressed. Your symptoms are classic. Your mother had depression. Your grandmother had depression. It's genetic. Take your medicine. Eventually you'll come out of it. Most people do.*

Maybe he was right. I did come out of it. Meds probably played a role.

But I think I was more right.

Nailing Jello to the Wall

The *Diagnostic and Statistical Manual of Mental Disorders* (DSM-5) devotes over 30 pages and a host of symptoms and diagnostic specifiers to the various permutations and combinations of human despair; that is, "major depressive disorder" (American Psychiatric Association [APA], 2013). When you look at it, these criteria are all over the map. There's no rationale for why certain things cluster. It's like nailing Jello to the wall. As a diagnosed person, it spawns an almost overwhelming urge to throw up my hands, stick my head in the sand, and turn over my future to someone else.

This is what makes the stress response so exciting to me. All I have is a lay understanding of stress. I'm pretty much totally self-taught at the level anyone can get by reading a bit of popular science. But if I combine that with a survival/trauma paradigm called "the defense cascade" that's emerging in the clinical literature, I can make sense of every symptom and subtype of depression based on my own experience of what happens in my own body. In fact, I can pretty much do this with the entire *DSM*.

This raises, for me, some important, troubling questions. By and large, most of society agrees we have a depression epidemic that affects millions of people each year. Everyone also pretty much agrees that suicide rates are disturbingly high. And yet, by and large, the mental health industry is still seeing and treating these concerns as biochemical and genetic in origin.

But the fact is, my body can turn this kind of stuff on and off, practically on command. Just in the course of writing this essay, I got to see, time and again, how all of this stuff eased or passed as the stress equation in me changed. Sometimes on, sometimes off. Sometimes many, sometimes just a few. On and on, over and over, in various patterns, depending on how, for me, the stress-cookie crumbled.

And, over the course of three months, I cycled through pretty much all the so-called "symptoms" of "major depressive disorder" as listed in the *DSM*— just based on how stressed I was, or wasn't, while writing this essay.

So, what does that say about the biogenetic, chemical imbalance theory and suggestions that depression is a lifelong illness and all I can do is take my meds?

In other words:

- What if we don't have a depression epidemic at all? What if we have a stress epidemic that's reaching traumatic/survival proportions?
- What if the reason a lot of us aren't feeling or getting any better is that we've been taught to believe we have a lifelong and incurable disease?
- What if we've been steered away from exploring our minds and bodies—learning how they actually work—into believing that our

attempts to survive and respond to traumatic, threatening real-life circumstances are "symptoms of mental illness"?

- What if a huge part of our distress is that we've been advised—by professionals, society, and everyone else in our known world—to just sit still and wait for "the experts" to fix us, and until then we're out of options?

As we will see, that kind of thinking—in and of itself—is a recipe for a state of "traumatic immobility" that explains away all the major indicators of *DSM*'s depression. No real disease needed—just the unpacking of a deceptive brain loop sold to us by Big Pharma, payola government, and the mental illness industry.

Introducing the Defense Cascade

The defense cascade is a framework trauma therapists have been working on. I have a cynical theory as to why. Obviously, recalling trauma can be upsetting. So upsetting, apparently, that some of us become unresponsive. It turns out that this can create quite a crisis. You might guess a crisis for the client, but it's actually for the clinician I suspect the concern is mostly about.

Suppose you're a therapist and the 50-minute session is over. So, you say to the client, "Your time is up." But they don't move. You say it again, but they still don't seem to hear you. So now you muster your most firm, directive clinical voice, *"Your time is up. I'll see you next week."*

Still nothing. Just dead air. It gets even worse because ethics prevent you from even patting the laggard's arm to get their attention. (Given that there is usually a second client in the waiting room whose session can't start until the first [current] client is removed, you can imagine how many therapists this scenario may have traumatized.)

Eventually, this phenomenon recurred enough times that it couldn't be written off. It had to be more than a pathetic, Hail Mary, end-of-session attention-seeking behavior by the first client. At that point, the professional world took some interest and some measurements.

What they found was fascinating (see Schauer & Elbert, 2010, p. 111).

The Defense Cascade
(Progression of Survival Defenses)

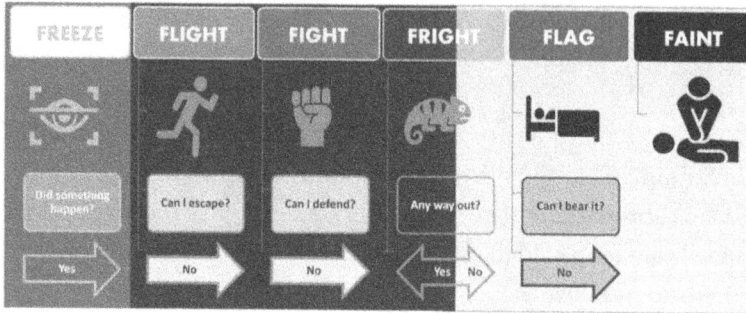

Figure 1: *The Defense Cascade*

As it turns out, the phenomenon we are talking about has a real name. It is the fourth defense in the diagram above: fright/tonic immobility. It also has measurable and observable physiological characteristics (Kozlowska et al., 2015; Schauer & Elbert, 2010; see also Roelofs, 2017).

Not only that, but it seems that there is a logical progression—and clear reasons in the mind and body—for when and why this phenomenon appears:

> [W]e propose that defense reactivity is organized to account for battlesomeness (chances to win a fight) of the threatened individual, that is, the appraisal of the threat by the organism in relation to its own power to counteract (age, gender, physical condition, defensive abilities, etc.) and, not least, for the threat-specifics (type of threat, type and speed of approach, context, threat involving blood loss, etc.). Whereas the dynamics of the defense cascade progresses in gradients of alternating ascending and descending activation, the various defense responses can be categorized into two general forms, namely active defense and immobility. (Schauer & Elbert, 2010, p. 110)

In other words, my body offers me two basic types of defenses (active/immobile) when I feel threatened. After a preliminary appraisal, I go with the approach I think offers me the best chance to survive. The type of defense I choose (active or immobile) depends on how threatened I feel.

In addition, both types (active, immobile) give me some sub-levels to choose from as the degree of threat changes. Different body systems are brought into play, in different combinations, based on the defense level I end up going with:

> Our model ... suggests six defense responses, notably *Freeze*, *Flight*, *Fight*, *Fright*, *Flag*, and eventually *Faint*, whereby during the two Fs *Flight* and *Fight* bodily responses are mainly regulated via the sympathetic branch ("uproar reactions") and the following three Fs, the second half of the cascade, are dominated by parasympathetic arousal, determining the spectrum of dissociative responding ("shut-down" reactions: *Fright*, *Flag*, and *Faint*). We thus may arrange the stages of the defense cascade in form of an inverted u-shaped arousal function with the alarming flight-fight responses on the ascent of the curve and the set of dissociative variants on the descent. (Schauer & Elbert, 2010, p. 111, emphasis in original)

A simple way of thinking about this is like a car. The active defenses—Fight and Flight—are controlled by the Gas Pedal (sympathetic) system. This system gets energy to my muscles and allows me to move. From there, it is a simple matter of direction:

- Fight is like barreling forward into the stuff I'm afraid of.
- Flight is like backing up and trying to get away.

Most people try to get away from scary stuff if they think that's an option (Schauer & Elbert, 2010). Freeze, Fright, Flag and Faint are all dominated by the Brake Pedal (parasympathetic) system of the car. If a Brake response comes on, it means that, for one reason or another, my body has decided that it's smarter to slow down or not move at all.

What is This Thing Called Fright?

Fright is a state of intense distress, equivalent to what my car would probably feel if I floored the Gas Pedal and slammed on the Brake Pedal at the same time. Like my car, the engine is all revved up and raring to go, but the energy it produces is totally jammed and blocked from taking me anywhere.

In humans, this dual activation of both the Gas Pedal (sympathetic) and Braking (parasympathetic) systems of our bodies is called "Fright." It typically occurs when intense fear or threat combines with a sense of being trapped or constrained (Schauer & Elbert, 2010).

Essentially, a threshold is reached where mental and physical arousal are skyrocketing. But there are no good options and, thus, no viable strategy for unleashing all that energy. It is no longer adaptive to run or fight (active defenses), so the body changes tactics and begins to shut down (immobile defenses).

In the prodromal period before complete shutdown, "[g]eneral fear symptoms are experienced, including dizziness, nausea, palpitation, drowsiness, lightheadedness, tension, blurred vision, feelings of irreality, numbing, and tingling appear" (Schauer & Elbert, 2010, p. 112).

As the lack of options is confirmed and hopelessness sets in, distress and activation jointly peak in a "peritraumatic 'panic-like' dual autonomic activation" (Schauer & Elbert, 2010, p. 113). This is the tipping point during which "sensation, perception, motor abilities, and speech behavior are dramatically altered" (Schauer & Elbert, 2010, p. 113).

A "'shut-down' reaction" occurs (Schauer & Elbert, 2010, p. 113):

- The Braking (parasympathetic) system powers on—forcing heart rate and blood pressure down and making active defenses all but impossible.
- The Gas Pedal (sympathetic) system goes into overdrive—muscles become "overly tense and rigid," and movements are "slow and

difficult" to the point where "overt behavioral actions are not an option" (p. 115).

- Normal channels of awareness and perception are blocked, and endogenous opioids flood the system.

In this dual Gas Pedal/Brake state, "various forms of dissociation appear" (p. 113):

- "Memory retrieval deficits" occur (p. 113).
- Consciousness alters, with a prevailing sensation of "alienation of oneself or the external world" and "a flattening of emotional experiences" (p. 113).
- There is failure, of both mind and body, to "deliberately control processes and take actions that can normally be influenced by an act of volition" (p. 113):

As a result, previously accessible information does not reach conscious awareness, and voluntary movements are not attempted (Schauer & Elbert, 2010).

Why Would I Ever Opt for Fright?

Fright is basically a strategic surrender when I'm overwhelmed and out of options. It buys me time to regroup—and, hopefully, I get hurt less:

> Tonic immobility [fright] is almost always displayed when the person is overwhelmed by threat and not allowed and not able to act aggressively against the threat. Thus immobility functions to suppress anger in the victim and acts bidirectionally to inhibit aggression. (Schauer & Elbert, 2010, p. 116)

To grasp what's going on, let's take a look at how this plays out in the wild. Suppose I'm a rabbit trying to avoid becoming a foxy meal. I've run my fastest, fought my hardest, but I've lost. So now the fox has me down by the neck, and it looks like I'm done for.

Not so fast! I still have one trick left up my sleeve: Play Dead. Next thing I know, the Brake slams on and overrides the Gas Pedal. Instant immobility.

Surprisingly, Fright may save my life. The Braking system so completely subdues me that I give no appreciable signs of life. The fox thinks I'm dead and loses interest or his appetite. The moment the fox is out of sight, the Brake lifts, and I floor the Gas Pedal back to my hole.

Time for the Spoiler

As you may have guessed, the Fright response is a big part of what I'm referring to here as "traumatic immobility." It's not the only factor, however.

Traumatic immobility also extends to stages 5 and 6 (Flag and Faint) of the defense cascade (see Figure 1). Flag and Faint largely result when Fright goes on too long, or when distress continues to rise. At that point, awareness of suffering loses adaptivity, so the Braking (parasympathetic) system shuts down consciousness even further, and Gas Pedal (sympathetic) arousal fades away. I end up just laying around—a sort of floppy, semi-comatose, helpless blob. That's Flag. If I become wholly unresponsive, that's Faint. Either way, no more faking it—this is true surrender. My mind and body have conceded defeat, and we're just waiting for the end.

Each of these variants on traumatic immobility has something to add to our discussion of depression. In fact, Fright, Flag and Faint all meet the *DSM* criteria for a Major Depressive Episode in their own right. In addition, they each neatly correlate with a specific depressive subtype (i.e., anxious, melancholic, and with catatonic features, respectively). The details of that deserve a chapter in its own right. Right now, it's time to dive deeper into traumatic immobility and the paradigm shift it points to.

It's *Not* All in My Head

When I came across the defense cascade, I could have kissed the researchers who wrote the article. Finally, I had some answers. Finally, I could explain experiences and deep moral conflicts that had been dogging me for 20 years. Finally, it wasn't all in my head.

Here are the basic components of traumatic immobility (Fright, Flag, Faint on the defense cascade).

1. Overwhelmed by threat
2. Out of options
3. Gas pedal (sympathetic) activation or shut-down
4. Brake (parasympathetic) shut-down
5. Reduced capacity to respond, mentally and physically, to compelling life circumstances

Here's how I applied that to make sense of my last major depression/*DSM* symptoms two years ago:

1. Felt constantly threatened (repeated job loss, poverty, homelessness, out of sync with mainstream and workplace values, relationship failure, social pariah): *low mood, worry, mental and physical activation, weird appetite and sleep*
2. Felt out of options (low physical, material and social resources; tired all the time, brain not functioning): *hopelessness, sadness, despair, indecision*
3. Gas pedal/sympathetic (constant pressure to do something to fix it): *worry, activation, insomnia, eating for energy*
4. Brake/parasympathetic (no clue how to fix it, where to turn or if it would ever get better): *low energy, low mood, low appetite and low interest in life; digestive troubles, stomach cramps, poor thinking and concentration; leaden limbs, sleeping a lot*
5. Life indefinitely stalled by Brake (wasting my life, leaving a legacy of suffering and pain, letting myself and others down): *worthlessness, emptiness, guilt, indecision, crying a lot, preoccupied with death and suicide*

So that's how what I was experiencing fit with what the *DSM* classifies as depression, including various symptoms and some of the subtype features.

When this nickel dropped, you might expect it to feel like a real "aha" moment. In reality, it was disappointing and anti-climactic. Painfully, the *DSM* criteria didn't come close to capturing the distress I was feeling—and they certainly didn't give me a clue as to why. I want to take some time and go into that now.

Where Did I Go?

For me, depression was like being in a constant state of grief over someone who was lost—except it was me. The person I had known myself to be wasn't there anymore—and, for all I could tell, was permanently gone. All that was left for me was to wait in bed and hope she would return. So, I just sat there watching as life passed me by and everything and everyone I had once cared about slipped away or left.

Then there it was—the reason in print:

> In order to enable a maximal defensive and "dead" appearance ("as if dead," "playing possum"), which provides survival advantage by complete giving in and cessation of fighting, *moving, perceptions and later emotions need to be switched off or deactivated*. To guarantee motionlessness in these highly perilous situations, *the organism should be unable and unwilling to use voluntary muscles and should feel neither anger nor pain, be finally emotionally numb*, as if anesthetized. (Schauer & Elbert, 2010, p. 113, emphasis added)

I found this weirdly reassuring. Knowing what was happening—and why—made me feel so much safer: *I'm not actually dying. I'm not even lost. Rather, a part of me is so scared—so in over my head about something gone wrong in my life—that my own body has shut me down. My very aliveness is being hidden from me (and others), deliberately, in response to the situation I am in.*

But how does my body make all of this seem so convincing? As it turns out, the way we perceive ourselves as being alive—and as actually present in our bodies—probably has something to do with the continual sensory feedback that our bodies give to our minds:

> A person's sensory processing (sight, hearing, smell, taste, and touch), of kinesthetic (perception of movement and muscular sense) and somesthetic (sensory data derived from skin, muscles, and body

organs) stimuli normally continuously serves the perceiving self as evidence that it resides "in" the physical body. (Schauer & Elbert, 2010, p. 117)

It probably also has a lot to do with our experiences of thinking and feeling. This is not just awareness of sensory information, but also the associations, emotions, and memories they generate—and all the mental processing our minds do about them. During traumatic immobility, the Brake system progressively shuts this down:

> Kinesthetic, somesthetic, nociceptive stimuli no longer seem to reach the central processing units, causing changes in body awareness and loss of control (depersonalization). Numbness prevails...Conscious processing of the events becomes limited, making meaning seems irrelevant.... emotional involvement fades away, that is, no action dispositions are assembled and memory consolidation becomes weak and later rehearsal more difficult. (Schauer & Elbert, 2010, p. 118)

Thus, access to the thoughts, feelings, and sensations that I experience as the essence of me is blunted or blocked. And so is my motivation and ability to address that. The resulting internal silence is deafening. I literally feel like I am dying—that the essence of "me" is gone, probably for good.

Am I Just Faking It?

The "Play Dead" response explains another thing that has really tortured me. I had this nagging sense, at the height of my depression, that *actually— I am faking it.* There was this odd internal turf war: Something deep inside me has dug in its heels *and insists it will not move*, while something else is whispering in my ear saying *You could do better if you tried.*

Well, there's an answer for that, too. Traumatic immobility isn't called the "Play Dead" response for nothing. A part of me knows there's still life inside somewhere. At the same time, the physiological changes that are taking place totally convince me otherwise.

With heartrate capped, digestion cramped, and righting reflex pulled out from under me, instinct commands that I lie down. Endogenous opioids (endorphins) swoop in. Communications crash, and it all gets very, very heavy. The rest is history.

Am I Morally Weak?

One of the hardest things about this state of mind and body was having to face myself: *Where did my integrity go? Why was I groveling in fear?*

There was no physical predator standing over me. I was being stalked by paperwork, bureaucracy, and poverty—not a lion or the Huns. I *knew* I was being irresponsible. I *knew* there was business to attend to. I *knew* there would be no rescue unless I created one.

But still, I couldn't do it. *Why, why, why?* Here's at least a partial answer: "*Tonic immobility guarantees negative or quiescent behavior even in the presence of massive aversive stimulation*, a stilled organism that makes no attempt to struggle for freedom or fight" (Schauer & Elbert, 2010, p. 115, emphasis added). The implication being that in this state of mind and body, survival instincts *override* the impulse toward "recuperative behavior" (p. 113).

Here is how that worked for me. I remember being hypnotically suggestible to some internal whisperer—*Stay still. Don't move. It's not safe enough yet. Getting up now will be certain disaster.* It seems ludicrous in retrospect. There were deadlines to meet, rent to pay, taxes to file, phone calls to make, forms to complete. But I just lay there waiting—desperately hoping for the odds to change.

Again, it helps to understand the physiology. The same "decoupling" we talked about above between body and brain likely affects our capacity for executive functioning—the ability to plan, prepare, and be disposed for action (Schauer & Elbert, 2010). It also affects the mirror neuron region of our brains, which helps us reflect and connect ourselves to the behavior of others. The joint effect is a vastly reduced ability to appreciate consequences, care about them, or mobilize the resources needed to address them.

The Dis-ease of Being Human

I don't know about you, but all of this helps me feel a heck of a lot more hominid and a heck of a lot less pathological or creepy. Instead of thinking of myself as having a brain disease, abnormal, defective, mentally ill, chemically deranged, mentally unscrewed, at the mercy of mysterious factors, randomly firing, or totally out of my control, I can just say to myself: *Oh, I'm having a rough time and my stress is too high. What do I need to change?* That shift alone brings the stress down several notches.

Imagine what that could do for other people too. Instead of those around me looking at me and saying: *Oh, what a weird freak. She's got this crazy, deranged brain thing going on that could make her flip out on me at any moment for no reason at all,* they can go: *Oh look, she's having a rough day, and her stress is too high. How can I be helpful?*

Suffice it to say, the stress response is a great leveler. It's vastly different that we're talking about something all of us can relate to—a genetic endowment we're all born into by virtue of being human. Call it the "human condition," if you will.

In a lovely, quirky way, it's both reassuring—and threatening—for everyone:

- We're *all* in this together.
- We're *all* genetically predisposed.

Now that we've come full circle, I'll happily concede this one to my doctor. After all, my mother was a mammal. My grandmother was a mammal. Their ancestors were mammals. They all got stressed too. *Aw shucks. I suppose I got it from them.*

Time to Brake

All of this can be a lot to digest. But I hope there's some good news just around the corner. For me, beginning to view these issues through the lens of stress and survival concerns has opened up a whole new way of working with them.

- If depression is a stress response, then it's potentially reversible. There's stuff I can do for myself, with or without the medical profession.
- If depression isn't a stress response, that still isn't the end of it. Stress affects virtually every system in our bodies (Sapolsky, 2004). Maybe I can free up some energy for coping or healing simply by learning more about how the stress response works and then tipping that balance in my favor.

To get the most out of this trauma-based model, however, I had to answer one final question: *Where is all this stress coming from?*

It's always tempting to blame the identified patient; for example, *you're not resilient enough, so work harder on your wellness tools.* But I'd like to push back a little. In modern times, it looks like depression and suicide rates have been rising for decades.

This suggests that these issues are not individual phenomena. They're more like something wrong with the culture—akin to rising sea levels in a world of human-created climate change. Accordingly, this begs the questions:

- Why are so many people in modern society stressed to the point of incapacity?
- Why are we feeling so helpless and hopeless that our bodies are concluding the best we can do is just lay down and die?
- What about modern society—and the options we are giving each other—is generating such resoundingly lethal impressions?

Once I started sincerely looking, the answers started rolling in (Knutson, 2020).

If you're like me, you may be surprised to realize how much you've been up against. Understanding that has helped a lot. I no longer feel like I'm doing something wrong or that breaking down is all about me.

Also, forewarned is forearmed. Now I can think more strategically about the defenses I use to protect myself and my future from some of the pitfalls of mainstream thinking and modern living.

Perhaps someday, together, we'll go one step further. Instead of blaming people for breaking down, we'll start changing the overwhelming odds— most of them socially created—that likely cause this.

References

American Psychiatric Association. (2013). *Diagnostic and statistical manual of mental disorders (DSM-5)*. American Psychiatric Publishing

Knutson, S. (2020). Stalked by Stress, Abandoned to Predation: The Appeal of Suicide in a Modern World. *Mad in America*.

Kozlowska, K., Walker, P., McLean, L., & Carrive, P. (2015). Fear and the defense cascade: clinical implications and management. *Harvard Review of Psychiatry, 23*(4), 263.

Roelofs, K. (2017). Freeze for action: neurobiological mechanisms in animal and human freezing. *Philosophical Transactions of the Royal Society B: Biological Sciences, 372*(1718), 20160206.

Sapolsky, R. M. (2004). *Why zebras don't get ulcers: The acclaimed guide to stress, stress-related diseases, and coping.* Holt paperbacks

Schauer, M., & Elbert, T. (2010). Dissociation Following Traumatic Stress. *Zeitschrift für Psychologie/Journal of Psychology, 218*(2), 109-127.

Exploring the Limits of Universal Human Needs in the Context of Mental Health: ADHD as a Case Example

Sofia Adam and Athanasios Koutsoklenis

Abstract: *This chapter critically assesses the analytical framework on universal human needs developed by Doyal and Gough (1991). This critical assessment focuses on the limitations associated with the endorsement of the biomedical model when addressing the basic need of health. We illustrate these limitations with particular reference to the case of Attention-Deficit/Hyperactivity Disorder (ADHD) which blurs the boundaries between physical and mental health. We move along three interrelated levels. First, we expose the deficiencies associated with the biomedical model. Second, we illustrate how the conceptualization of mental health within this model affects the form and content of appropriate health care and education. Third, we question the dual strategy based on the expert codified and user's experiential knowledge. The main intention is to defy allegations of scientific neutrality in social policy formation and open up new research directions which allow for alternative systems of social provisioning.*

Introduction

Theories of human needs have a long history. Their explicitly interdisciplinary object of inquiry is manifested in the various contributions stemming from social theory, political science, development studies, social policy, philosophy, and psychology (Springborg, 1981). A major demarcating line between the various theoretical contributions concerns the universal or relative character of human needs.

The universal camp intends to ground an objective as opposed to subjective understanding of well-being and universal as opposed to relative criteria for distributive justice. According to this framework, all humans irrespective of time and place share some basic or fundamental needs

(Doyal and Gough, 1991; Max-Neef, 1989) or core capabilities (Nussbaum, 2011). Divergences emerge with regard to the hierarchical — or not — nature of these needs as well as their fixity across space and time.

This chapter critically assesses the analytical framework developed by Doyal and Gough (1991) on universal basic needs, intermediate needs, and their satisfiers. In particular, we highlight the limitations associated with the endorsement of the biomedical model with particular reference to mental health disorders and the case of Attention-Deficit/Hyperactivity Disorder (ADHD).

We engage with the analytical framework developed by Doyal and Gough (1991) because it bridges thin and thick theories of human needs (Dean, 2009); differentiates between needs, satisfiers and preconditions; engages with both the content of basic needs and the procedural conditions for their optimum fulfillment; offers concrete directions for policy interventions; and informs recent contributions toward a sustainable eco-social welfare (Gough, 2017; Koch et al., 2016; Koch et al., 2017; Lindellee et al., 2021) for addressing the current poly- and permacrisis (The Conversation, 2022). We selected the case of ADHD because it blurs the distinction between physical and mental health and because it is ever-expanding as a diagnosis to unprecedented levels.

The critical assessment moves along three interrelated levels. First, we assess the uncritical endorsement of the biomedical model in order to ground health as a basic need. Second, we provide critical insights which problematize the content of appropriate health care and education in the case of persons diagnosed with ADHD. Third, we expose the limits of the procedural conditions proposed by Doyal and Gough (1991) as a dual strategy linking the codified expert knowledge and the experiential knowledge of relevant users. In the concluding section, we summarize the main critical points in order to shed light on the social production of needs and their modes of satisfaction.

Addressing the universal basic need for health through the biomedical model: the case of ADHD

Doyal and Gough (1991) structure their theory of universal basic needs in a systematic manner. They first distinguish between needs and wants. Human needs are objective/extensional, non-substitutable, and satiable whereas wants are subjective/intentional, substitutable, and insatiable. In addition, human needs are plural; they cannot be summarized and accounted for by a single dimension (Gough, 2017). All humans have common basic needs irrespective of space and time. In order to define these basic needs, they associate human welfare with the avoidance of serious harm. Serious harm is in turn defined as the impaired participation in any form of life.

Towards this goal, all humans have the basic needs of physical health and individual autonomy.[1] Physical health is defined according to the biomedical model as the lack of disease, and this is considered a solid basis enabling transcultural comparison. Individual autonomy is dependent on three variables: understanding, mental health, and opportunities. Understanding is the outcome of appropriate learning mechanisms. Mental health is manifested as practical rationality and responsibility. Opportunities refer to the potential of an actor to engage in new and significant actions, namely performing significant social roles as parent, householder, worker, or citizen. Finally, critical autonomy is introduced as the potential to follow a different rather than the dominant mode of life.

The definition of health as the absence of disease suffers from all the deficiencies of the biomedical model. These involve the mechanistic and compartmentalized understanding of the human body, which is analyzable into separate parts, the inherent reductionism of illness to a physical, biological disease neglecting socio-economic factors, and the sharp distinction between physical and mental health (Rocca and Anjum, 2020). Adhering to this problematic distinction is also evident in the way mental

---

[1] In subsequent works, Gough introduces as a separate basic need social participation (Gough, 2017). This brings a circularity in the original definition since social participation is deemed as a precondition in order to achieve social participation.

health is conducive to autonomy while physical health stands on its own as a basic human need.

In the field of mental health, the most accredited world-wide expert professional association is the American Psychiatric Association (APA) with the associated *Diagnostic and Statistical Manual of Mental Disorders (DSM)* as the main instrument for the establishment and diffusion of codified expert knowledge in the field of mental health. The huge influence of the *DSM* is captured concisely by Horwitz (2021: ix):

> [I]ts diagnoses define what mental disorders are considered legitimate, how patients conceive of their problems, who receives government benefits, and which conditions psychotropic drugs target and insurance companies will pay to treat. They also delineate the curriculum that is taught to psychiatrists and other mental health professionals, the diagnoses that researchers and epidemiologists explore, and the psychic problems that public policies attempt to remedy.

From the publication of the third edition of the *DSM* in 1980 and onward, the APA has replaced dynamic psychiatry with a biomedical framework (Horwitz, 2002). This paradigm shift was not based on promising scientific discoveries but on consensus among experts (Davies, 2013; Horwitz, 2002; Stier, 2013). For example, fundamental to the biomedical model is the assumption that biological discoveries will eventually establish the somatic etiology of separate and independent mental diseases (Jacobs and Cohen, 2012). Despite intense efforts and large investments, reliable diagnostic biomarkers or pathophysiologies for mental disorders are still not available (Frisch, 2021; Hyman, 2021; Schleim, 2022).

Conceptualizing mental disorders through a biomedical framework cast those diagnosed as governed by genetic or neurochemical abnormalities which can in turn provoke negative social attitudes and dehumanization (Lebowitz and Ahn, 2014). This suggests that biological explanations might significantly decrease the clinician's empathy, a very important parameter for clinical outcomes (Lebowitz and Ahn, 2014).

The preferment of biogenetic explanations may also induce pessimism and set the stage for self-fulfilling prophecies that could hamper recovery from psychological problems (Haslam and Kvaale, 2015; Kvaale et al., 2013a). Moreover, those endorsing biological explanations for mental disorders perceive affected persons as more dangerous and demand more distance from them (Kvaale et al., 2013b).

Nevertheless, the biomedical conceptualization of mental disorder (Thyer, 2015) keeps expanding both horizontally (encompassing qualitatively new forms of human distress and suffering) and vertically (encompassing quantitatively less severe phenomena) (Haslam, 2016). By the time of publishing *DSM-5*, the continuous medicalization[2] of human behavior became increasingly critiqued both within and outside the confines of the biomedical model.

ADHD is selected as an exemplary case in addressing the deficiencies of the biomedical model because the very definition of the disorder blurs the distinction between physical and mental health. More importantly, the estimated prevalence of ADHD is ever-expanding as ADHD diagnosed U.S. children and adolescents increased from 6.1% in 1997-1998 to 10.2% in 2015-2016 (Xu et al., 2018).

The ADHD 'epidemic' is not exclusive to the U.S.A.; for example, in France the ADHD diagnosis among children and adolescents increased by 96% between 2010 and 2019 (Ponnou and Thomé, 2022). However, ADHD is one of the most contested diagnoses as it has been under ontological, epistemological, and axiological debate since its introduction in the second edition of *DSM* (Laurence and McCallum, 1998).

One strand of skepticism stems from within the dominant biomedical model. Allen Frances, an eminent psychiatrist, worked on *DSM-III* and later became the chairperson of the *DSM-IV* Task Force. In 2013, he published a critical book highlighting the changes in the diagnostic thresholds and diagnostic criteria of *DSM-5* which have made diagnoses

---

[2] The process 'by which nonmedical problems become defined and treated as medical problems, usually in terms of illnesses or disorders' (Conrad, 1992: 209).

'loose' leading to overdiagnosis and excessive medication (Frances, 2013). Posner et al. (2020) reviewed the state-of-the-art knowledge about the causes, pathophysiology, diagnosis, epidemiology, and treatment of ADHD. They also stress the constant changes of the very definition of ADHD by stating that:

> Attention-deficit hyperactivity disorder (ADHD), like other psychiatric syndromes, has been refined and developed over the past 50 years, from its first contemporary description (second edition; DSM-II) as a hyperkinetic reaction of childhood to its current inclusion in DSM-5 as a lifespan neurodevelopmental condition. (Posner et al., 2020: 1)

After reviewing the available evidence from a biomedical perspective, the authors concluded that despite the cumulative evidence pointing towards an understanding of ADHD as a continuum with variations in degree rather than in kind, clinical practice still rests on a categorical diagnosis with arbitrary clinical boundaries with regard to the number and severity of symptoms, degree of impairment, and needs for intervention (Posner et al., 2020: 8-9).

Even *DSM-5-TR* authors admit that at least some of their fundamental presumptions are not well-grounded in science. ADHD is placed within the *DSM-5-TR*'s chapter on Neurodevelopmental Disorders characterized as "developmental deficits or differences in brain processes that produce impairments of personal, social, academic, or occupational functioning" (APA, 2022: 36) even though evidence confirming the neurodevelopmental basis has not yet materialized. In particular, *DSM-5-TR* authors state that "no biological marker is diagnostic for ADHD" and that "meta-analysis of all neuroimaging studies do not show differences between individuals with ADHD and control subjects" (APA, 2022: 73).

Outside the confines of the biomedical model, criticism is blunter given that the association between biological dysfunctions or causes and mental health difficulties in general is not established (Moncrieff, 2022). *DSM* authors are confined to a descriptive approach towards diagnosis solely based on behavioral indicators called symptoms without the requirement to understand nor identify any presumed underlying causes or dynamics of the behavior in question (Kirk et al., 2013). Such behavioral indicators-symptoms are then rebranded as diagnostic criteria which in the absence of a solid biomedical cause-effect explanatory framework are necessarily ambiguous, arbitrary, redundant, and subjective while they are themselves subject to decontextualization, de-agentilization and ableism (Honkasilta and Koutsoklenis, 2022, 2023).

ADHD conceptualization is subject to a number of logical fallacies. First, as already mentioned, ADHD is defined:

> [A]s a neurodevelopmental disorder defined by impairing levels of inattention, disorganization, and/or hyperactivity-impulsivity. Inattention and disorganization entail inability to stay on task, seeming not to listen, and losing materials necessary for tasks, at levels that are inconsistent with age or developmental level. Hyperactivity-impulsivity entails overactivity, fidgeting, inability to stay seated, intruding into other people's activities, and inability to wait— symptoms that are excessive for age or developmental level. (APA, 2022: 37)

This definition follows a circular logic; that is, if an individual has attention-deficit/hyperactivity disorder, it is because he is inattentive, distracted, and hyperactive-impulsive; and if an individual is inattentive, distracted and hyperactive-impulsive, it is because he has ADHD. The resulting definitional inaccuracy is inevitable until diagnostic criteria are grounded on something other than descriptive wording (Jacobs and Cohen, 2012).

The second type of fallacy is called affirming the consequent; if the second part of the logical construction is true, then this proves the antecedent (Tait, 2009). For example, according to the diagnostic criteria, if the child is "often acting as if 'driven by a motor'", "often has difficulty waiting his or her turn" and so on, then the child has ADHD.

The third type of fallacy is called appeal to authority. The international consensus statement on ADHD (Barkley et al., 2002) is probably the most notable example of the drive to establish the dominant position by stating that those who critique ADHD as a valid disorder are "similar to those declaring the earth flat, the laws of gravity debatable, and the periodic table in chemistry a fraud" (Barkley et al., 2002: 90). This quest for settling once and for all the debate is not based on the best available evidence but in relation to the large number of prominent authors who signed it. But "weight of numbers, in the absence of satisfactory supporting evidence, is no argument at all" (Tait, 2009: 247). Scientific knowledge is (or more accurately should be) established by evidence rather than authority.

Finally, ecological fallacy refers to the erroneous belief that average group findings can be applied on an individual level. Studies that use aggregate measures of attributes, such as the size of the brain, are very limited in what they can infer about individuals in the population under examination (te Meerman et al., 2022). For example, Hoogman et al. (2017: 2) came to the conclusion "that patients with ADHD have altered brains; therefore ADHD is a disorder of the brain."

However, Batstra et al. (2017) reminded that biological differences do not automatically imply pathology while, Dehue et al. (2017: 438) remarked that:

> Hoogman and colleagues only found average differences with small effect sizes. This finding implies considerable overlap between groups and significant within-group variation. Consequently, there is no point in conveying that a child with ADHD has a brain disorder. Brain scans can only differ and never tell which characteristics should count as a disorder.

To sum up, the biomedical model suffers from many deficiencies in the definition of health, the conceptualization of mental health, and the arbitrary classification of different human conditions as disorders as the case of ADHD illustrates. This conceptualization affects the form and content of intermediate needs such as appropriate health care and education, to which we now turn.

Addressing intermediate needs: the form and content of appropriate health care and education in the case of ADHD

Doyal and Gough (1991) bridge thin (general, universal) and thick (particular, relative) theories of human needs through the introduction of intermediate needs or universal satisfier characteristics. These intermediate needs include: adequate nutritional food and water, adequate protective housing, non-hazardous work environment, non-hazardous physical environment, appropriate healthcare, security in childhood, significant primary relationships, physical security, economic security, safe birth control and child-bearing, and appropriate education.

The target of policy interventions is to secure the optimum satisfaction of basic needs through the minimum satisfaction of intermediate needs (minopt level[3]). Overall, basic need satisfaction is dependent on the existence of four societal preconditions: production, reproduction, cultural transmission, and authority. These societal preconditions are also presented in transcultural terms meaning that every society should fulfill these functions in order to ensure basic need satisfaction. This conceptualization, however, is subject to a number of limitations as will be shown in the following.

The individual level of analysis is retained from the level of basic need definition to the definition of intermediate needs and of particular satisfiers (Clifford, 1984). The societal preconditions intend to rectify this, but they do not allow for the conceptualization of another system of social provisioning. More importantly, they keep intact the distinction between production and reproduction while the latter's content is restricted to procreation and infant-care and socialization.

---

[3] The minopt level of intermediate needs' satisfaction is explained in the following: "Thus the crucial task in constructing indicators of need-satisfaction is to ascertain *the minimum quantity of intermediate need-satisfaction required to produce the optimum level of basic need-satisfaction* measured in terms of the physical health and autonomy of individuals. In the spirit of Rawls, we could call this level the *minimum optimorum.*" (Doyal and Gough, 1991, pp. 162-163).

However, social reproduction theorists have clearly demonstrated that labor producing commodities and labor producing people are both parts of the systemic totality of capitalism, and they should not be differentiated either spatially (points of production versus points of reproduction) or functionally (material versus symbolic) (Bhattacharya, 2017; Fraser, 1989). That is, despite the rhetoric of universality, human needs are framed in accordance with a restrictive understanding of the existing society while the horizon for their satisfaction is within the contours of the existing society.

According to the Doyal and Gough (1991) framework, individuals should have appropriate healthcare and appropriate education among others. The case of ADHD exposes antagonistic views in the proposed form and content of these intermediate needs within the contours of the dominant mental health care and educational paradigm.

The biomedical model prioritizes the technical aspects of health care as the diagnosis allows rational choice of the appropriate technical intervention regardless of whether pharmaceutical or psycho-social treatment is selected (Timimi, 2014). In terms of pharmaceutical interventions, a 2016 national parent survey for children 2–17 years of age estimated that 62% of ADHD diagnosed children were on medication (Danielson et al., 2022). What is more, 69% of the DSM-5 task force members reported having ties to the pharmaceutical industry (Cosgrove and Krimsky, 2012).

However, the critical question is not the financial dependence of the dominant psychiatry on the industry but that "psychiatry exists as a medical subspecialty in part because industry has been able to co-opt the lack of biological markers to its own advantage" (Cosgrove and Wheeler, 2013: 98). In terms of diagnosis-based psycho-social interventions, Timimi (2014: 213) remarks that:

> By importing the diagnostic model from general medicine, we end up miss-selling and under-utilizing the unique skills the profession of psychiatry brings to healthcare by the "dumbing down" of what we do into simplistic, diagnosis-driven protocols that have more to do with successful consumer culture marketing than with science.

Indeed, the evidence shows that common factors (i.e., factors that all therapeutic endeavors have in common) are way more important in determining outcomes than therapeutic techniques targeting specific diagnoses (Duncan et al., 2009; Miller et al., 2008; Wampold, 2015). The focus on technical aspects of psycho-social interventions has little impact on outcomes in comparison to the relational and contextual aspects (Timimi, 2017).

Such aspects become central in non-diagnostic, outcome-oriented models of psycho-social interventions such as Outcome Orientated Child and Adolescent Mental Health Services (OO-CAMHS) that have been developed by a community team in the United Kingdom (Timimi, 2013). Central to this model is the incorporation of systematized feedback from the users on the progress and the consolidation of an alliance between the service user and the service provider.

In the field of education, the interconnection of the educational system with the establishment and expansion of the ADHD diagnosis is manifold. Education policies leave teachers little choice but to find diagnostic categories for "disorderly" students to fit in (Hinshaw and Scheffler, 2014). Teachers play an important role in the diagnostic process; they have been found to "pre-label" disruptive children (McMahon, 2012) and to be the first to imply a diagnosis of ADHD (Gesser-Edelsburg and Boukai, 2019).

Several school-related variables appear to affect the likelihood of students to receive an ADHD diagnosis, including being among the younger in class (Koutsoklenis et al., 2019), having a relatively older teacher (Schneider and Eisenberg, 2006) or living in a state with strict school accountability policies (Hinshaw and Scheffler, 2014). ADHD diagnosis is used as an instrument of institutional governance resulting in a top-down process of distributing and directing educational resources according to information communicated via the diagnosis (Honkasilta and Koutsoklenis, 2022). For example, in the USA laws and policies related to school accountability and the push for performance give schools the incentive to direct parents toward seeking diagnoses in order to attract resources needed to raise students' performance (as measured in test scores) and to exempt low achieving students from lowering the district's overall achievement ranking (Hinshaw and Scheffler, 2014).

When schools promote diagnoses nurturing a "special educational need," education professionals are inclined to distance themselves from the responsibility of adequately meeting that need since the diagnosis itself is considered a legitimate biomedical proof that the problem lies within the child (Honkasilta and Koutsoklenis, 2022). This approach can lead to segregated school environments as in the case of Sweden with classes specifically designed for ADHD students (Malmqvist and Nilholm, 2016). In this context, the main priority of the educational system is to control ADHD related symptoms mainly through pharmaceutical interventions (Malmqvist, 2018). Such findings become particularly alarming when taking into account the lack of robust evidence regarding the long-term effectiveness of pharmaceutical treatments for ADHD (Cortese et al., 2018; Santos et al., 2021; Schweren et al., 2018).

Furthermore, Hjörne and Säljö (2019) studied classroom interactions in eight ADHD classes via video recordings during a period of seven years. They reached the conclusion that "it is difficult to see how the learning will improve when placed in these segregated settings where the role expectations are so limited and where they differ in such obvious manners from mainstream classrooms" (Hjörne and Säljö, 2019: 236).

Addressing the procedural conditions towards social needs satisfaction: the dual strategy in the case of ADHD

Doyal and Gough (1991) propose a dual strategy for the specification of the particular satisfiers of intermediate needs based upon the codified expert knowledge and grounded experiential knowledge through consultation with the relevant users. These are the procedural conditions towards the satisfaction of basic human needs in specific societies.

This dual strategy links externally as two distinct pillars: codified expert knowledge and grounded experiential knowledge (Doyal and Gough, 1991; Gough, 2017, 2020). It is based on the explicit intention to allow for cultural variation in the definition and measurement of basic needs' satisfiers and to avoid accusations of paternalism. However, this dual strategy is subject to serious limitations in general and with reference to the case of ADHD.

The term codified expert knowledge denotes that there is a state-of-the-art knowledge in every domain addressing basic human needs that should guide social policy formation. However, in manifold domains of social policy, we detect fierce debates concerning the organization and delivery of appropriate services. In this regard, codified expert knowledge may easily be equated with the dominant approach to the exclusion of alternative conceptualizations and policy suggestions while projecting an alleged epistemological neutrality. The argument put forward by Doyal and Gough (1991) that this codified expert knowledge evolves over time does not suffice to allow for the ongoing antagonisms not following a linear progress towards the establishment of truth claims.

Evidence-based practice has derived in analogy from its parent movement—evidence-based medicine (Gomory, 2013). In the case of ADHD, the literature promoting evidence-based practice privileges specific types of evidence produced by experimental research and particularly from Randomized Control Trials (RCTs). RCT studies are generally considered either as the *best* source of evidence or even as the *only* source of evidence (Koutsoklenis and Gaitanidis, 2017). In the following, we highlight four major areas of concern regarding the bias stemming from this particular research methodology.

First, evidence-based practice in the case of ADHD is *per se* diagnosis driven. As such, it is formulated on the basis of the diagnosis, and conveys the certainty that the diagnosis is valid and accurate despite the proliferation of evidence questioning the validity and accuracy of the diagnosis itself. For a RCT to be valid, the selection of participants must be random from a population of individuals who all have the same underlying disease; this is highly unlikely given the lack of validity and accuracy plus the heterogeneity of the population diagnosed with ADHD (Koutsoklenis and Gaitanidis, 2017).

Second, experience, values, agency, meaning and other contextual factors are either excluded as irrelevant or reduced to observable behaviors that can be controlled and technically manipulated. What is missing is that individuals' response to mental health interventions does not only depend on the intervention's specifications but also on how individuals interpret and construe the intervention (Koutsoklenis and Gaitanidis, 2017).

Third, the prioritization of a particular research methodology stipulates in advance what is to be ascertained. If it is pre-decided that RCTs must be used for research to climb up the "credibility hierarchy" (Hammersley, 2001: 545), many research questions would be omitted and thus left unexplored and ultimately unanswered. For example, Bjornstad and Montgomery (2005) reviewed the effectiveness of family therapy for children with ADHD for the prestigious Cochrane Database of Systematic Reviews. In their review, they only included RCT studies, discrediting in this way all other evidence based on different research methodologies as less valuable or important. Ten years later, the aforementioned review received the highest rate in a meta-analysis carried out by Watson et al. (2015). In this way, the scientific bias feeds on itself.

Fourth, RCTs use group aggregated averages in the data analysis. This means that by default they do not intend to explore the particular needs of specific persons in their settings which however is the ultimate goal of mental health interventions (Gomory, 2013).

With regard to the other pillar of the procedural conditions, the experiential knowledge of the relevant users, the concept of user involvement fits well with the dual strategy proposed by Doyal and Gough (1991). However, in the framework of the managerialist-consumerist model of welfare, user involvement "represents a kind of intelligence gathering/market research activity, with origins in the philosophies of the market and managerialism and their stated interest in cost-effectiveness and effective control and rational decision-making" (Beresford, 2013: p. 143).

In addition, the organization of focus groups with the involvement of users often leads to the "professionalization" of users as consultants and trainers (Clifford, 1984; Cowden and Singh, 2007). The interpolation of public administration and public deliberative action is multidirectional (Fraser, 1989). As Wetherly (1996) has noted, the dual strategy presupposes a quest for consensus. The potential of such social audits and fora to elucidate critical insights on behalf of the concerned users rests upon the Habermasian framework of communicative action and the decolonization of the public sphere. In this framework, consensus is expected to be the product of an unconstrained discussion under conditions of freedom, equality, and fairness.

Unfortunately, such loci of social interaction are not given, and they cannot be constructed through social engineering. No matter how benevolent the intentions, these public spaces are not free from hierarchies of all sorts— and this does not only refer to the co-existence of experts and service users, but to the differing positions among users themselves (Dean, 2009). As Fraser (1989) has rightly pointed out, there are opposing social movements with conflicting interpretations of social needs. A consensual approach to social policy formation does not do justice to the competing quests for health care and education provision in this regard.

The organization CHADD is of particular relevance. CHADD was founded in Florida (USA) in 1987 by Dr. Harvey Parker, a clinical psychologist, and Fran Gilman and Carol Lerner, in their role as parents, in order "to provide support and to share information about ADHD."[4] Its goals and priorities are "to serve as a clearinghouse for evidence-based information on ADHD," "as a local face-to-face family support group for families and individuals affected by ADHD," and as "an advocate for appropriate public policies and public recognition in response to needs faced by families and individuals with ADHD."[5] Therefore, CHADD could serve as an illustrative example of an organization based on the dual strategy supported by Doyal and Gough (1991).

In practice, CHADD promotes a particular, uncritical view of ADHD. For example, CHADD states that "ADHD is medically and legally recognized as a treatable yet potentially serious disorder, affecting up to nine percent of all children, and approximately four percent of adults."[6] This is the result

---

[4] https://chadd.org/adhd-weekly/chadd-marks-30-years-supporting-the-adhd-community/
[5] https://chadd.org/about/#history
[6] https://chadd.org/about/

of the organization being established based on diagnosis and taking as self-evident the diagnostic validity and accuracy of ADHD as well as its treatment organized around this biomedical framing.

At the same time, there are other examples of users' organizations who do not organize based on the diagnoses while still demanding the satisfaction of the mental health needs of their members. For example, the organization Stichting Pill[7] supports that drugs-based mental health practice entails major risks for the users as drugs are increasingly prescribed too quickly, too much, and/or for too long. This does not mean that they succumb to a similarly uncritical denial of mental suffering and/or drug treatment but that they strive to build an active platform in order to empower people seeking assistance. Therefore, there is not a representative case of a user organization out there or a consensus on the specific form and content of appropriate services.

Concluding remarks

This chapter addresses the analytical framework of universal human needs given a renewed interest in the formation of social policy and public interventions to better able address social welfare in a sustainable manner. Despite the benevolent intentions to found objective grounds for an effective social policy, these proposed grounds are not solid and may actually be disempowering for transformative social policy design and implementation on a number of fronts.

The endorsement of the biomedical model rests upon the assumption of scientific neutrality through alignment with the dominant biomedical model in the definition of health. This model, however, has been highly questioned even within its own confines, especially with regard to the definition of mental health disorders as the case of ADHD has clearly manifested—let alone voices which criticize the construction of diagnostic categories.

The conceptualization of mental health disorders affects to a great extent the form and content of health care and education for the persons

---

[7] https://www.stichting-pill.nl/

diagnosed as such. It entails a self-feeding process whereby labeling substitutes the examination of a persons' context and, in turn, the design of support in accordance with contextual factors. It fosters over-prescriptions of drugs, even for diagnostic categories whose neurophysiological basis is not proven as in the case of ADHD.

More importantly, it builds on the individual rectification through technical interventions leaving aside the community and context of affected persons. These limitations are not resolved by the addition of users' voice as a supplement to the codified expert knowledge. This strategy does not allow for conflicting views to emerge in both camps, experts and users alike. In other words, this consensual approach can be problematic and disempowering.

There is antagonism within and between both sides (experts and users). The role of social scientists is to illuminate these competing quests and claims, to explicitly state the assumptions holding them apart, and choose sides on the basis of explicit premises (i.e., theories which represent those whose needs are unmet; Clifford, 1984) without disregarding the urgency of social needs satisfaction.

The assessed analytical framework of universal human needs suffers epistemologically from a confinement within the paradigm of alleged scientific neutrality; this does not allow for the critical examination of the social production and satisfaction of needs in alternative settings. In other words, it does not explore social practices and institutions able to produce alternative definitions of social needs. It would also explicitly allow for the advancement of collective modes for the satisfaction of social needs which alter both their form and content.

Doyal and Gough (1991) do acknowledge that satisfiers are not necessarily addressed at the individual level, but they do not systematically explore how the collective satisfaction of social needs might entail social practices beyond the dominant socio-economic and scientific paradigm.

References

American Psychiatric Association (2022) *Diagnostic and Statistical Manual of Mental Disorders, 5th edn, Text Revision*. Washington, DC: American Psychiatric Association.

Batstra L, te Meerman S, Conners K, Frances A (2017) Subcortical brain volume differences in participants with attention deficit hyperactivity disorder in children and adults. *Lancet Psychiatry* 4(6): 439.

Barkley RA (2002) International consensus statement on ADHD. *Clinical Child and Family Psychology Review* 5: 89–111.

Beresford P (2013) From 'other' to involved: user involvement in research: an emerging paradigm. *Nordic Social Work Research*, 3(2): 139–148, DOI: 10.1080/2156857X.2013.835138

Bhattacharya T (ed.) (2017) *Social Reproduction Theory: Remapping Class, Recentering Oppression*. Pluto Press.

Bjornstad GJ. and Montgomery P (2005) Family therapy for attention-deficit disorder or attention-deficit/hyperactivity disorder in children and adolescents. *Cochrane Database of Systematic Reviews* 2: 1–26.

Clifford D (1984) Concept formation in radical theories of need: a comment on Doyal and Gough's A Theory of Human Needs. *Critical Social Policy* 4(11): 147–150.

Conrad P (1992) Medicalization and Social Control. *Annual Review of Sociology* 18: 209–232.

Cortese S, Adamo N, Del Giovane C, Mohr-Jensen C, Hayes AJ, Carucci S, Atkinson LZ, Tessari L, Banaschewski T, Coghill D, Hollis C, Simonoff E, Zuddas A, Barbui C, Purgato M, Steinhausen HC, Shokraneh F, Xia J, Cipriani A (2018) Comparative efficacy and tolerability of medications for attention-deficit hyperactivity disorder in children, adolescents, and adults: a systematic review and network meta-analysis. *Lancet Psychiatry* 5(9): 727–738.

Cosgrove L and Krimsky S (2012) A comparison of DSM-IV and DSM-5 panel members' financial associations with industry: A pernicious problem persists. *PLoS Medicine* 9(3): e1001190.

Cosgrove L and Wheeler EE (2013) Industry's colonization of psychiatry: Ethical and practical implications of financial conflicts of interest in the DSM-5. *Feminism & Psychology* 23(1): 93–106.

Cowden S and Singh G (2007) The 'User': Friend, foe or fetish?: A critical exploration of user involvement in health and social care. *Critical Social Policy* 27(1): 5–23.

Davies J (2013) *Cracked. The Unhappy Truth about Psychiatry.* New York: Pegasus Books.

Dean H (2009) Critiquing capabilities: the distractions of a beguiling concept. *Critical Social Policy* 29(2): 261–273.

Dehue T, Bijl D, de Winter M, Scheepers F, Vanheule S, van Os J, Verhaeghe P, and Verhoeff B (2017) Subcortical brain volume differences in participants with attention deficit hyperactivity disorder in children and adults. *Lancet Psychiatry* 4(6): 438–439.

Doyal L and Gough I (1991) *A theory of human need.* New York: Guilford Press.

Frances A (2013) *Saving normal: an insider's revolt against out-of-control psychiatric diagnosis, dsm-5, big pharma, and the medicalization of ordinary life.* William Morrow.

Fraser N (1989) *Unruly Practices: Power, Discourse, and Gender in Contemporary Social Theory.* Minnesota: University of Minnesota Press.

Frisch S (2021) Why biological psychiatry hasn't delivered yet–and why neurology knows. *Psychiatry Investigation* 18: 1145–1148.

Gesser-Edelsburg A and Boukai RH (2019) Does the education system serve as a persuasion agent for recommending ADHD diagnosis and medication uptake? A qualitative case study to identify and characterize the persuasion strategies of Israeli teachers and school counselors. *BMC Psychiatry* 19(153).

Gomory T (2013) The limits of evidence based medicine and its application to mental health evidence-based practice (Part One). *Ethical Human Psychology and Psychiatry* 15(1): 18–34.

Gough I (2020) Defining floors and ceilings: the contribution of human needs theory. *Sustainability: Science, Practice and Policy* 16(1): 208–219.

Gough I (2017) *Heat, Greed and Human Need*. Chetenhalm: Edward Elgar Publishing.

Hammersley M (2001) On 'systematic' reviews of research literatures: a 'narrative' response to Evans & Benefield. *British Educational Research Journal* 27: 543–554.

Haslam N (2016) Concept creep: Psychology's expanding concepts of harm and pathology. *Psychological Inquiry* 27(1): 1–17.

Haslam N and Kvaale EP (2015) Biogenetic explanations of mental disorder: The mixed-blessings model. *Current Directions in Psychological Science* 24(5): 399–404.

Hinshaw SP and Scheffler RM (2014) *The ADHD Explosion: Myths, Medication, Money, and Today's Push for Performance*. Oxford: Oxford University press.

Hjörne E and Säljö R (2019) Teaching and learning in the special education setting: agency of the diagnosed child. *Emotional and Behavioural Difficulties* 24(3): 224–238.

Honkasilta J and Koutsoklenis A (2023) ADHD in the making: From "identifying" symptoms to "symptomatic" identities. In: Maisel E. (ed) Deconstructing ADHD: Mental Disorder or Social Construct? (pp. 370-399). The Ethics International Press.

Honkasilta J and Koutsoklenis A (2022) The (un)real existence of ADHD—Criteria, functions, and forms of the diagnostic entity. Frontiers in Sociology 7: 814763.

Hoogman M, Bralten J, Hibar DP, et al. (2017) Subcortical brain volume differences in participants with attention deficit hyperactivity disorder in children and adults: a crosssectional mega-analysis. *Lancet Psychiatry* 4: 310–319.

Horwitz AV (2021) *DSM: A History of Psychiatry's Bible*. Baltimore: John Hopkins University.

Horwitz AV (2002) *Creating Mental Illness*. Chicago: The University of Chicago Press.

Huth EJ, King K and Lock S (1988) Uniform requirements for manuscripts submitted to biomedical journals. *British Medical Journal* 296(4): 401–405.

Hyman SE (2021) Psychiatric disorders: grounded in human biology but not natural kinds. *Perspectives in Biology and Medicine* 64: 6–28.

Kirk SA, Gomory T and Cohen D (2013) *Mad Science: Psychiatric Coercion, Diagnosis, and Drugs*. New Brunswick, NJ: Transaction.

Koch M, Buch-Hansen H and Fritz M (2017) Shifting Priorities in Degrowth Research: An Argument for the Centrality of Human Needs. *Ecological Economics* 138: 74–81.

Koch M, Gullberg A T, Schoyen M A and Hvinden B (2016) Sustainable welfare in the EU: Promoting synergies between climate and social policies. *Critical Social Policy* 36(4): 704–715.

Koutsoklenis A and Gaitanidis A (2017) Interrogating the effectiveness of educational practices: A critique of evidence-based psychosocial treatments for children diagnosed with Attention-Deficit/Hyperactivity Disorder. *Frontiers in Education* 2: 11.

Koutsoklenis A and Honkasilta J (2023) ADHD in the DSM-5-TR: What has changed and what has not. *Frontiers in Psychiatry* 13: 1064141.

Koutsoklenis A, Honkasilta J, and Brunila K (2020) Reviewing and reframing the influence of relative age on ADHD diagnosis: beyond individual psycho(patho)logy. *Pedagogy, Culture and Society* 28: 165–181.

Kvaale EP, Haslam N and Gottdiener WH (2013a) The 'side effects' of medicalization: a meta-analytic review of how biogenetic explanations affect stigma. *Clinical Psychology Review* 33(6): 782-794.

Kvaale EP, Gottdiener WH and Haslam N (2013b) Biogenetic explanations and stigma: A meta-analytic review of associations among laypeople. *Social Science & Medicine* 96: 95–103.

Laurence J and McCallum D (1998) The myth-or-reality of attention-deficit disorder: a genealogical approach. *Discourse: Studies in the Cultural Politics of Education* 19: 183–200.

Lebowitz MS and Ahn W (2014) Effects of biological explanations for mental disorders on clinicians' empathy. *PNAS 111*(50): 17786–17790.

Lindellee J, Alkan Olsson J, and Koch M (2021) Operationalizing sustainable welfare and co-developing eco-social policies by prioritizing human needs. *Global Social Policy* 21(2): 328–331.

Malmqvist J (2018) Has schooling of ADHD students reached a crossroads? *Emotional and Behavioural Difficulties* 23(4): 389–409.

Malmqvist J and Nilholm C (2016) The antithesis of inclusion? The emergence and functioning of ADHD special education classes in the Swedish school system. *Emotional and Behavioural Difficulties* 21(3): 287–300.

Max-Neef M (1989) *Human scale development: An option for the future. Development Dialogue* 1(1): 5–80.

McMahon SE (2012) Doctors diagnose, teachers label: the unexpected in pre-service teachers' talk about labelling children with ADHD. *International Journal of Inclusive Education* 16(3): 249–264.

Miller S, Wampold B, and Varhely K (2008) Direct comparisons of treatment modalities for youth disorders: A meta-analysis. *Psychotherapy Research* 18: 5–14.

Moncrieff, J (2010) Psychiatric diagnosis as a political device. *Social Theory & Health* 8(4): 370–382.

Nussbaum MC (2011) *Creating Capabilities: The Human Development Approach.* Cambridge, MA: Harvard University Press.

Ponnou S and Thomé B (2022) ADHD diagnosis and methylphenidate consumption in children and adolescents: A systematic analysis of health databases in France over the period 2010–2019. *Frontiers in Psychiatry* 13: 957242.

Posner J, Polanczyk GV, and Sonuga-Barke E (2020) Attention-deficit hyperactivity disorder. *Lancet* 395: 450–462.

Rocca E and Anjum RL (2020) Complexity, Reductionism and the Biomedical Model. In: Anjum RL, Copeland S and Rocca E (eds) Rethinking Causality, Complexity and Evidence for the Unique Patient. Cham: Springer, pp. 75-94.

Santos GM, Santos EM, Mendes GD, Fragoso YD, Souza MR, and Martimbianco ALC (2021) A review of Cochrane reviews on pharmacological treatment for attention deficit hyperactivity disorder. *Dementia & Neuropsychologia* 15(4): 421–427.

Schleim S (2022) Why mental disorders are brain disorders and why they are not: ADHD and the challenges of heterogeneity and reification. *Frontiers in Psychiatry.* 13: 943049.

Schneider H and Eisenberg D (2006) Who receives a diagnosis of Attention-Deficit/ Hyperactivity Disorder in the United States elementary school population? *Pediatrics* 117(4): 601–609.

Schweren L, Hoekstra P, van Lieshout M., Oosterlaan J, Lambregts-Rommelse N, Buitelaar J, Franke B, and Hartman C (2018) Long-term effects of stimulant treatment on ADHD symptoms, social-emotional functioning, and cognition. *Psychological Medicine* 49(2): 217–223.

Springborg P (1981) *The Problem of Human Needs and the Critique of Civilisation*. London: Allen & Unwin.

Stier M (2013) Normative preconditions for the assessment of mental disorder. *Frontiers in Psychology* 4:611.

Tait G (2009) The logic of ADHD: a brief review of fallacious reasoning. *Studies in Philosophy and Education* 28(3): 239–254.

te Meerman S, Freedman JE and Batstra L (2022) ADHD and reification: Four ways a psychiatric construct is portrayed as a disease. *Frontiers in Psychiatry* 13:1055328.

Timimi S (2017) Non-diagnostic based approaches to helping children who could be labelled ADHD and their families. *International Journal of Qualitative Studies on Health and Well-Being* 12(sup1) 1–18.

Timimi S, Moncrieff J, Jureidini J, Leo J, Cohen D, Whitfield C, et al. (2004) A critique of the international consensus statement on ADHD. *Clinical Child and Family Psychology Review* 7: 59–63.

Timimi S, Tetley D, Burgoine W, and Walker G (2013) Outcome Orientated Child and Adolescent Mental Health Services (OO-CAMHS): A whole service model. *Clinical Child Psychology and Psychiatry* 18: 169–184.

The Conversation (2022) Permacrisis: what it means and why it's word of the year for 2022 https://theconversation.com/permacrisis-what-it-means-and-why-its-word-of-the-year-for-2022-194306

Thyer BA (2015) The DSM-5 Definition of Mental Disorder: Critique and Alternatives. In: Probst B. (ed) *Critical Thinking in Clinical Assessment and Diagnosis. Essential Clinical Social Work Series*. Cham: Springer, pp. 45–68.

Wampold BE (2015) How important are the common factors in psychotherapy? An update. *World Psychiatry* 14(3): 270–277.

Watson SM, Richels C, Michalek AM, and Raymer A (2015) Psychosocial treatments for ADHD: a systematic appraisal of the evidence. *Journal of Attention Disorders* 19: 3–10.

Wetherly P (1996) Basic needs and social policies. *Critical Social Policy* 16(46): 45–65.

Xu G, Strathearn L, Liu B, Yang B, Bao W (2018) Twenty-year trends in diagnosed Attention-Deficit/Hyperactivity Disorder among US children and adolescents, 1997-2016. *JAMA Network Open* 3(1):e181471.

An Alternative Framework for Assessing Psychiatric Genetics Research

Jay Joseph and Mary Boyle

Abstract: *Jay Joseph's first book,* The Gene Illusion: Genetic Research in Psychiatry and Psychology, *was published in 2004. It was a detailed critique of genetic research on "schizophrenia," IQ, and criminality, and concluded that there was little if any scientifically valid evidence in support of genetic influences on human behavioral differences. Following the publication of his fourth book on this topic,* Schizophrenia and Genetics: The End of An Illusion *(Joseph, 2023), psychologist/author Mary Boyle invited Jay for an interview to discuss the changes that have occurred in behavioral science genetic research over the last 20 years, and whether his earlier conclusions still stand.*

Acknowledgement: A version of this chapter was first published by Mad in America on June 22, 2023.

Mary Boyle: Your many publications and your latest book, *Schizophrenia and Genetics: The End of An Illusion,* show that a lot has happened in psychiatric and behavioral genetics research since you first published in that area. We'll be talking about what has and hasn't changed and how you see the implications. But first, tell us how you became interested in this area and what keeps you engaged with it.

Jay Joseph: I became interested in the "genetics of schizophrenia" topic as a U.S. clinical psychology graduate student in the mid-1990s. The arguments fascinated me, and because I saw the genetic argument as weak, it was stunning to hear that the debate had been largely closed in favor of genetics by the 1980s. My desire to learn more about genetic research led me to the writings of critics of the mental health system and the medical model. I discovered several authors who had written critically about genetic research in psychiatry and psychology (including your work [Boyle, 2002]). Their writings inspired me to look more closely at the original studies. I've been publishing analyses of genetic research and theories in the social and behavioral sciences continuously since the late 1990s,[1] including a doctoral dissertation, four books, several book chapters, peer-reviewed journal articles, and online articles.[2]

A lot has changed in the past 20 or so years, but the problematic fundamentals have not. For example, the unjustified production of heritability estimates based on environmentally confounded twin studies of behavior continues (*heritability* is itself a disputed concept [Moore & Shenk, 2016]). Behavioral gene discovery claims also continue, but as in 2004, such claims are based on gene-behavior associations (correlations) that most likely are spurious or non-causative because they are based on chance findings, false assumptions, and/or systematic error. The mainstream media usually ignores these significant problems and often reports new behavioral twin studies or gene discovery claims as "landmarks" or "breakthroughs." The authors of these media reports believe that twin study assumptions are valid (they aren't, as I'll describe later) and write as if decades of false-alarm gene discovery claims had never happened.

Boyle: Psychiatric diagnostic concepts have been increasingly criticized by service users, professionals, and researchers. Many psychologists—and some psychiatrists—don't use them, including the label "schizophrenia." Has this had any impact on genetic research?

Joseph: Not much, because genetic researchers in psychiatry must continue to use these disputed labels to define the diagnoses they study. Although establishing both the reliability and validity of psychiatric conditions is a prerequisite for any attempt to search for genes or genetic influences, the literature shows both are questionable (Frances, 2012).

Nevertheless, psychiatric diagnoses are presented as illnesses or even "diseases" in mainstream textbooks, journal articles, media outlets, and at websites including those run by the UK National Health Service (NHS), mainstream psychiatry organizations, the U.S. National Institute of Mental

---

[1] https://jayjoseph.net/publications/
[2] https://www.madinamerica.com/author/jjoseph/

Health (NIMH), and many other influential and respected sites. The organizations behind these and other websites assume that DSM or ICD psychiatric diagnoses are valid medical conditions, and that heredity plays a key role in causing them.

Boyle: There have been significant changes in research techniques and theories of genetic influence over the last twenty or thirty years. What do you see as the most important?

Joseph: The main molecular genetic research methods in the 1990s and 2000s were the *linkage* and *candidate gene association* study methods. There were countless gene discovery claims based on these methods in that era (e.g., Cloninger, 2002 and Elkin et al., 2004). However, by the 2010s, the initial early-1990s excitement had given way to the crushing realization that all researchers had found was genetic fool's gold in psychiatry (Farrell et al., 2015), IQ research (Chabris et al., 2012), and other areas.

Some of us argued back in 2004-2005 that claims then being made about discoveries of "genes for behavior" and "genes for psychiatric disorders" were based on a genetic mirage. For example, in a 2005 exchange with leading psychiatric genetic researcher Kenneth Kendler in the *American Journal of Psychiatry*, I wrote that we should consider "the possibility that genes for the major psychiatric disorders do not exist" (Joseph, 2005, p. 1985). Kendler pointed to several "positive" psychiatric linkage and candidate gene results in response (Kendler, 2005).

It subsequently developed that the critics had been right all along about the genetic mirage. As Jonathan Flint, Kendler, and a colleague wrote in the 2020 (2nd) edition of *How Genes Influence Behavior*, "Literally thousands of papers reporting the results of physiological candidate gene association tests. ... are now considered to be false positives" (Flint et al., 2020, p. 60). This discovery led them to conclude that "it's not too harsh to say simply that these studies have taught us nothing useful about the genetic basis of psychiatric disease" (p. 60). In his 2018 book *Blueprint: How DNA Makes Us Who We Are*, top behavioral geneticist Robert Plomin called behavioral candidate gene research a "flop," a "fiasco," and an "approach [that] failed everywhere" (Plomin, 2018, p. 234).

Another research area focuses on rare genetic variants, such as *copy number variants* or "CNVs," accompanied by many claims of gene association. However, as Flint and colleagues wrote in *How Genes Influence Behavior*, "the early hope that CNVs would reflect the 'royal road' to understanding molecular genetic effects on schizophrenia has been disappointing" (Flint et al., 2020, p. 98).

Currently, *genome-wide association studies* (GWAS) and calculations of *polygenic risk scores* (PRS) derived from GWAS results are a major focus of attention. These methods involve the idea that many genetic variants each make a small contribution to a characteristic or "disorder." The GWAS era began in 2005-2007.

A GWAS, CNV, or PRS study might find an *association* (correlation) between genetic variants and a given diagnosis or behavioral characteristic (IQ, for example). But these methods don't provide evidence that genes play a role in *causing* the diagnosis or characteristic. Correlations and PRS "predictions" are not causes and may be spurious and/or the result of systematic error, as earlier behavioral linkage and candidate gene researchers learned the hard way. In 2022, Thomas Insel, the biologically oriented former director of the NIMH, recognized that "in contrast to the mutations discovered for cancer or rare diseases, none of the genetic variants associated with mental illness can be considered causal" (Insel, 2022, p. 132).

Other GWAS/PRS major problem areas include the questionable validity of psychiatric diagnoses and behavioral characteristics such as IQ and personality, population stratification confounds (Charney, 2022; Coop & Przeworski, 2022), a lack of individual predictive value, the practice of increasing a sample size to find statistically significant gene associations, the frequent inability to replicate gene associations in independent samples, low PRS generalizability across global populations, that "variation explained by" does not mean "caused by," and the potential "fishing expedition" aspect of "hypothesis-free" studies in which researchers base their conclusions on statistically significant yet chance associations.

GWAS publications have reported all kinds of improbable gene associations ("hits") in the past few years, including characteristics such as getting concussions (Kim et al., 2020), self-reported childhood maltreatment (Dalvie et al., 2020), crying habits,[3] ice cream flavor preferences,[4] loneliness (Day et al., 2018), musical beat synchronization (Niarchou et al., 2022), regular attendance at a sports club, pub, or religious group (Van De Vegte et al., 2020), and white wine liking (Pirastu et al., 2015). I see these "discoveries" as giant GWAS red-flag warnings of systematically biased research, and they bear an uncanny resemblance to earlier candidate gene association study red flags (see, for example, Fowler & Dawes, 2008).

For the past 15 years, genetic researchers have been struggling with what they call a "missing heritability" problem, that is, the gap between (misleading) heritability estimates from twin studies (see below) and the disappointing results of molecular genetic research (Maher, 2008). The most likely explanation for the missing heritability problem in psychiatric genetic research is that causative genes are "missing" because they do not exist. I said as much in *The Gene Illusion*, in my 2006 book *The Missing Gene: Psychiatry, Heredity, and the Fruitless Search for Genes*, and in a 2012 article (Joseph, 2012). I continue to hold this view in 2023.

Boyle: How have researchers responded to what seem like unpromising outcomes?

Joseph: They often respond by implying that GWAS-identified associations constitute gene discoveries, and that better methods and larger samples will produce more discoveries and increased "GWAS heritability" in the future. Although researchers and the media announce new behavioral gene "discoveries" almost daily, the failed behavioral candidate gene era provides a telling example of how a widely promoted scientific structure can produce thousands of gene-discovery claims over two-plus

---

[3] https://blog23andme.wpengine.com/wp-content/uploads/2014/10/ASHG2014_Chao_CryEasily-1.pdf
[4] https://blog.23andme.com/articles/genes-scream-for-ice-cream

decades and then come crashing down upon the discovery that the structure produced only false-positive non-findings (Border et al., 2019).

The best example is the frequently cited claim that people experiencing "stressful life events" are more likely to be diagnosed with depression if they carried a 5-HTTLPR gene variant. Despite the publication of at least 450 research papers about this variant, by 2019 or so it became clear that the 15-year-old 5-HTTLPR depression story did not hold up (Yong, 2019). "There Is No 'Depression Gene,'" read the title of a 2019 article published in *Science* (Lowe, 2019). (My review of the "genetics of major depression" literature here.[5])

In his 2014 book *Misbehaving Science: Controversy and the Development of Behavior Genetics*, sociologist Aaron Panofsky described behavioral geneticists' "coping strategy" of "technological optimism" in the face of gene discovery failures. By this, he meant the "optimism that the next level of technology will overcome past disappointments" (Panofsky, 2014, p. 177). Disappointing results from PRS studies, including a study of "educational attainment" (Okbay et al., 2022) based on three million individuals, suggest that currently employed "next level" methods such as GWAS and PRS will suffer a fate similar to the earlier failed linkage and candidate gene methods in psychology, psychiatry, and related fields.

Psychiatric Genomics Consortium co-founder Patrick Sullivan concluded in 2017 that the "historical candidate gene studies" he and many others had previously promoted (e.g., Sullivan, 2005) "didn't work, and can't work," (Sullivan, 2017, p. 2) and he "strongly suggest[ed] that we abandon candidate gene guesswork…as they have only provided false directions and wasted effort" (Sullivan, 2017, p. 4). It is likely that the authors of future publications will arrive at similar evaluations of psychiatric genetic CNV, GWAS, and PRS research.

Boyle: You mentioned twin studies earlier. These and adoption studies have been especially influential in research on areas such as "schizophrenia," IQ, "personality," "bipolar disorder" and criminal behavior. Yet you and other critics have forensically shown that they don't

---

[5] https://www.madinamerica.com/2022/08/depression-genetics-pillar/

support genetic explanations. You devote several chapters of your new book to them as well as your 2015 book *The Trouble with Twin Studies: A Reassessment of Twin Research in the Social and Behavioral Sciences*. Why do you think it's so important to keep these studies – some of which are now 90 and more years old – in the limelight?

Joseph: It is important to keep twin studies in the limelight because they (and, to a lesser extent, adoption studies) continue to supply the evidence most often cited in support of substantial genetic influences on a wide range of behavioral characteristics, and because twin study heritability estimates guide molecular genetic research (Hagenbeek et al., 2023). Support for twin studies is seen in journal articles, textbooks, websites, and across social and traditional media.

Yet twin studies are based on accepting a key assumption that is clearly wrong, and adoption studies have their own set of problem areas. Neuroscientist/geneticist Kevin Mitchell wrote in 2009, "Familiality and twin concordance data are the bedrock on which all psychiatric genetics, including GWAS, is based and justified" (Mitchell & Porteous, 2009, p. 740). What Mitchell saw as bedrock is more like quicksand.

Most twin studies find that reared-together MZ (monozygotic, identical) twin pairs behave more similarly than do reared-together same-sex DZ (dizygotic, fraternal) twin pairs. These findings are rarely disputed. What *is* disputed is what these findings mean. Twin researchers interpret their findings genetically by assuming that MZ and DZ environments are similar, and that the only behaviorally relevant factor distinguishing these pairs is their differing degrees of *genetic* relationship to each other (100% vs. an average 50%).

Critics, on the other hand, have argued since the 1930s that the MZ-DZ "equal environment assumption" (EEA) as it relates to behavioral twin studies is false because, when compared with same-sex DZ pairs, MZ pairs grow up experiencing (1) more similar treatment by parents and others; (2) more similar physical and social environments; (3) more similar treatment by society due to their sharing a very similar physical appearance; (4) a much greater tendency to spend time together, to have common friends and peer influences, and to model their behavior on each other; and (5) identity confusion and a much stronger level of emotional attachment to each other.

Even though the evidence overwhelmingly shows that MZ environments are much more similar than DZ environments, psychology, psychiatry, and other behavioral science areas continue to endorse genetic interpretations of twin study results. Nevertheless, twin study MZ-DZ comparisons cannot be interpreted genetically because such comparisons are unable to disentangle the potential influences of genes and environments. Behavioral twin researchers, it seems, have been engaged in a century-long scientific folly of epic proportions.

Turning to so-called "twins reared apart" studies—a method still recovering from the Cyril Burt scandal of the 1970s[6]—I showed in a 2022 analysis (Joseph, 2022a) that the actual result of the famous 1990 "Minnesota Study of Twins Reared Apart" (MISTRA) article published in *Science* was a failure[7] to find genetic influences on IQ (0% heritability).

The Minnesota researchers arrived at their conclusion in favor of 70% IQ heritability by using methods that included (1) suppressing their DZ-apart full-sample *control group* IQ correlations (which have never been published), (2) counting environmental influences as genetic influences, (3) failing to acknowledge that most twin pairs they studied were only *partially* reared apart, (4) keeping their raw data off-limits to independent reviewers, and (5) mistakenly assuming the non-existence of behavior-shaping cohort influences experienced by two people of the same sex who are born and grow up at the same time in the same historical era (Rose, 1982). Twin study results never speak for themselves; interpretation is everything.

Boyle: In your new book, you situate psychiatric genetics research within the context of the replication crisis and questionable research practices in

---

[6] https://www.madinamerica.com/2018/04/leon-j-kamin-nemesis-genetic-determinism/
[7] https://www.madinamerica.com/2022/05/debunking-minnesota-study-twins-reared-apart/

the behavioral sciences. What do you think this adds to our understanding of what's going on in this area?

Joseph: There is a growing realization that the scientific research/ publication process is in crisis. It is known as the *replication crisis*, meaning a crisis brought about by later independent analysts' discovery that they could not replicate some key scientific research findings (Open Science Collaboration, 2015). The original findings were probably non-findings[8] resulting from poorly performed research or from data and conclusions manipulated by researchers to match their own or their funding sources' expectations.

A wise person once said, "Data don't tell stories; scientists tell stories." Previously accepted stories researchers told us about their data are receiving increasing attention and scrutiny, and we can now evaluate behavioral and psychiatric genetic research using replication crisis concepts and terms such as the *questionable research practices* (QRPs) described by behavioral scientist Leslie John and colleagues in 2012. These researchers found that the use of QRPs as reported anonymously by academic psychologists was "surprisingly high" (John et al., 2012, p. 524).

An aspect of the QRP concept is *p-hacking*, which describes the practice of researchers consciously or unconsciously manipulating definitions and data, either openly or behind the scenes, to transform non-findings into publishable career-enhancing "findings" that reach the conventional .05 level of statistical significance (Head et al., 2015). P-hacking is a significant problem in behavioral research (the MISTRA, for example) and extends into the molecular genetic realm.

In 2016, behavioral geneticist Eric Turkheimer wrote that "genome-wide association [research] is unapologetic, high-tech p-hacking," (Turkheimer, 2016, p. 27) where if "no significant results are discovered the first time around, the process is repeated with even larger samples, continuing until something significant finally emerges" (Turkheimer, 2016, p. 27).

---

[8] https://www.bps.org.uk/psychologist/reproducibility-replication-and-open-science

As I described in detail in *Schizophrenia and Genetics*, the famous schizophrenia adoption studies performed in Denmark between 1968 and 1994 by American researchers Seymour Kety, David Rosenthal, Paul Wender and their Danish colleagues provide a disturbing example of how psychiatry, psychology, and other behavioral science fields continue to pass off massively flawed studies as "landmark" research.

To match their genetic confirmation biases and to achieve statistically significant results in the genetic direction, the Danish-American adoption investigators (1) dismissed or minimized the impact of environmental confounds such as selective placement, late separation, and late placement; (2) openly manipulated data and temporarily removed diagnostic categories from key comparisons; (3) called one of their studies "preliminary" and decided to collect data past the study's data collection stop-point; (4) changed key group comparisons; and (5) broadened the definition of schizophrenia "as widely as it may have ever been reasonably conceived before" (Rosenthal, 1975, p. 19), and then re-narrowed the definition, over 26 years.

For Rosenthal and Kety (1968), concluding that heredity did not contribute to schizophrenia was unacceptable. Far from objectively evaluating their results, they reasoned that if their data showed no evidence of assumed genetic causes—as it did at several key points—there must be something wrong with the data, or with the study design, that they needed to fix. That's not how science is supposed to work.

The language developed since the early 2010s to describe unsound research practices has enabled those of us with perspectives that differ from mainstream behavioral science positions to tell *our* stories in new and better ways. The Danish-American schizophrenia adoption studies are perhaps the longest-running example of openly p-hacked research ever seen in the behavioral sciences and constitute a half-century-long scientific deception in psychiatry that should not survive the replication crisis.

The current behavioral science research/publication system provides an open invitation for researchers to engage in QRPs and p-hacking. In his 2020 book *Science Fictions: How Fraud, Bias, Negligence and Hype Undermine the Search for Truth*, psychologist Stuart Ritchie acknowledged that "the system of peer review and journal publication" is "badly broken" (Ritchie, 2020, p. 6). The system is broken in part because it allows researchers—behind the scenes and before submitting their manuscripts to academic journals—to collect data, analyze results, and reach conclusions consistent with their confirmation biases.

The replication crisis has led to increasing calls to require research *preregistration* in behavioral research, where investigators would submit their research rationale, hypotheses, design and analytic strategy, and planned data collection stop-point to a journal for peer review *before* collecting and analyzing data (Nosek et al., 2018). Preregistration methods in the form of *register reports* have been adopted by hundreds of scientific journals in the past decade (Chambers & Tzavella, 2021). Research preregistration alone cannot fix a broken system, but it's a good place to start.

Boyle: In *Schizophrenia and Genetics*, you discuss two well-known family studies: the "Genain Quadruplets," all of whom were diagnosed as "schizophrenic" and the Galvin family (discussed in the book *Hidden Valley Road)*, where six boys were given that diagnosis. You show how researchers and commentators have downplayed or even ignored the horrific abuse and trauma these children suffered in favor of a genetic explanation. These are extreme examples but are there other ways researchers keep genetics in the foreground in the face of a weak evidence base?

Joseph: Yes. For example, Robert Plomin argued in *Blueprint* that most environmental influences on behavior are actually genetic influences, and that the remaining true environmental influences are "mostly random—unsystematic and unstable—which means that we cannot do much about them" (Plomin, 2018, p. xii). By this logic, because society "cannot do much about" the environment and cannot do much about heredity either, there is no need to spend millions of dollars on behavioral genetic research.

Plomin justified counting most environmental influences as genetic influences by arguing that "we select, modify and even create our experiences in part on the basis of our genetic propensities" (Plomin, 2018,

p. ix)," meaning that "children make their own environments, regardless of their parents" (Plomin, 2018, p. 83). Similar faulty arguments have been put forward by others about childhood maltreatment, implying that children partly "create" family environments containing physical, sexual, and emotional abuse (Dalvie et al., 2020).

Do people who suffer from racism and other oppressive aspects of society create their suffering? Are some people genetically less bothered by these adversities (Sharma & Ressler, 2019)? In any case, environmental influences are environmental influences, not genetic influences. (My review of *Blueprint* was published in 2022 [Joseph, 2022b].)

Despite poor returns, molecular genetic researchers in psychiatry and psychology also help keep genetics in the foreground by using language that is often optimistic, including phrases such as "spectacular advances," "momentum of genomic science," "revolutionary genetic research," "golden post-genomic era," and "the future looks bright." As seen in *Blueprint*, public statements of excitement, optimism, and discovery by leading researchers are at times accompanied by private feelings of disappointment and failure.

Boyle: There's a lot of talk now about conflicts of interest in medical and psychiatric research, and especially about the role of pharmaceutical companies. There's not yet much public discussion about vested interests and conflicts of interest in genetic research. How much of an issue is this and should we be worried about it?

Joseph: Conflicts of interest are a major issue we should be concerned about since there is a symbiotic relationship[9] between psychiatry, psychiatric genetics, supporters of neoliberal political policies, and drug companies. All have a vital and mutual interest in convincing the public that "mental disorders" are individual-based and largely genetic brain diseases in need of medication "like other diseases."

---

[9] https://www.madinamerica.com/2021/09/anatomy-industry-commerce-payments-psychiatrists-betrayal-public-good/

However, the evidence for neurotransmitter or genetic causes, even for diagnoses like schizophrenia[10] and major depression,[11] is weak. A leading group of neuroscientists concluded in 2022, "Despite three decades of intense neuroimaging research, we still lack a neurobiological account for any psychiatric condition" (Nour et al., 2022, p. 2524).

There's a gold rush aspect of psychiatric molecular genetic research. Drug companies still believe they can design and patent drugs targeted at a person's genotype and stand to profit even more in the future. Other ways genes can be monetized include the development of patented diagnostic tests, direct-to-consumer (DTC) genetic tests such as 23andMe, and products aimed at marital partners and post-conception embryo selection.

There are frequent declared and non-declared conflicts of interest in psychiatric molecular genetic research. It's difficult for researchers, institutions, and academic journals to remain objective when salaries, "consulting fees,"[12] grants, endowments, profits, royalties, advertising revenues, potential patent fortunes,[13] and scientific recognition are at stake.[14]

As in 2004-2005, psychiatric genetic researchers continue to discover only "gene association" fool's gold, most likely because that's all there is to discover. But as long as the system keeps going and staves off a candidate-gene-style GWAS/PRS/CNV collapse, the insiders will continue to profit. More and more, the entire enterprise resembles a smaller scientific version of the U.S. "military-industrial complex."

Boyle: What you're saying suggests that genetic research in the behavioral sciences, and the ways it's communicated, is something we should be

---

[10] https://www.madinamerica.com/2019/06/genetic-models-schizophrenia-explain-little-researchers-find/

[11] https://www.madinamerica.com/2022/08/depression-genetics-pillar/

[12] https://www.nytimes.com/2008/06/08/us/08conflict.html

[13] https://patents.google.com/patent/US20040185468A1/en

[14] https://www.broadinstitute.org/news/650-million-commitment-stanley-center-broad-institute-aims-galvanize-mental-illness-research

concerned about not just as researchers, service-users or professionals, but as citizens…

Joseph: We should be very concerned because we are being fed a false and harmful narrative. The mainstream story about the genetics of most areas of human behavior follows a seven-step corrupted process, which goes something like this:

1. Academic researchers in the fields of behavioral genetics and psychiatric genetics produce unsound research (accompanied by misleading heritability estimates [Robette et al., 2022]) based on false assumptions and/or genetically misinterpreted data, which is then accepted for publication by peer-reviewed scientific journals.

2. Researchers producing unsound research are often rewarded and even honored,[15] which motivates them to produce even more unsound research.

3. Respected academic fields and government agencies (including health-related agencies such as the NHS and the NIMH) endorse and promote this unsound research in textbooks, websites, and other publications.

4. The mainstream media reports on and promotes unsound research, often in the form of articles and news reports of supposed new discoveries based mainly on twin studies, including selectively reported[16] stories about individual pairs of reunited "separated twins" supposedly displaying "spooky" behavioral similarities (for example, the "Jim Twins"[17]).

5. The mainstream media regularly reports on supposedly exciting new molecular genetic behavioral gene discoveries as if five decades of false-alarm claims had never happened.

---

[15] https://www.thecrimson.com/article/1999/9/29/kety-awarded-prize-for-medical-research/

[16] https://www.madinamerica.com/2016/03/bewitching-science-revisited-tales-of-reunited-twins-and-the-genetics-of-behavior/

[17] https://www.mirror.co.uk/news/us-news/twins-separated-birth-find-each-28960150

6. Books (e.g., *Hidden Valley Road*[18] and *The Gene: An Intimate History*[19]), videos, online articles, and social media posts by journalists and some highly respected researchers and authors promote and celebrate unsound research, while the works of critics are usually ignored, distorted, or dismissed.

7. Students and teachers in the academic world, political policy makers, and the general public are convinced by the above process that what are in fact unsound studies and false-alarm or non-causative behavioral gene association claims are actually sound studies and causative gene discoveries.

The above process describes how corporations, the mainstream media, and the politically powerful attempt to "manufacture consent" in the area of human behavioral differences just as they manufacture consent for their domestic and especially foreign policy positions and actions. The process encourages people to accept and possibly promote various related political, social policy, scientific, and social-relations viewpoints.

The process also supports practices such as psychiatric genetic counseling programs, selective adoption placements, producing genetic risk profiles, prioritizing funding of genetic over environmental research, and even the promotion of eugenic interventions that involve selecting for "desirable traits." People diagnosed with "schizophrenia" or another "mental disorder" may worry that they are carrying faulty genes they might pass on to their children. Others may fear that they harbor predisposing genes if other family members are diagnosed. These are important ethical issues that don't get nearly enough attention.

Boyle: How do you see psychologists' and others' responsibilities and influence in this area?

Joseph: Psychologists and other behavioral scientists should ensure that the research they cite and endorse is methodologically sound and is based

---

[18] https://www.madinamerica.com/2023/01/hidden-valley-road-schizophrenia-genes/
[19] https://www.madinamerica.com/2019/12/twin-studies-and-ken-burns-upcoming-documentary-on-the-gene-an-intimate-history/

on well-founded assumptions. Unfortunately, the replication crisis has demonstrated that we cannot rely on the peer-review process to prevent the publication of methodologically unsound research based on false assumptions and QRPs (e.g., candidate gene association studies and twin research).

Psychologists and psychiatrists should be willing to challenge psychiatric and behavioral genetic claims that their fields have integrated into their consensus positions. We all understand that a field's consensus views are not always correct, especially in the politically charged social and behavioral "soft sciences."

By necessity, critical analysis of behavioral and psychiatric genetic research includes consulting the works of critics of these fields, giving their arguments due consideration, and exploring alternatives to diagnosis and medicalization. We are responsible for ensuring that teaching curricula include critical analyses of genetic research (which may be omitted from standard textbooks) and that this informs our discussions with clients, colleagues, teachers, students, and the media.

Boyle: Some, maybe many, readers may be saying at this point, "But surely our genetic endowment must have some impact on our mental life and behavior, and we need to research this." What would you say to them?

Joseph: I would say to them that although genes are, of course, involved in most aspects of human functioning, focusing on genetics to understand who we are, psychologically, and how humans differ, behaviorally, is a mistaken approach lacking scientific support.

Psychiatric and behavioral geneticists argue that heredity plays an important role in producing "individual differences in behavior." To understand how these differences arise, they say we should focus on reared-together twins, reared-apart twins, adoptees, brains, genes, IQ scores, biological-relative IQ correlations, "personality," a range of statistical modeling techniques, "mental disorders," crime statistics, GWAS hits, polygenic risk scores, and heritability estimates.

Supporters of this approach sometimes depict those who focus on environmental causes of behavioral differences as suggesting that people are born as psychological "blank slates." Steven Pinker attributed this view to environmentalists in his 2002 book *The Blank Slate: The Modern Denial of Human Nature* and it has continued since then.

However, so-called "blank slatism" is a straw man because few who focus on environments hold such views as they relate to cognitive and other abilities and temperament. They usually argue that while there may well be inborn differences among people in these areas, it is perinatal, family, social, cultural, religious, educational, geographical, and political environments (including oppression) that together play a decisive role in shaping human behavior and abilities, and that focusing on "individual differences" and problematic heritability estimates implies limited changeability and distracts our attention from the need to improve or radically change these environments.

Instead, those of us who focus on environments point to the many characteristics, potentials, needs, desires, biological similarities, and abilities *we all share*–and prioritize progressive policies and programs related to healthcare, education, jobs, housing, nutrition, disease prevention, maternity/paternity leave, anti-discrimination, poverty alleviation, wealth redistribution, war prevention, and so on.

Regarding DSM and ICD "mental disorders," although many people see it as axiomatic that disordered genes are an important underlying cause of major psychiatric diagnoses such as schizophrenia, bipolar disorder, ADHD, and depression, there is no scientifically valid evidence supporting the direct role of genes, even if genes play some role in differences in abilities and temperament.

After decades of research, the psychiatric and behavioral genetics fields have produced no findings beneficial to the human condition as they relate to the major psychiatric diagnoses and psychological characteristics such as IQ and personality. In various ways, though, they have produced harm.

The psychiatric genetics field has harmed people not only because of its eugenic ("racial hygiene") history and origins but because it diverts our attention from evidence-backed causes of human suffering and dysfunction (Joseph & Wetzel, 2012). The behavioral genetics field's misplaced emphasis on genes and supposedly high within-group "IQ heritability" is sometimes cited by "race scientists" to claim that "races" and classes differ genetically[20] in "measured intelligence," and is also cited in support of regressive political policies.

Supporters of psychiatric and behavioral genetic research need to explain how these fields are contributing valid information that benefits society. If a better world finds no one funding or engaging in "genes for behavior" research, I doubt any of us would suffer from it.

Further Reading

Boyle, M., & Johnstone, L. (2020). *A Straight Talking Introduction to the Power Threat Meaning Framework: An Alternative to Psychiatric Diagnosis*. PCCS Books.

Kirk, S. A., Gomory, T., & Cohen, D. (2013). *Mad Science: Psychiatric Coercion, Diagnosis, and Drugs*. Routledge.

Panofsky, A. (2014). *Misbehaving Science: Controversy and the Development of Behavior Genetics*. University of Chicago Press.

Richardson, K. (2022). *Understanding Intelligence*. Cambridge University Press.

References

Border, R., Johnson, E. C., Evans, L. M., Smolen, A., Berley, N., Sullivan, P. F., & Keller, M. C. (2019). No support for historical candidate gene or candidate gene-by-interaction hypotheses for major depression across multiple large samples. *American Journal of Psychiatry, 176*(5), 376–387. https://doi.org/10.1176/appi.ajp.2018.18070881

Boyle, M. (2002). *Schizophrenia: A scientific delusion? (2nd ed.). Routledge.*

---

[20] https://twitter.com/jayjoseph22/status/1649123405336281089?s=20

Chabris, C. F., Hébert, B., Benjamin, D. J., Beauchamp, J. P., Cesarini, D., Van Der Loos, M. J. H. M., Johannesson, M., Magnusson, P. K. E., Lichtenstein, P., Atwood, C. S., Freese, J., Hauser, T. S., Hauser, R. M., Christakis, N. A., & Laibson, D. (2012). Most reported genetic associations with general intelligence are probably false positives. *Psychological Science, 23(11), 1314–1323.* https://doi.org/10.1177/0956797611435528

Chambers, C., & Tzavella, L. (2021). The past, present and future of registered reports. *Nature Human Behaviour, 6(1), 29–42.* https://doi.org/10.1038/s41562-021-01193-7

Charney, E. (2022). The "golden age" of behavior genetics? *Perspectives on Psychological Science, 17(4), 1188–1210.* *https://doi.org/10.1177/17456916211041602*

Cloninger, C. R. (2002). The discovery of susceptibility genes for mental disorders. *Proceedings of the National Academy of Sciences of the United States of America, 99(21), 13365–13367.* https://doi.org/10.1073/pnas.222532599

Coop, G., & Przeworski, M. (2022). Lottery, luck, or legacy. A review of "The genetic lottery: Why DNA matters for social equality." *Evolution, 76(4), 846–853.* https://doi.org/10.1111/evo.14449

Dalvie, S., Maihofer, A. X., Coleman, J. R. I., Bradley, B., Breen, G., Brick, L. A., Chen, C. Y., Choi, K. W., Duncan, L., Guffanti, G., Haas, M., Harnal, S., Liberzon, I., Nugent, N. R., Provost, A. C., Ressler, K. J., Torres, K., Amstadter, A. B., Austin, S. B., . . . Nievergelt, C. M. (2020). Genomic influences on self-reported childhood maltreatment. *Translational Psychiatry, 10(1).* https://doi.org/10.1038/s41398-020-0706-0

Day, F. R., Ong, K. K., & Perry, J. R. B. (2018). Elucidating the genetic basis of social interaction and isolation. *Nature Communications, 9(1).* https://doi.org/10.1038/s41467-018-04930-1

Elkin, A., Kalidindi, S., & McGuffin, P. (2004). Have schizophrenia genes been found? *Current Opinion in Psychiatry, 17(2), 107–117.*

Farrell, M. S., Werge, T., Sklar, P., Owen, M. J., Ophoff, R. A., O'Donovan, M., Corvin, A., Cichon, S., & Sullivan, P. F. (2015). Evaluating historical candidate genes for schizophrenia. *Molecular Psychiatry, 20(5), 555–562.* https://doi.org/10.1038/mp.2015.16

Flint, J., Greenspan, R. J., & Kendler, K. S. (2020). *How genes influence behavior (2nd ed.). Oxford University Press.*

Fowler, J. H., & Dawes, C. T. (2008). Two genes predict voter turnout. *The Journal of Politics, 70(3), 579–594.* https://doi.org/10.1017/s0022381608080638

Frances, A. J. (2012, October 30). DSM 5 field trials discredit APA. *Psychology Today.* https://www.psychologytoday.com/us/blog/dsm5-in-distress/201210/dsm-5-field-trials-discredit-apa

Hagenbeek, F. A., Hirzinger, J. S., Breunig, S., Bruins, S., Kuznetsov, D., Schut, K., Odintsova, V. V., & Boomsma, D. I. (2023). Maximizing the value of twin studies in health and behaviour. *Nature Human Behaviour, 7(6), 849–860.* https://doi.org/10.1038/s41562-023-01609-6

Head, M. L., Holman, L., Lanfear, R., Kahn, A. T., & Jennions, M. D. (2015). The extent and consequences of P-Hacking in science. *PLOS Biology, 13(3), e1002106.* https://doi.org/10.1371/journal.pbio.1002106

Insel, T. (2022). *Healing: Our path from mental illness to mental health.* Penguin.

John, L. K., Loewenstein, G., & Prelec, D. (2012). Measuring the prevalence of questionable research practices with incentives for truth telling. *Psychological Science, 23(5), 524–532.* https://doi.org/10.1177/0956797611430953

Joseph, J. (2005). Research paradigms of psychiatric genetics. *American Journal of Psychiatry, 162(10), 1985.* https://doi.org/10.1176/appi.ajp.162.10.1985

Joseph, J. (2012). The "missing heritability" of psychiatric disorders: Elusive genes or Non-Existent genes? *Applied Developmental Science, 16(2), 65–83.* https://doi.org/10.1080/10888691.2012.667343

Joseph, J. (2022a). A reevaluation of the 1990 "Minnesota Study of Twins Reared Apart" IQ study. *Human Development, 66(1), 48–65.* https://doi.org/10.1159/000521922

Joseph, J. (2022b). A blueprint for genetic determinism. *American Journal of Psychology, 135(4), 442–454.* https://doi.org/10.5406/19398298.135.4.13

Joseph, J. (2023). *Schizophrenia and Genetics: The End of an Illusion.* Routledge.

Joseph, J., & Wetzel, N. A. (2012). Ernst Rüdin: Hitler's racial hygiene mastermind. *Journal of the History of Biology, 46(1), 1–30.* https://doi.org/10.1007/s10739-012-9344-6

Kendler, K. S. (2005). Dr. Kendler replies. *American Journal of Psychiatry, 162(10), 1985–1986.* https://doi.org/10.1176/appi.ajp.162.10.1985-a

Kim, S. K., Roche, M., Fredericson, M., Dragoo, J. L., Horton, B., Avins, A., Belanger, H. G., Ioannidis, J. P. A., & Abrams, G. D. (2020). A genome-wide association study for concussion risk. *Medicine and Science in Sports and Exercise, 53(4), 704–711.* https://doi.org/10.1249/mss.0000000000002529

Lowe, D. (2019, March 10). *There is no "depression gene." Science. https://www.science.org/content/blog-post/there-no-depression-gene*

Maher, B. A. (2008). Personal genomes: The case of the missing heritability. *Nature, 456(7218), 18–21.* https://doi.org/10.1038/456018a

Mitchell, K. J., & Porteous, D. J. (2009). GWAS for psychiatric disease: is the framework built on a solid foundation? *Molecular Psychiatry, 14(8), 740–741.* https://doi.org/10.1038/mp.2009.17

Moore, D. S., & Shenk, D. (2016). The heritability fallacy. *WIREs Cognitive Science, 8(1–2).* https://doi.org/10.1002/wcs.1400

Niarchou, M., Gustavson, D. E., Sathirapongsasuti, J. F., Anglada-Tort, M., Eising, E., Bell, E., McArthur, E., Straub, P., Aslibekyan, S., Auton, A., Bell, R. K., Bryc, K., Clark, S., Elson, S. L., Fletez-Brant, K., Fontanillas, P., Furlotte, N. A., Gandhi, P., Heilbron, K., . . . Gordon, R. L. (2022). Genome-wide association study of musical beat synchronization demonstrates high polygenicity. *Nature Human Behaviour, 6(9), 1292–1309.* https://doi.org/10.1038/s41562-022-01359-x

Nosek, B. A., Ebersole, C. R., DeHaven, A. C., & Mellor, D. T. (2018). The preregistration revolution. *Proceedings of the National Academy of Sciences of the United States of America, 115(11), 2600–2606.* https://doi.org/10.1073/pnas.1708274114

Nour, M. M., Liu, Y., & Dolan, R. J. (2022). Functional neuroimaging in psychiatry and the case for failing better. *Neuron, 110(16), 2524–2544.* https://doi.org/10.1016/j.neuron.2022.07.005

Okbay, A., Wu, Y., Wang, N., Jayashankar, H., Bennett, M. H., Nehzati, S. M., Sidorenko, J., Kweon, H., Goldman, G., Gjorgjieva, T., Jiang, Y., Hicks, B., Tian, C., Hinds, D. A., Ahlskog, R., Magnusson, P. K. E., Oskarsson, S., Hayward, C., Campbell, A., . . . Young, A. I. (2022). Polygenic prediction of educational attainment within and between families from genome-wide association analyses in 3 million individuals. *Nature Genetics, 54(4), 437–449.* https://doi.org/10.1038/s41588-022-01016-z

Open Science Collaboration. (2015). Estimating the reproducibility of psychological science. *Science, 349(6251).* https://doi.org/10.1126/science.aac4716

Panofsky, A. (2014). *Misbehaving science: Controversy and the development of behavior genetics. University of Chicago Press.*

Pirastu, N., Kooyman, M., Traglia, M., Robino, A., Willems, S. M., Pistis, G., Amin, N., Sala, C., Karssen, L. C., Van Duijn, C. M., Toniolo, D., & Gasparini, P. (2015). Genome-wide association analysis on five isolated populations identifies variants of the HLA-DOA gene associated with white wine liking. *European Journal of Human Genetics, 23(12), 1717–1722.* https://doi.org/10.1038/ejhg.2015.34

Plomin, R. (2018). *Blueprint: How DNA makes us who we are. MIT Press.*

Ritchie, S. (2020). *Science fictions: How Fraud, Bias, Negligence, and Hype Undermine the Search for Truth. Metropolitan Books.*

Robette, N., Génin, E., & Clerget-Darpoux, F. (2022). Heritability: What's the point? What is it not for? A human genetics perspective. *Genetica, 150(3–4), 199–208.* https://doi.org/10.1007/s10709-022-00149-7

Rose, R. J. (1982). Separated twins: Data and their limits. *Science, 215(4535), 959–960.* https://doi.org/10.1126/science.215.4535.959

Rosenthal, D. (1975). "The Spectrum Concept in Schizophrenic and Manic-Depressive Disorders," in D. Freedman (Ed.), *Biology of the Major Psychoses* (pp. 19-25), New York: Raven Press.

Rosenthal, D. & Kety. S. S. (Eds.). (1968). *The transmission of schizophrenia.* Pergamon Press.

Sharma, S. K., & Ressler, K. J. (2019). Genomic updates in understanding PTSD. *Progress in Neuro-Psychopharmacology and Biological Psychiatry, 90, 197–203.* https://doi.org/10.1016/j.pnpbp.2018.11.010

Sullivan, P. F. (2005). The genetics of schizophrenia. *PLOS Medicine, 2(7), e212.* https://doi.org/10.1371/journal.pmed.0020212

Sullivan, P. F. (2017). How good were candidate gene guesses in schizophrenia genetics? *Biological Psychiatry, 82(10), 696–697.* https://doi.org/10.1016/j.biopsych.2017.09.004

Turkheimer, E. (2016). Weak genetic explanation 20 years later. *Perspectives on Psychological Science, 11(1), 24–28.* https://doi.org/10.1177/1745691615617442

Van De Vegte, Y. J., Said, M. A., Rienstra, M., Van Der Harst, P., & Verweij, N. (2020). Genome-wide association studies and Mendelian randomization analyses for leisure sedentary behaviours. *Nature Communications, 11(1).* https://doi.org/10.1038/s41467-020-15553-w

Yong, E. (2019, May 17). A waste of 1,000 research papers. *The Atlantic.* https://www.theatlantic.com/science/archive/2019/05/waste-1000-studies/589684/

The Art of Involving the Person: The Existential Fundamental Motivations as Structure of the Motivational Process

Alfried Längle

Abstract: *Seen from an existential point of view, motivation consists essentially in moving the will, the human's way of realising one's freedom. To come to terms of a responsible motivation, it is necessary to refer to one's personhood into the decisions of the ego. Motivation as a process emerges in dialogical steps starting from the given reality towards what the person resonates with, and the ego intends. Seen in this light, motivation is an expression of the (mostly unconscious) human intention to come to existence. To be able to do so, the fundamental themes of existence must be referred to. Thus, motivation is related fundamentally to the structure of existence. As for its operating tools, holistic and responsible motivation relates to the (spiritual or noetic) power of the person as described in the Personal Existential Analysis (PEA). The intention of this paper is to show the relation between the structure of existence and the motivational process. According to the "four cornerstones of existence," the individual first must come to terms with his being in the world, then with his own life and with his own identity. Subsequently, he is open for and prone to enter relationships with a greater context, from which personal meaning derives. This has been found in our phenomenological empirical research in the 1990s. Moreover, these four fundamental aspects of existence form a matrix for the psychopathological understanding of psychic disorders and provide a background for clinical interventions. They represent the structural (or content) model of modern Existential Analytical Psychotherapy.*

What Makes for Motivation?

Talk about motivation is ubiquitous in social sciences such as psychology, psychotherapy, pedagogics, sociology, politics as well as in marketing and economics. It seems obvious that we need good motivation for the achievement of our life tasks, for creativity, growth, social functioning, and personal fulfillment.

But there a substantial question arises from the very beginning about the nature of motivation: do we really need to *become motivated from outside* or are we already and *originally motivated* due to our nature and humanness? Is the essence of what we call "motivational process" an act of *receiving* something? Or does the motivational process merely consist in shaping this process of being primordially, constantly, and generally moved? Then motivating someone would simply mean to provide a theme for that pre-established energy.

This would mean that we do not help people to be motivated but help them to find *what for* they can best implement the existent motivational force for their lives. The motivational process would provide a direction for the intentional power, a reason for the decision, and show the value of the particular action for one's life. In other words, motivating someone would be to help find possibilities, values, authenticity, and meaning for what one does.

Alfred Adler and George Kelly (cf. Brunner et al. 1985) took the position that humans are originally motivated by their nature and need not be moved from outside. So did Viktor Frankl, one of Adler's disciples or let us, rather say, an adherent of his circle. This position was also taken by the "potentialists" of the humanistic psychology movement like Carl Rogers (1961): if the circumstances are favorable for activity, humans develop all their activities and potentials of their own.

Frankl's "Will to Meaning"

For Frankl, we are indeed motivated by *biological* and *social* drives, but primarily and, most profoundly, we are motivated by our personal "Will to Meaning." This means that any person is fundamentally moved by a *spiritual* striving for a deeper *understanding* of what one experiences or does. This motivational force is regarded to be a direct result of the essence of human "nature." It is seen in the personal (= noetic or spiritual) dimension of man, and the will to meaning is rooted in this dimension.

In Frankl's theory (1973, XVIII ff.; 1959, 672), this spiritual dimension is marked by the three basic human potentials[1] which consist of ("psychological") spirituality, freedom, and responsibility. The quest for meaning and, with it, the primary motivational process can therefore be understood as a concomitant necessity inherent in this dimension. It basically consists in the challenge created by our freedom.[2]

Freedom paradoxically brings along a compulsion of choice – being free means that we are forced to choose. A prerequisite of any real choice is the notion of the content and the understanding of the context in which the decision has to be made. The intentional goal of the will arises from this horizon and, if adopted by the subject, it turns out to be a value—probably the highest value one can see in the given situation. These are the elements of *existential meaning*: the greatest (or highest or deepest) value in the given situation, which can be seen and understood by the individual to be within the reach of his abilities. Frankl's primary motivation thus turns out to be an immediate consequence of the realisation of the person's will, the human expression of freedom.

Frankl developed this logotherapeutic concept of motivational theory in an era that was dominated by determinism, reductionism, subjectivism and monadology,[3] all of which he fervently combated. His education took place in that period and, hence, his thinking was exposed to some of these ideas. Frankl's personal and scientific accomplishment was certainly the overcoming of these tendencies in his overall concept of logotherapy. He achieved this especially with his concepts of meaning and of self-transcendence, both cornerstones of his anthropology.

---

[1] Frankl calls them also "existentials" – referring to Heidegger's term "Existentialien."
[2] "Psychological spirituality" explains what is meant. It captures the meaning of the situation and activates the person's potential of being free. Responsibility, on the other hand, is also related to freedom: it imposes itself only there where humans are free. Seen from these practical aspects, freedom reveals itself as the decisive factor of the spiritual dimension. The importance of freedom explains why it is more often treated in philosophical and psychological theories than meaning and responsibility.
[3] Theory that sees the human being as a "monade" (from Greek monos - alone, sole), i.e. isolated from the world like wrapped in a cocoon (*G.W. Leibnitz, 1720*).

But it seems to me that in the motivational angle of his theory, he may have adopted some individualistic thinking by tracing back the concept of existential motivation to the concept of will. He even reinforced the pertaining concept by naming it "will" to meaning. Frankl himself explained the decision of calling his motivational concept "will" to meaning by his intention to formulate a counterweight to Nietzsche's "Will to Power." At the same time, he wanted to define the "true" content by replacing the instrumental value of "power" by the more spiritual value of "meaning."

The Modern Quest for Meaning

In our times, it is not the theme of freedom that dominates the discussion of social problems, of psychopathologies, and the scientific discourse. Freedom was a big question in the 1960s and 1970s because of the genetic discoveries bringing up neo-Darwinian discussions like seeing human behaviour as just evolutionary adaptation. The theme of freedom was covered by biological "necessities" which dominate. The year 1968 was a year of revolutionary outburst of free will against the social repression and rigid conformism. These are no longer the themes of our time.

Nowadays, different problems are predominant: marital and family life have widely evolved into broadly accepted forms of single life; the communities, social experiments and sexual promiscuity of the 70s have turned to fantasy games in virtual worlds, TV-channel-hopping, or internet surfing. For sexuality, the open acceptance of homosexuality and diverse gender-feelings is broadly achieved.

The social cohesion in politics and economy has been loosened in favor of a high degree of individualism, of liberal economic concepts with competition and rivalry, of a new feeling of freedom by utilizing and challenging the resources of the individual to the utmost degree. This new feeling of freedom brings along more isolation not only for the older people, but also for entire cultures.

The *"schizophrenic aspect" of our times* is that we have the best structures of communication mankind has ever had, that we travel more internationally—more than any generation before us—but that we feel lonelier and there is probably less real exchange between the cultures than before. The increase in contact between people of different cultures has led to a consumption of the pleasant aspects of cultures, but doubtfully to a true dialogue. This lack of profound dialogue and, consequently, lack of understanding provokes anxiety of alienation and of loss of identity.

This phenomenon can be observed in tourism and immigration. The increase of speed has brought along a decrease of contact, the increase of information has led to a decrease of communication, and the increase of traffic has destroyed much of personal encounter. September 11 can be seen as an example: it shows the huge and frightening failure in communication and encounter between different cultures.

Existential Paradigm

As children of our time and faced with its specific problems, we have to adapt our theories to the needs and sufferings of today. We have, therefore, further elaborated the motivational concept in Existential Analysis into an approach that is by no means less humanistic or personal. Our new concept follows a different paradigm. As a complement to the individualistic one of freedom and personal will, which laid ground to the development of this postmodern era, we now need as a counterweight to the shadow of freedom an *interpersonal paradigm*.

This is the line we have adopted in modern Existential Analysis. We have enlarged our motivational concept by basing it on likely most original activity of personhood: on our being essentially dialogical, prone to and directed towards exchange with others. Being oneself, finding oneself needs the field of tension of the "inter-", the "between", the "aida" as the Japanese say (Kimura 1982; 1995,103ff.).

This spiritual need for communication and dialogue is also underlined by the numerous personality disorders related to the loss of self! There is no "me" without a "you," as Buber and Frankl stated. Being oneself as a person means being in communication, being in a continuous inner and outer exchange of contents, fine-tuning the outer with the inner reality and, vice versa, oneself with the objective meaning of the situation. Motivation

is understood as engaging in that continuous flow which is established by
nature between the person and his world. They are inseparably connected
and interrelated, in uninterrupted reciprocal action. Or as Heidegger has
defined it: being a person, "Dasein," means "being-in-the-world," means
dealing with "otherness."

Existential Concept of Motivation

From an existential point of view, dialogue (or "communication" as Jaspers
says) is an essential constituent in human psychology and in the
understanding of the essence of human existence. If we take the capacity
for *dialogue as a characteristic* of being a person (i.e., a being with mind and
spirit and a potential for decision-making), then humans are always
waiting for their completion by a "partner" in the broadest sense. As
dialogical beings, we expect and look for something or someone
"speaking" to us, calling us, needing us, talking to us, looking for us,
challenging us.

We get the necessary *provocation* through everything we are confronted
with—that we have in front of us, that we are dealing with. At exactly that
moment, the object before us starts "speaking" to us. Being provoked
means being called. This provocation is the *starting point of any motivation.*

In other words, seen from an existential point of view *motivation means
involvement of the person,* initiating the personal processes by provocation in
some kind of vis-à-vis. Of course, the best vis-à-vis is a partner speaking to
us. This processual capacity of the person is described in the theory of the
method of "Personal Existential Analysis (PEA)" (Längle 1994c). This
method is an application of this concept with the goal of engaging personal
potentials in a process of dealing with information and encounter.

This model, which is fundamental for any kind of involvement of the
person, helps to distinguish three steps within the motivational process:

1. Recognizing something in its worth or value, in as far as it speaks
    to us. This is often a challenge demanding action on our part. To

see what a situation provokes in us means to recognize the situational meaning involved.

2. Harmonizing and bringing the perceived value, challenge or meaning into accordance with the inner reality. That is, examining the consistency with the rest of our values, with attitudes, abilities, and capabilities and with our conscience.

3. The final step in the development of motivation is the inner consent to one's own active involvement. This consent and the act of harmonizing the new value with one's personal reality leads to the presence of one's inner person in one's actions, and to the integration of the new value and the person himself into a wider context (meaning).

Without this involvement of the person in the motivational process, we would not deal with a question of motivation. Instead, there would be a sort of reflex or of reaction, but no "action." Any act, any deed, is defined as a *decided* act and is, therefore, *voluntary* and free.

If we take motivation as a *free* decision to act, then we must also take into consideration the concept of *will*. Frankl (1970, 37-44; 1987, 101-104) saw meaning as the moving part in free will. An existential view of will takes it as the anthropological axis of existence. A *processual description* of will, however, relies on the fundamentals of existence and, therefore, shows more than just meaning as being basic for constituting will. Free and realistic will is based on three more elements:

1. on the real ability and capacity of the subject;
2. on the emotional perception of the situational value;
3. on the inner permission and leave for that act, emerging from an agreement with one's concepts of life and morality.

Before we go into this, let us conclude this part of the exposition dealing with the structure of motivation by adding a reflection on the initial problem of the two basic concepts of motivation: do people need to be motivated from *outside*, or can the motivation only be shaped and canalized because people are *intrinsically* motivated? Our theory is that this existential concept results in forming a bridge between two opposite positions:

a) it is the *interrelation* with the vis-à-vis from which motivation emerges. Being touched and provoked, as well as understanding the situation, is like *being called* on by something or someone. This appeal activates the constitutional "being-in-the-world" because of a recognition or understanding of what this particular situation is about. This equals the recognition of the situational or existential meaning. Furthermore, this means that we *receive an impulse* from the recognition of the essential message from our vis-à-vis (outer world, but also body, feeling, thoughts).

b) By our *understanding* of the context and by our inner agreement, motivation gets its shape and receives its content.

Seen in that light, the notion of "being-in-the-world" provides the grounds on which the personal forces are activated. This happens by a perceptive encounter with some form of otherness or with oneself.

Let us now have a closer look at the four fundamental motivations for a fulfilled existence.

The four Fundamental Conditions for a Fulfilling Existence

In the first part we have elaborated the crucial point for motivation, which lies in attaining the *dialogical potential* of the subject. Its "pro-*vocation*" can be taken as the starting point for any motivation. The need and the ability for dialogue are seen as the dynamic essence of the person (with subsequent potentials like freedom and will). This dialogue (with the world and with oneself) is a prerequisite for building up motivation.

We have pointed out that for this reason there is *no motivation without cognition, accordance, bringing into harmony, inner consent and meaning.* For the aspect of freedom in motivation—seeing it as moving a person towards a *free* act within the world—the structure of will has to be taken in account. Will is fundamentally related to the structure of existence, which in turn is shaping the motivation substantially. This—the provocation into dialogue and the relation to the fundamental structure of existence—is the *central hypothesis* of this chapter.

If we look more closely, we see that this concept of motivation implies a dialogical *confrontation* with the given facts of our existence. All preconditions of existence can be summarized in four fundamental structures—the "cornerstones of existence":

- the *world* in its factuality and potentiality
- *life* with its network of relationships and its feelings
- *being oneself* as a unique, autonomous *person*
- the *wider context* where to place oneself = *development* through one's activities, opening one's *future*

Existence in our understanding needs a continuous *confrontation* and a dialogical *exchange* with each of these four dimensions. It is on this basis that the subject forms his specific notions about reality. These four realities challenge the person to give his response—they ask for his inner consent, activate his inner freedom.

But they are not only challenging dimensions—they are also structures which, at the same time, allow to entrust oneself to each of these given realities. Their facticity is the fundament of what we call existence. As such, they fundamentally move our existence and can be called "fundamental existential motivations" (Längle 1992a, b; 1994a; 1997a, b; 1998c).

The World – Dealing with Conditions and Possibilities

The first condition arises from the simple fact that I am here at all, that I am in the world. But where to go from here? Can I cope with my being there? Do I understand it? I am there, and as an old German saying from the 12th century goes in free translation: "I don't know where I am from, I don't know where to, I wonder why I am so glad."

I am there, there is me—how is that even possible? Questioning this seemingly self-evident fact can go to great depth once I go into it. And if I really think about it, I realize that I cannot truly comprehend this. My existence appears like an island in an ocean of ignorance and of connections that surpass me. The most adequate and traditional attitude towards the incomprehensible is one of astonishment. Basically, I can only be astonished that I am there at all.

But I am there, which puts *the fundamental question of existence* before me: *I am – but can I be?* For making this question practical I may apply it to my own situation. Then, I may ask myself: Can I claim my place in this world under the conditions and with the possibilities I have? This demands three things: *protection, space, and support.*

- Do I enjoy *protection*, acceptance, do I feel at home somewhere?
- Do I have enough *space* to be there?
- Where do I find *support* in my life?

If this is not the case, the result will be restlessness, insecurity, and fear (cf. Längle 1996). But if I *do* have these three things, I will be able to feel trust in the world and confidence in myself, maybe even faith in God. The sum of these experiences of trust is the fundamental trust, the trust in whatever I feel as being the last support in my life.

But, in order to be there, it is not enough to find protection, space and support—I also have to *seize* these conditions, to make a *decision* in their favor, to *accept* them. My *active* part in this fundamental condition of being there is to accept the positive sides and to endure the negative sides. To *accept* means to be ready to occupy the space, to rely on the support and to trust the protection; in short "to be there" and not to flee.

To *endure* means the force to let be whatever is difficult, menacing, or unalterable and to "support" what cannot be changed. Life imposes certain conditions on me, and the world has its laws to which I must bend myself. This idea is expressed in the word "subject" in the sense of "not independent." On the other hand, these conditions are reliable, solid, and steady. To let them be, to accept them as given, is only possible if I can be at the same time.

Therefore, to accept means to let each other be because there is still *enough space* for me, and the circumstances do not menace me anymore. Man procures himself the space he needs with his ability to tolerate and to accept conditions. If this is not the case, psychodynamics takes over the guidance in the form of coping *reactions*, which are to secure life (Längle 1998a).

Life – Dealing with Relationships and Emotions

Once someone has his space in the world, he can fill it with life. Simply being there is not enough. We want our existence to be *good* since it is more than a mere fact. It has a "pathic dimension," which means that it does not simply happen, but that we experience and suffer or enjoy it. Being alive means to cry and to laugh, to experience joy and suffering, to go through pleasant and unpleasant things, to be lucky or unlucky, and to experience worth and worthlessness. As much as we can be happy, as deeply can we suffer. The amplitude of emotionality is equal in both directions, whether this suits us or not.

Therefore, I am confronted with the *fundamental question of life*: I am alive — do I *like* this fact? Is it good to be there? It is not only strain and suffering that can take away the joy of life. It may as well be the shallowness of daily life and the negligence in one's lifestyle that make life stale. In order to seize my life, to love it, I need three things: *relationship, time and closeness*. In verifying the presence of life in one's own situation we may ask ourselves questions like this:

- Do I have *relationships* in which I feel closeness, for which I spend time and in which I experience community?
- What do I take *time* for? Do I take time for valuable things, worthy to spend my time for? To take time for something means to give away a part of one's life while spending it with someone or something.
- Can I feel close and maintain *closeness* to things, plants, animals, and people? Can I admit the closeness of someone else?

If relationships, closeness, and time are lacking, *longing* will arise, then *coldness* and finally depression. But if these three conditions are fulfilled, I experience myself as being in *harmony with the world and with myself* and I can sense the depth of life. These experiences form the fundamental value, the most profound *feeling for the value* of life. In each experience of a value, this fundamental value is touched upon, it colors the emotions and affects and represents our yardstick for anything we might feel to be of worth. This is what our theory of emotion as well as the theory of values relate to.

Still, it is not enough to have relationships, time, and closeness. My own consent, my active participation is asked for. I *seize* life, engage in it, when I *turn to* other people, to things, animals, intellectual work or to myself— when I go towards it, get close, get into touch or pull it towards me. If I turn to a loss, *grief* arises. This "to turn to" will make life vibrate within me. If life is to make me move freely, my consent to being touched (to feeling) is necessary.

Being a Person – Dealing with Uniqueness and Conscience

As pleasant as this emotional swinging may be, it is still not sufficient for a fulfilling existence. In spite of my being related to life and to people, I am aware of my being separate, different. There is a singularity that makes me an "I" and distinguishes me from everybody else. I realize that I am on my own, that I must master my existence myself and that, basically, I am alone and maybe even solitary. But, besides, there is *so much more* that is equally singular. The *diversity, beauty, and uniqueness* in all of this makes me feel respect.

In the midst of this world, I discover myself unmistakably—I am *with* myself, and I am given *to* myself. This puts before me the *fundamental question of being a person*: I am myself—*may* I be like this? Do I feel free to be *like that*? Do I have the *right* to be what I am and to behave as I do?

This is the plane of identity, of knowing oneself and of ethics. To succeed here, it is necessary to have experienced three things: *attention, justice, and appreciation*. Again, one can verify this third cornerstone of existence in one's own existence by asking:

- By whom am I *seen*?
- Who considers my uniqueness and respects my *boundaries*?
- Do people do me *justice*?
- For what am I *appreciated*–for what can I appreciate myself?

If these experiences are missing, *solitude* will be the result, *hysteria* as well as a need to hide behind the *shame*. If, on the contrary, these experiences have been made, I will find myself, find my authenticity, my relief, and my self-respect. The sum of these experiences builds *one's own worth*, the profoundest worth of what identifies my own self at its core: the self-esteem.

To be able to be oneself, it is not enough to simply experience attention, justice, and appreciation. I also have to say, "yes to myself." This requires my *active* participation: to *look* at other people, to encounter them and, at the same time, to delimitate myself and to stand by my own but to refuse whatever does not correspond to myself.

Encounter and *regret* are the two means by which we can live our authenticity without ending up in solitude. Encounter represents the necessary bridge to the other, makes me find his essence as well as my own "I" in the "you." Thus, I create for myself the appreciation requisite for feeling entitled to be what I am.

Meaning – Dealing with Becoming, Future and Commitment

If I can be there, love life and find myself therein, the conditions are fulfilled for the fourth fundamental condition of existence: the recognition of what my life is all about. It does not suffice to simply be there and to have found oneself. In a sense, we must transcend ourselves if we want to find fulfillment and to be fruitful. Otherwise, we would live as if in a house where nobody ever visits.

Thus, the transience of life puts before us *the question of the meaning of our existence*: I am there—*for what* is it good? For these three things are necessary: *a field of activity, a structural context, and a value to be realized in the future.* For a practical application we can ask ourselves questions of the following type:

- Is there a *place* where I feel *needed*, where I can be productive?
- Do I see and experience myself in a *larger context* that provides structure and orientation to my life? Where I want to be integrated?
- Is there anything that *should still be realized* in my life?

If this is not the case, the result will be a feeling of *emptiness, frustration, even despair* and, frequently, *addiction*. If, on the contrary, these conditions are met, I will be capable of *dedication* and *action* and, finally, of my own form of *religious belief*. The sum of these experiences adds up to the meaning of life and leads to a sense of fulfillment.

But it does not suffice to have a field of activity, to have one's place within a context, and to know of values to be realized in the future. Instead, the *phenomenological attitude* is needed which we spoke about at the beginning. This attitude of openness represents the *existential access* to meaning in life; that is, dealing with the questions put before me in each situation (Frankl 1973, XV, 62).

"What does this hour want from me, how shall I respond?" The meaningful thing is not only what *I* can expect from life, but, in accordance with the dialogical structure of existence, it is equally important what *life wants from me*, what the moment expects *from me*, and what *I* could and should do *now* for others as well as for myself. My *active* part in this open attitude of openness is to bring myself into *agreement* with the situation, to examine whether what I am doing is really a good thing: for others, for myself, for the future, for my environment. If I act accordingly, my existence will be fulfilling.

Viktor Frankl (1987, 315) once defined meaning as "a possibility against the background of reality." In another context (Frankl 1985, 57), he referred to the potentialities underlying the meaning:

> The potentialities of life are not indifferent possibilities; they must be seen in the light of meaning and values. At any given time only one of the possible choices of the individual fulfills the necessity of his life task.

This notion of valuable possibilities endorsed with the theory of the fundamental existential motivations defines meaning even more concretely as "the *most valuable, realistic* possibility of the given situation, for which I feel I should decide myself." *Existential meaning* is, therefore, what is possible *here and now* based on facts and reality, what is possible *for me,* may it be what I need now or what is the most pressing, valuable or interesting alternative now. To define and redefine this continually is an extremely complex task for which we possess an inner organ of perception capable of reducing this complexity to livable proportions: our sensitivity as well as our moral conscience.

Besides this existential meaning, there is an *ontological meaning*. This is the overall meaning in which I find myself and which does not depend on me. It is the philosophical and religious meaning, the meaning the creator of the world must have had in mind. I can perceive it in divination and in faith (cf. Längle 1994b for the differentiation between the two forms of meaning).

There is a story that Frankl used to tell and that illustrates in a simple way the importance of the ontological meaning for understanding life (cf. Längle 2002, 60ff). With this story I intend to end my presentation:

It was at the time when the cathedral at Chartres was being built. A traveler came along the way and saw a man sitting at the roadside, cutting a stone. The traveler asked him astonished what he was doing there. "Don't you see? I am cutting stones!" Nonplussed, the traveler continued on his way. Around the next bend, he saw another man, also cutting stones. Again, he stopped and asked the same question. "I am cutting cornerstones," was the reply. Shaking his head, our man traveled on. After a while he met a third man who was sitting in the dust and cutting stones, just as the others had been. Resolutely he walked up to him and asked: "Are you also cutting cornerstones?" The man looked up at him, wiped the sweat from his brow and said, "I am working at a cathedral."

References

Brunner R, Kausen R, Titze M (Eds) (1985) Wörterbuch der Individualpsychologie. München: Reinhardt

Frankl VE (1959) Grundriß der Existenzanalyse und Logotherapie. In: Frankl V, v Gebsattel V, Schultz JH (Eds) Handbuch der Neurosenlehre und Psychotherapie. München: Urban & Schwarzenberg, vol III, 663-736

Frankl VE (1970) The Will to Meaning. Foundations and Applications of Logotherapy. New York: New American Library

Frankl VE (1973) The Doctor and the Soul. From Psychotherapy to Logotherapy. New York: Random House. (German: Ärztliche Seelsorge. Wien: Deuticke [1946] 1982. After 1987: Frankfurt: Fischer)

Frankl VE (1985) Psychotherapy and Existentialism. Selected papers on Logotherapy. New York: Washington Square Press

Frankl VE (1987) Ärztliche Seelsorge. Grundlagen der Logotherapie und Existenzanalyse. Frankfurt: Fischer

Kimura B (1982) The phenomenology of the between: on the problem of the basic disturbance in schizophrenia. In: de Koning et al (Eds) Phenomenology and Psychiatry. London, 173-185

Kimura B (1995) Zwischen Mensch und Mensch. Strukturen japanischer Subjektivität. Darmstadt: Wissenschaftliche Buchgemeinschaft

Längle A (1992a) Was bewegt den Menschen? Die existentielle Motivation der Person. Vortrag bei Jahrestagung der GLE in Zug/Schweiz. Published (1999) Die existentielle Motivation der Person. In: Existenzanalyse 16, 3, 18-29

Längle A (1992b) Ist Kultur machbar? Die Bedürfnisse des heutigen Menschen und die Erwachsenenbildung. In: Kongreßband „Kulturträger im Dorf", Bozen: Auton. Provinz, Assessorat für Unterricht und Kultur, 65-73

Längle A (1994a) Lebenskultur-Kulturerleben. Die Kunst, Bewegendem zu begegnen. Bulletin 11, 1, 3-8

Längle A (1994b) Sinn-Glaube oder Sinn-Gespür? Zur Differenzierung von ontologischem und existentiellem Sinn in der Logotherapie. In: Bulletin der GLE 11, 2, 15-20

Längle A (1994c) Personal Existential Analysis. In: Psychotherapy East and West. Inte-gration of Psychotherapies. Seoul: Korean Acadamy of Psychotherapists 1995, 348-364

Längle A (1996) Der Mensch auf der Suche nach Halt. Existenzanalyse der Angst. In: Existenzanalyse 13, 2, 4-12

Längle A (1997a) Das Ja zum Leben finden. Existenzanalyse und Logotherapie in der Suchtkrankenhilfe. Wien: Facultas, 13-33

Längle A (1997b) Modell einer existenzanalytischen Gruppentherapie für die Suchtbehandlung. Wien: Facultas, 149-169

Längle A (1998a) Verständnis und Therapie der Psychodynamik in der Existenzanalyse. In: Existenzanalyse 15, 1, 16-27

Längle A (2002) Sinnvoll leben. Logotherapie als Lebenshilfe. Freiburg: Herder; 5. Aufl.

Rogers CR (1961) On Becoming a Person. A Therapist's View of Psychotherapy. Houghton Mifflin Co – German: Entwicklung der Persönlichkeit. Stuttgart: Klett-Cotta, 1988, 49

Comparing Buddhist, Stoic, and Existential Analysis Frameworks to Enrich Philosophy as a Way of Life: Towards a Common Factors Approach

Kate Hammer and William Van Gordon

Abstract: *As a contribution to critical psychiatry and critical psychology, this chapter surveys Philosophy as a Way of Life (PWL) as a source for different conceptions of the self which can inform clinical practice. Three frameworks – Buddhism, Stoicism, and existential analysis – are considered. Relevant psychometric scales are discussed as a means for determining empirically if common factors underlie facets of these frameworks. The Buddhist-derived Ontological Addiction Theory, Terror Management Theory and an existential analytic conception of addiction are considered. The Mental Illness-Health Matrix is then proposed as an organizing tool for investigating common factors underlying the three frameworks. Finally, the discussion is situated in relation to process-based therapy and the rise of idiographic approaches to care.*

Acknowledgements: With thanks to Alfried Längle, M.D., Ph.D. for his review of this manuscript.

Introduction: Philosophy as a Way of Life

Historian and classicist Pierre Hadot portrays ancient philosophy as "a mode of existing-in-the-world, which had to be practiced at each instant, and the goal of which was to transform the whole of the individual's life" (Hadot, 1995, p. 265). It was, according to Hadot, "a method for training people to live and to look at the world in a new way," (p. 107). Writing specifically of Stoicism, Hadot characterized its fundamental "spiritual attitude" (p. 84) as a form of attention that "allows us to respond immediately to events, as if they were questions asked of us all of the sudden" (p. 85). Hadot further states "we are not dealing with mere knowledge, but with the transformation of our personality" (p. 85). It is for Hadot, thus, "a real existential commitment" (Sharpe, 2016, p. 412).

Philosopher Matthew Sharpe draws on Hadot's conception of Philosophy as a Way of Life (PWL) in his collaboration with cardiology researcher Robert P. Nolan. They propose for inclusion in palliative counselling activities that Hadot would characterize as "spiritual exercises" (Sharpe & Nolan, 2023). Their proposal is framed in terms of medicine's long-standing relationship with philosophy, which they document citing primary philosophical texts from ancient Greece and Rome and contemporary classicists. Their primary contention is "that the meta-philosophical approach of PWL, as developed by Hadot, is consistent with efforts to re-establish an effective dialogue between the science and philosophy of well-being" (p. 1175).

The present chapter contributes to a parallel effort by asking what PWL brings to the discipline of psychology. Is it just the techniques themselves (which have been taken up by Cognitive Behavioral Therapy [CBT] and Rational Emotive Behavioral Therapy [REBT])? Or can the ontologies PWL foregrounds bring something to clinical conceptions of individuals and their suffering?

The present excursion aims to contribute to a "post-technological psychiatry" and clinical psychology incorporating both empirical science and psychotherapeutic techniques while framing them in new ways (Bracken et al., 2012, p. 432). Specifically, this chapter considers the conceptions of self and of well-being in three frameworks: a religion (Buddhism), an ancient philosophy (Stoicism), and an existential psychotherapeutic approach elaborated by Alfried Längle.

Table 1 (see Appendix A) summarizes key features of Buddhism, Stoicism, and Länglean Existential Analysis. A further framework, a psychosocial theory called Terror Management Theory (TMT), provides a bridge between them. Where the frameworks overlap, corresponding notions are drawn to the fore and the question posed: do common factors exist across them and what implications might a common-factors approach have for clinical work?

A Religion: Buddhism

Buddhism's presence in psychotherapeutic practice is evident across various therapeutic principles, particularly mindfulness (Kabat-Zinn, 1991). While there exist many subdivisions of Buddhist thought and practice, a closer look at the metaphysics of Buddhism allows a clearer conception of its power to contribute to clinical work (see summary in Table 1 in Appendix A).

Buddhist metaphysics underpins Meditation Awareness Training (MAT), an 8-week intervention pioneered in the United Kingdom that "focuses on cultivating penetrating insight into the nature of selfhood and reality" (Barrows & Van Gordon, 2021, p. 6). Insight of a metaphysical nature is gained through teaching, contemplation, and direct experience (Dalai Lama, 2018). At the heart of MAT is the idea: "the self is a construction of the mind and that there are no credible grounds for believing that there is an inherently existing 'I' that operates independently of everything else" (Barrows & Van Gordon, 2021, p. 7). Shonin et al. (2016) situate this idea in a three-phase treatment:

1. Becoming aware of self
2. Deconstructing the imputed self
3. Reconstructing a dynamic and non-dual self

According to Barrows and Van Gordon (2021), this treatment addresses the inner process of Ontological Addiction (OA; Van Gordon et al., 2018). Ontology means "being" and thus the phrase "ontological addiction" provocatively refers to an over-investment in "I, me, mine" to the exclusion of otherness and impermanence. The definition of OA given in Shonin et al. (2013) is "the unwillingness to relinquish an erroneous and deep-rooted belief in an inherently existing 'self' or 'I' as well as the 'impaired functionality' that arises from such a belief" (p. 64).

A key principle of Ontological Addiction Theory (OAT) is not to pathologize anyone who does not subscribe to the Buddhist metaphysical view. Instead, OAT foregrounds a culturally prevalent egoistic conception of self as individualistic (Watkins, 1992). As elucidated further below, a key facet of OA can be illuminated by discussing defenses against death anxiety.

A Psychosocial Theory: Terror Management Theory

Terror Management Theory (TMT) is a theoretical and empirical research framework for elucidating how people respond to mortality. The premise is that human cultures have developed buffers that protect people from existential terror and that legacies are an "immortality project" insofar as "a working level of narcissism is inseparable from self-esteem" (Becker, 1973, p. 9, p. 24).

While many TMT empirical studies use Western, educated people from industrialized, rich, developed nations (WEIRD; Henrich et al., 2010), TMT's relevance to clinical populations is borne out. The presence of death anxiety in treatment-seeking individuals (across diagnostic categories) has been empirically established (Menzies et al., 2019) and the case advanced for death anxiety as a transdiagnostic construct for psychopathology (Iverach et al., 2014; Menzies & Menzies, 2023).

TMT stipulates that a defended "symbolic self" forms to diffuse anxiety about death's inevitability. This symbolic self is characterized by "a sense of personal value that is obtained by believing (a) in the validity of one's cultural worldview and (b) that one is living up to the standards that are part of that worldview" (Pyszczynski et al., 2004, pp. 436-437). The cultural worldview refers to outer reality and self-esteem characterizes the introjection of standards in the inner reality. Read through the lens of Self-Determination Theory, TMT's model implies "contingent self-esteem" that results in "unstable self-worth" (Ryan & Deci, 2018, p. 255). Ryan and Deci characterize TMT as "a deficit-need theory, since the motivations it has in focus are primarily defensive and reactive in nature" (p. 92).

How does the "symbolic self" fare in terms of ontological addiction? OAT stipulates: "individuals reify their sense of self to a point that they relate to themselves as the centerpiece in a world in which all other lifeforms, objects, and concepts are deemed to be peripheral" (Van Gordon et al., 2018, p. 893). Ontological addiction, then, is a form of over-extended self-esteem. The peripherization of all that is non-self might be comparable to the infrahumanization process studied by Cuddy et al. (2007) and Leyens et al. (2007).

In infrahumanization, outgroups are imputed to experience less exclusively human emotion and are likened to animals. Leyens et al. (2001) investigates the attribution of emotion to outgroup members by ingroup members to further an understanding of how attribution of essence (as in, the essence of human beings) features in exclusionary dynamics. Such essentialism corresponds to the reification of self. A reified self as a source of infrahumanization links essentialism to the defensive worldview. When enacted as patriotism, warmongering, and xenophobia, the reified self has profound effects at a societal level (Greenberg et al., 2001; Greenberg et al., 2014; Legendre et al., 2022; Tjew-A-Sin & Koole, 2019).

For individuals managing their death fear through symbolic defenses or through philosophical or spiritual practice, there are two forms of death salience: impersonal and personal. Impersonal death reminders are oblique and generalized; words like "grave" or images like a skull or tombstone. By contrast, other death reminders are personal; one feels confronted by one's own mortality rather than by finitude in general. These different mortality cues are linked to inner processes; impersonal cues are associated with unconscious processing and personal cues with conscious awareness.

Moreover, according to TMT, unconscious processing of death cues mobilizes self-esteem concepts and defensive cultural worldviews (see Dar-Nimrod, 2022, for a summary of the literature). A new scale, the Death Anxiety Beliefs and Behaviours Scale (DABBS; Menzies et al., 2022), usefully distinguishes clinically significant death anxiety and distress. The 24-point Ontological Addiction Scale (OAT-24; Barrows et al., 2022; see Table 2) can be used to survey individuals high on death anxiety and holding defensive worldviews. Ontologically addicted individuals may be too self-involved to consciously receive and react to death reminders because the defended self seeks invincibility and so responds with suppression or denial, as TMT posits. Perhaps unconscious processing will reveal their susceptibility to death fears, although this needs to be born out in future empirical investigation.

#1 Felt you needed to receive more attention or affection from a person you care about?

#2 Thought about how others see you?

#3 Thought about how you could avoid experiencing discomfort?

#4 Felt the need for more attention or recognition?

#5 Felt uplifted when you were praised?

#6 Felt superior to others?

#7 Felt uplifted when you experienced financial or material gain?

#8 Felt good when you experienced fewer challenges?

#9 Felt you needed to try harder in order to receive praise or avoid criticism?

#10 Felt you needed to do better in order to avoid shame or humiliation?

#11 Felt you needed more money or material possessions?

#12 Felt an increasing need to occupy yourself to avoid being on your own?

#13 Found it hard to accept your mistakes and shortcomings?

#14 Found it hard to overcome rejection?

#15 Found it hard to give something away?

#16 Found it hard to live more simply?

#17 Felt low when you were criticized?

#18 Felt inferior to others?

#19 Felt low when you encountered financial or material loss?

#20 Felt low when you encountered difficult circumstances?

#21 Stopped being kind to somebody you care about because they offended you?

#22 Felt worried about not being recognized after having acted in others' interests?

#23 Stopped helping others because it was causing discomfort or inconvenience?

#24 Felt regret about giving something away?

Table 2: *Ontological Addiction measured on a 24-item instrument using a 5-point Likert Scale.*

Stoicism: A Philosophical Response to Finitude

Terror Management Theory describes a cultural and psychological orientation in response to death's inevitability. The theme of inescapable mortality is also central to the ancient philosophy, Stoicism. The metaphysics of Stoicism is summarized in Table 1 (Appendix A). Stoicism is familiar to clinicians because of its re-expression in Cognitive Behavioral Therapy (CBT; McGlinchey, 2004; Menzies & Whittle, 2022; Robertson, 2018). Le Bon (2023) goes so far as to say that while Stoicism is the framework for cultivating flourishing and resilience, and CBT is for mental health problems, he anticipates a further "third-wave CBT" which draws not only on mindfulness and values clarification (as do Acceptance & Commitment Therapy [Hayes et al., 2006]; Compassion Focused Therapy [Gilbert, 2014]; and Mindfulness Based Cognitive Therapy [Segal et al., 2013]) but is more expressly Stoic in nature.

Should this arise, therapeutic Stoic training might be analogous to MAT's mobilization of Buddhist wisdom, although to date studies of Stoic training evaluations have been few in number (Brown et al., 2022; Hammer & Van Gordon, 2023; MacLellan & Derakshan, 2021). Working with clinical psychologists at University of London Royal Holloway, Le Bon has developed a psychometric screening tool called Stoic Attitudes and Behaviours Scale (SABS; Le Bon, 2018) for use alongside psychopathology and positive psychology instruments. SABS permits researchers (and participants) to measure "how Stoic" an individual is before and after an intervention. Here, capital-S Stoicism refers to the ancient philosophy, not the repression of emotional expression or pain affect.

Stoic practice, as understood by Pierre Hadot (2001), consists of an "armamentarium" of spiritual exercises that make personal death proximal, conscious, and the focus for active contemplation. Their application cultivates a more virtuous character and social nature. SABS items such as "If things don't go well for me/my family/friends, I can't live a good life," "I need to be well thought of by others in order to be happy," "I need quite a lot of money in order to be happy" — and, in the negative, "I care about the suffering of others," "I do not act on urges when it would be unwise to act on them," and "Every day I spend some time thinking about how I can best face challenges in the day ahead" — point to an overlap with OAT-24.

Alongside Stoic practice, direct contemplation of one's own death is also activated by near-death experiences. Studying near-death experiences, Cozzolino theorized how individuals process death via either a personalized existential system or an abstract, categorical one (2006). Theoretically, and later empirically (Cozzolino & Blackie, 2013; Cozzolino et al., 2014), Cozzolino posited that the personal existential system of processing mortality revealed a self that differed from the defended and symbolic self-predicated by TMT.

Indeed, here the personal self is constituted by self-concept clarity (including self-acceptance), internal locus of control, self-realization, and existential well-being (Cozzolino, et al., 2014). The actualized self-described by Cozzolino neither avoids nor fears death. It is not ontologically addicted. Placing the frameworks side-by-side—whether a person pursues a life of Buddhist practice, Stoic practice or existential-personal engagement—the movement in general is away from a defended, rigid, self-separating "sovereign" self towards a place of more humility and greater openness towards the cosmos.

Existential Analysis: A Relational Self, Addressing the World

A phenomenological depth psychotherapy developed by Viennese medical doctor and psychotherapist Alfried Längle called Existential Analysis brings a useful conception of self to the current discussion. Länglean Existential Analysis (LEA) builds on the philosophical anthropology conceived by psychiatrist Viktor Frankl.[1] In LEA, the self is understood as a socially embedded and evolving construction connected (or disconnected, in cases of maladaptation or developmental derailment) from the deep person (*nous*) (see Table 1 in Appendix A). Although LEA does not reference Heinz Kohut, LEA's conception resembles Kohut's self "as a *system* that embodies a *relationship*" (Strozier et al., 2022, p. 42). Kohut's understanding of relationality derives from philosopher Edmund Husserl's concept of intersubjectivity (pp. 44-45), and phenomenology lies at the heart of LEA.

Personhood (the ability to be oneself) stands in a polarity between One's Own and the Other engaged in a perpetual dialectical process, according

---

[1] Viktor Frankl was a student of Alfred Adler, whose conception of "will to power" was referenced by Ernest Becker (1973) in his formulation of self-esteem as a mortality defense (Längle, 2019).

to LEA (Längle, 2021). "Self" according to Längle emerges as a representation of the deep person accepted by the ego, encompassing the objects of self-reflection and the totality of identifications emerging from engagement in inner contemplation and outer engagement (Längle, 2021). Self is not, in a word, an essence. In LEA, my re-flection is understood as the process of mirroring back at me from the outside (through the behavior of others, through relationships, through accomplishments and the effects of my actions) and from the inside, through noticing how I experience myself and contemplating all that I receive.

Self-worth induction begins from the outside when I receive attention, justice (in correspondence with my essence as it shows in expression, gestures, deeds), and appreciation (that the other evaluates me as valuable) (Längle, 2021). LEA's account covers the ground of attachment theory; but also designates internal processes that the individual, as they develop, can take up on their own behalf as they mature. Attention, when given by the individual to themselves, becomes the capacity to self-distance. To do justice to oneself is to take oneself seriously, a process that germinates into moral conscience and ethical awareness from within, which differs from rule compliance referring to external sources of authority. Finally, appreciating oneself gives rise to the cognitive capacity to self-assess, which again fosters critical distance (Längle, 2021).

When I find my own person, according to LEA, I encounter myself, I listen intimately as I meet myself, I can stand-with-myself as I am withstanding judgements of important others. This parallels the wisdom Hadot envisaged as the goal of ancient philosophy, striving towards "the domain of consciousness and lucidity" (1995, p. 103). There is no craving, I am authentic in my encounter: I with myself, open to the world. This conception of the existentially open self resonates with OAT:

A less-pronounced sense of self fosters clarity of perceptive and cognitive processes and allows the individual to construct a sense of self that is dynamic, inseparable from its environment, and that is full and complete due to experiencing that all things are "empty" (Van Gordon et al., 2018, p. 895).

According to LEA, an individual's self-worth dialogues with the world continually. It is not sealed off, indiscriminate, or over-bearing. A fully dialogical self cannot be ontologically addicted. This becomes evident in LEA's conception of addiction, which is elucidated further below.

Addiction, Viewed Existentially

According to Muir (2015), an existential analytic psychotherapist trained by Längle:

> "[B]ehind every addiction lies a neediness, an emptiness, a seemingly insatiable hunger. Addiction simulates greediness for life by gulping in pseudo external nourishment because the addict/person is unable to find that nourishment from within" (Muir, 2015, pp. 111-112).

Muir (2015) likens the "false, temporary sense of fullness" (p. 112) to a colander emptying with each bout. Muir further designates addiction a "temporal disorder; it offers a shameful past, a fettered present, and a seemingly hopeless future" (p. 112). The individual's capacity to resist the imperative is weak due to recognizable attitudes: an attitude of wishfulness distanced from reality; an intolerance for frustration and pain; and the view that suffering has no worth (Längle, 2023).

> In Existential Analysis (EA), we see addiction as the simultaneous experience of an imperative that has a powerful driving character, which forces an attraction to an object or substance, while simultaneously offering the affected individual an experience of powerlessness in the face of a subjective deficit (Muir, 2015, p. 111).

The suffering comprises a loss of freedom and a-personal behavior because the craving for the addictive "stuff" effects an alienation. The addicted person's will has been severed from their personal values and, consequently, their will is confused. The part of the addicted person who reviles their own greedy dependency and/or the stuff's harmful effects feels guilt, shame, and embarrassment. While an addicted individual may feel disgust at their greediness for the stuff, they lack strength to break the compulsive cycle (Längle, 2023). This gives rise to "the illusion that they have no will. They feel compelled to use/act addictively" (Muir, 2015, p. 113).

Admission of powerlessness, as encoded in the First Step of the 12-Step Alcoholics Anonymous program, plays a role in LEA's addiction treatment process (Längle, 2023). But so, too, does self-acceptance of their craving. Helping a client "choose to use is existentially healthier than abdicating responsibility for [their] actions" (Muir, 2015, p. 113). In addiction's grip, the voice of the deep person (*nous*) is muffled (Längle, 2023). Muir has taken Miller and Rollnick's Motivational Interviewing framework and used it to "open an arena for a dual dialogue" that gives space to the voice of the person and the voice of the addict "so that we can see [these two voices] are diametrically opposed" (2015, p. 112). In this way, ambivalence is openly engaged in existential analytic therapy.

The addicted person has lost (or never grasped) their relationality to a wider horizon of meaning, to a wider world. Meaninglessness can precede addiction, according to LEA. The individual struggles to answer questions such as: "Is there a place where I feel needed, where I can be productive? Do I see and experience myself in a larger context that provides structure and orientation to my life? Where I want to be integrated? Is there anything that should still be realized or accomplished in my life?" (Längle, 2003, p. 34). According to this theoretical model, the addicted person is capable of little self-distance, experiences self-transcendence rarely if at all, and their personal freedom and responsibility is curtailed.

The Existence Scale (Längle et al., 2003) surveys these dimensions with items such as "Things are only meaningful to me as far as they meet my own desires," "The fulfillment of one's own wishes has priority," "I'm only interested in a situation that meets my wishes," and "Life has betrayed me because it has not fulfilled my wishfulness," suggesting that an association may be found between OAT-24 scores and Existence Scale scores. Clearly, empirical research is needed to evaluate this, but anecdotal reports indicate that convergence on these scales may be empirically borne out. For example, based on more than 12,500 hours of therapy, Muir observed that no client has ever presented "stand-alone, sui generis addiction"; rather "in every case there has been some concurrent disorder" (2015, p. 112).

Personality Disorders: Shocks of Selfhood and Clinical Presentations

LEA understands personality disorders as arising from a persistent reaction to distance from unbearable pain or deprivation. The reaction pattern in personality disorders leads "to persistent, profound imbalances and inner-psychic tensions, [giving rise] to a persistent and constant self- and other-damaging behavior" (Längle, 2000, p. 1). At the level of disorder (rather than neurosis), personality disorder is marked by an "adrift (uncontrollable, inwardly disconnected) reaction, decoupled by stimuli, with ingrained, stereotyped psychodynamics" which takes form as "impulsive lashing out" (pp. 1-2) amid which the individual cannot access their deep person (*nous*).

Hollowness, lack of feeling, and dissociation are modes of experience arising when contact with the deep person is blocked (Längle, 2011). Personality disorders of selfhood (known in the diagnostic literature as histrionic, borderline, narcissistic, dissocial, paranoid, paraexistential, and immature personality) often externalize in response to pains of constriction and pressure (giving rise to mental anguish), pain of woundedness (giving rise to disgust and dread) and pain of being left alone (giving rise to agony) (Längle, 2011).

OAT has also considered personality disorders including borderline personality disorder (BPD), which is understood to be an "extreme form of suffering emerging from ontological addiction" (Ducasse et al., 2020, p. 944). Ducasse et al. (2020) further posit that "self-grasping ignorance" may manifest differently and warn against "an oversight in respect of the common grasping at inherent existence which appears to underlie most categorial diagnoses, including BPD" (p. 944). Death anxiety was found by Menzies et al. (2019) to be present across diagnostic categories. If, like death anxiety, OA is also widespread in treatment-seeking populations, how do we conceptualise it in clinical work?

New Matrix for Mental Health and Mental Illness

If OA is common because of contemporary western culture's structures and reward systems, OAT throws into question the opposition of mental health and mental illness. Individuals can be free from mental illness but, considering their defensive, symbolic self and its preoccupation with "I, me, mine," they may not possess mental health.

Lomas and Vanderweele (2023) propose the Mental Illness Health (MIH) matrix, the core idea of which is that health is more than the absence of illness (Keyes, 2005). The matrix serves as a container for data pertaining to mental health and mental illness, allowing the co-presence (or co-absence) of mental health and mental illness to be visualized; and for changes over time in either parameter to be mapped. At its simplest form, it presents a 2x2 grid (see Table 3).

Status of Mental Health	Status of Mental Illness	Called
Mentally healthy	No mental illness	Thriving
Mentally healthy	Mentally ill	Struggling
No mental health	Mentally ill	Faltering
No mental health	No mental illness	Languishing

Table 3: *The quadrants of the Mental Illness Health Matrix (Lomas & Vanderweele, 2023)*

The status of an individual with a defended symbolic self, fearful and avoidant of death might be rendered as languishing in a MIH matrix; for while there may be no mental illness *per se*, they may live with an absence of mental health. Conversely, when an existentially-engaged individual (leveraging PWL) experiences mental illness, their mental *health* may protect them from languishing even as they struggle with mental *illness*. Addiction recovery might entail a shift from faltering to struggling as the individual becomes more mentally healthy insofar as the compulsive lust and greed for the addictive substance is still felt.

To apply the MIH matrix, clinicians and researchers can determine what measures of specific health and illness states should be used, converting any scale into a score on (for example) a 10-point range so that all instrument scores can be placed on the matrix. The arithmetic conversion retains the meaning of symptoms below clinical thresholds whereas categorial assignments erase them. Thus, the MIH supports factor analytic research, including along the lines of investigation suggested in this chapter, into the overlap (or not) between ontological addiction, Stoicism, and existentiality via the psychometric instruments discussed.

The clinical application of MIH as a record over time of treatment informed by one or more of the frameworks discussed here supports an idiographic approach to care. Idiographic approaches to clinical treatment depend on dimensions rather than diagnostic categories (Gutiérrez et al., 2020; Hopwood et al., 2017). The rise of testable models, mediation and moderation studies harkens a new era Hofmann and Hayes call "process-based therapy" (PBT; 2019, p. 42). PBT is "the contextually specific use of evidence-based therapeutic processes linked to evidence based therapeutic procedures to help solve the problems and promote the prosperity of an individual" (Hayes et al., 2019, p. 41).

Can a treatment pursued in terms of one PWL framework give rise to changes measured in another? Addressing this question will show clinicians how philosophical systems embed into work with clients. McGlinchey (2004) observed that philosophy can show us "where current psychotherapy theory and practices arose" (p. 52) but, perhaps, also (two decades on) where they are heading. If the common factor approach sketched here is, in due course, borne out empirically, the historical and cultural base of PWL widens and PWL's clinical relevance will be substantially enriched.

References

Barrows, P., & Van Gordon, W. (2021). Ontological Addiction Theory and Mindfulness-Based Approaches in the Context of Addiction Theory and Treatment. Religions, 12(586), 1–10. https:// doi.org/10.3390/rel12080586

Barrows, P., Shonin, E., Sapthiang, S., Griffiths, M. D., Ducasse, D., & Van Gordon, W. (2022). The Development and Validation of the Ontological

Addiction Scale. *International Journal of Mental Health and Addiction, 21*(6), 4043–4070. https://doi.org/10.1007/s11469-022-00840-y

Becker, E. (1973). *Denial of death.* Souvenir Press.

Bracken, P., Thomas, P., Timimi, S., Asen, E., Behr, G., Beuster, C., Bhunnoo, S., Browne, I., Chhina, N., Double, D., Downer, S., Evans, C., Fernando, S., Garland, M. R., Hopkins, W., Huws, R., Johnson, B., Martindale, B., Middleton, H., Moldavsky, D., Moncrieff, J., Mullins, S., Nelki, J., Pizzo, M., Rodger, J., Smyth, M., Summerfield, D., Wallace, J. & Yeomans, D. (2012). Psychiatry beyond the current paradigm. *The British Journal of Psychiatry, 201,* 430-434. https://doi.org/10.1192/bjp.bp.112.109447

Brown, M. E. L., MacLellan, A., Laughey, W., Omer, U., Himmi, G., LeBon, T., & Finn, G. M. (2022). Can Stoic training develop medical student empathy and resilience? A mixed-methods study. *BMC Medical Education, 22*(1), Article 340. https://doi.org/10.1186/s12909-022-03391-x

Cozzolino, P. J. (2006). Death contemplation, growth, and defense: Converging evidence of dual-existential systems? *Psychological Inquiry, 17*(4), 278–287. https:// doi.org/10.1080/10478400701366944

Cozzolino, P. J., & Blackie, L. E. (2013). I die, therefore I am: The pursuit of meaning in the light of death. In J. Hicks & C. Routledge (Eds.), *The experience of meaning in life: Classical perspectives, emerging themes, and controversies* (pp. 31–45). Springer.

Cozzolino, P. J., Blackie, L. E., & Meyers, L. S. (2014). Self-related consequences of death fear and death denial. *Death Studies, 38*(6), 418–422.

Cuddy, A. J. C., Rock, M. S., & Norton, M. I. (2007). Aid in the Aftermath of Hurricane Katrina: Inferences of Secondary Emotions and Intergroup Helping. *Group Processes & Intergroup Relations, 10*(1), 107–118. https://doi.org/10.1177/1368430207071344

Dalai Lama. (2018). *An Introduction to Buddhism.* Snow Lion Publications.

Dar-Nimrod, I. (2022). Death awareness and Terror Management Theory. In Menzies, R. G., Menzies, R. E. & Dingle G., Eds. *Existential Concerns and Cognitive-behavioral Procedures: An integrative approach to mental health* (pp. 35-55). Springer Nature.

Ducasse, D., Van Gordon, W., Brand-Arpon, V., Courtet, P., & Olié, E. (2020). Borderline personality disorder: From understanding ontological addiction to psychotherapeutic revolution. *European Archives of Psychiatry and Clinical Neuroscience, 270,* 941–945. https://doi.org/10.1007/s00406-019-01029-6

Gilbert, P. (2014). The origins and nature of compassion focused therapy. *British Journal of Clinical Psychology, 53*(1), 6–41. https://doi.org/10.1111/bjc.12043

Greenberg, J., Schimel, J., Martens, A., Solomon, S., & Pyszcznyski, T. (2001). Sympathy for the devil: Evidence that reminding whites of their mortality promotes more favorable reactions to white racists. *Motivation and Emotion, 25*(2), 113–133. https://doi.org/10.1023/A:1010613909207

Greenberg, J., Vail, K., & Pyszczynski, T. (2014). Terror Management Theory and research: How the desire for death transcendence drives our strivings for meaning and significance. In *Advances in Motivation Science* (Vol. 1, pp. 85–134). Elsevier. https://doi.org/10.1016/bs.adms.2014.08.003

Gutiérrez, F., Ruiz, J., Peri, J. M., Gárriz, M., Vall, G. & Cavero, M. (2020). Toward an integrated model of pathological personality traits: Common hierarchical structure of the PID-5 and the DAPP-BQ. *Journal of Personality Disorders, 34*(Supplement C), 25-39. https://doi.org/10.1521/pedi_2019_33_431

Hadot, P. (1995). *Philosophy as a Way of Life*. Trans. M. Chase. Blackwell.

Hadot, P. (2001). *The Inner Citadel: The* Meditations *of Marcus Aurelius*. Trans. M. Chase. Harvard University Press.

Hammer, K., & Van Gordon, W. (2023). Joyful Stoic Death Writing: An Interpretative Phenomenological Analysis of Newcomers Contemplating Death in an Online Group. *Journal of Humanistic Psychology,* 00221678231178051. https://doi.org/10.1177/00221678231178051

Hayes, S. C., Hofmann, S. G., Stanton, C. E., Carpenter, J. K., Sanford, B. T., Curtiss, J. E., & Ciarrochi, J. (2019). The role of the individual in the coming era of process-based therapy. *Behaviour Research and Therapy, 117,* 40–53. https://doi.org/10.1016/j.brat.2018.10.005

Hayes, S. C., Luoma, J. B., Bond, F. W., Masuda, A., & Lillis, J. (2006). Acceptance and Commitment Therapy: Model, processes and outcomes. *Behaviour Research and Therapy, 44*(1), 1–25. https://doi.org/10.1016/j.brat.2005.06.006

Henrich, J., Heine, S. J., & Norenzayan, A. (2010). The weirdest people in the world? *Behavioral and Brain Sciences, 33*(2-3), 61-83.

Hofmann, S. G., & Hayes, S. C. (2019). The future of intervention science: Process-based therapy. *Clinical Psychological Science, 7*(1), 37–50. https://doi.org/10.1177/2167702618772296

Hopwood, C. J., Kotov, R. , Krueger, R.F., Watson, D., Widiger, T. A., Althoff, R. R., Ansell, E. B., Bach, B., Bagby, R. M., Blais, M. A., Bornovalova, M. A., Chmielewski, M., Cicero, D. C., Conway, C., De Clerq, B., De Fruyt, F., Docherty, A. R., Eaton, N. R., Edens, J. F., Forbes, M. K., Forbush, K. T., Hengartner, M. P., Ivanova, M. Y., Leising, D., Livesley, W. J., Lukowitsky22, M. R., Lynam, D. R., Markon, K. E., Miller, J. D., Morey, L. C., Mullins-Sweatt, S. N., Ormel, J. H., Patrick, C. J., Pincus, A. L., Ruggero, C., Samuel, D. B., Sellbom, M., Slade, T., Tackett, J. L., Thomas, K. M., Trull, T. J., Vachon, D. D., Waldman, I. W., Waszczuk, M. A., Waugh, M. H., Wright, A. G. C., Yalch, M. M., Zald, D. H., & Zimmermann, J. (2017). The time has come for dimensional personality disorder diagnosis. *Personality and Mental Health,* 18, 82-86. https://doi.org/10.1002/pmh.1408

Iverach, L., Menzies, R. G., & Menzies, R. E. (2014). Death anxiety and its role in psychopathology: Reviewing the status of a transdiagnostic construct. *Clinical Psychology Review, 34*(7), 580-593. https://doi.org/10.1016/j.cpr.2014.09.002

Kabat-Zinn, J. (1991). *Full Catastrophe Living.* Delta.

Keyes, C. L. M. (2005). Mental illness and/or mental health? Investigating axioms of the complete state model of health. *Journal of Consulting and Clinical Psychology,* 73(3), 539–548. https://doi.org/10.1037/0022-006X.73.3.539

Längle, A. (2000). Lexical short description of personality disorder. GLE-International.

Längle, A. (2003). The art of involving the person: Fundamental existential motivations as the structure of the motivational process. *European Psychotherapy* 4(1), 25-36.

Längle, A. (2011). Hysteria: Understanding and therapy of hysteria and of personality disorders. Trans. D. Trobisch. GLE-International.

Längle, A. (2019). The history of logotherapy and existential analysis. In E. van Deurzen, E. Craig, A. Längle, K.J. Schneider, D. Tantam & S. du Plock (Eds.), *The Wiley World Handbook of Existential Therapy, First Ed.* (pp. 309-323). Wiley.

Längle, A. (2021). The third fundamental motivation: The fundamental condition for personhood and the ability to be oneself. Student Manual, 10th Edition. GLE International.

Längle, A. (2023, May 18-21). Private seminar on addiction. GLE-UK. London, England.

Längle, A., Orgler, C., & Kundi, M. (2003). The Existence Scale: A new approach to assess the ability to find personal meaning in life and to reach existential fulfilment. *European Psychotherapy*, 4(1), 135-151.

Le Bon, T. (2018, December 14). Stoic week 2018 report part 3: Impact on well-being by Tim LeBon. *Blog Post.* https://modernstoicism.com/stoic-week-2018-report-part- 3-impact-on-well-being-by-tim-lebon/

Le Bon, T. (2023, September 23). Stoicism and well-being: Your practical Stoic toolkit [Conference presentation]. *Stoic Icons: The legacy of Seneca, Epictetus, Cicero, and Marcus Aurelius*, London, United Kingdom.

Legendre, T. S., Yu, H. (Chandler), Ding, A., & Matera, J. M. (2022). Boycotting Asian restaurants: The effect of mortality salience, contagion name, and media exposure on boycotting. *International Journal of Hospitality Management, 107.* https://doi.org/10.1016/j.ijhm.2022.103333

Leyens, J.-P., Rodriguez-Perez, A., Rodriguez-Torres, R., Gaunt, R., Paladino, M.-P., Vaes, J., & Demoulin, S. (2001). Psychological essentialism and the differential attribution of uniquely human emotions to ingroups and outgroups. *European Journal of Social Psychology, 31*(4), 395–411. https://doi.org/10.1002/ejsp.50

Leyens, J.-P., Demoulin, S., Vaes, J., Gaunt, R., & Paladino, M. P. (2007). Infra-humanization: The Wall of Group Differences: Infra-humanization. *Social Issues and Policy Review, 1*(1), 139–172. https://doi.org/10.1111/j.1751-2409.2007.00006.x

Lomas, T. & VanderWeele, T. J. (2023). The Mental Illness – Health Matrix and the Mental State Space Matrix: Complementary meta-conceptual frameworks for evaluating psychological states. *Journal of Clinical Psychology, 79*(8), 1902-1920. https://doi.org/10.1002/jclp.23512

MacLellan, A., & Derakshan, N. (2021). The effects of Stoic training and adaptive working memory training on emotional vulnerability in high worriers. *Cognitive Therapy and Research, 45*(4), 730–744. https://doi.org/10.1007/s10608-020-10183-4

Menzies, R. E. & Menzies, R. G. (2023). Death anxiety and mental health: Requiem for a dreamer. *Journal of Behavior Therapy and Experimental Psychiatry 78*. https://doi.org/10.1016/j.jbtep.2022.101807

Menzies, R. E., Sharpe, L. & Dar-Nimrod, I. (2019). The relationship between death anxiety and severity of mental illnesses. *British Journal of Clinical Psychology, 58*(4), 452-467. https://doi.org/10.1111/bjc.12229

Menzies, R. E., Sharpe, L., & Dar-Nimrod, I. (2022). The development and validation of the Death Anxiety Beliefs and Behaviours Scale. *British Journal of Clinical Psychology, 61*(4), 1169–1187. https://doi.org/10.1111/bjc.12387

Menzies, R. E., & Whittle, L. F. (2022). Stoicism and death acceptance: Integrating Stoic philosophy in cognitive behaviour therapy for death anxiety. *Discover Psychology, 2*(1), 11. https://doi.org/10.1007/s44202-022-00023-9

McGlinchey, J. B. (2004, Spring). On Hellenistic philosophy and its relevance to contemporary CBT: A response to Reiss (2003). *The Behavior Therapist,* 51-52.

Muir, B. (2015). Addiction and meaning. *Existenzanalyse, 32*(2), 111-115.

Pyszczynski, T., Greenberg, J., Solomon, S., Arndt, J., & Schimel, J. (2004). Why Do People Need Self-Esteem? A Theoretical and Empirical Review. *Psychological Bulletin, 130*(3), 435–468. https://doi.org/10.1037/0033-2909.130.3.435

Robertson, D. (2018). *The Philosophy of Cognitive-Behavioural Therapy (CBT): Stoic philosophy as rational and cognitive psychotherapy.* Routledge.

Ryan, R. M. & Deci, E. L. (2018). *Self-determination Theory: Basic psychological needs in motivation, development, and wellness.* Guilford Press.

Segal, Z. V., Williams, J. M. G., & Teasdale, J. D. (2013). *Mindfulness-Based Cognitive Therapy for Depression, 2nd Ed.* Guilford Press.

Sharpe, M. (2016). Socratic Ironies: Reading Hadot, reading Kierkegaard. *Sophia, 55,* 409-435. https://doi.org/10.1007/s11841-016-0512-6

Sharpe, M. & Nolan, R. P. (2023). Philosophy as a way of life, spiritual exercises, and palliative care. *Journal of Evaluation in Clinical Practice, 29,* 1171-1179. https://doi.org/10.1111/jep.13902

Shonin, E., Van Gordon, W., & Griffiths, M. D. (2016). Ontological Addiction: Classification, Etiology, and Treatment. Mindfulness, 7(3), 660–671. https://doi.org/10.1007/s12671-016-0501-4

Shonin, E., Van Gordon, W., & Griffiths, M. D. (2013). Buddhist philosophy for the treatment of problem gambling. *Journal of Behavioral Addictions,* 2,63–71.

Strozier, C. B., Pinteris, K., Kelley, K., & Cher, D. (2022). *The New World of Self: Heinz Kohut's transformation of psychoanalysis and psychotherapy.* Oxford University Press.

Tjew-A-Sin, M., & Koole, S. L. (2018). Terror Management in a Multicultural Society: Effects of Mortality Salience on Attitudes to Multiculturalism Are Moderated by National Identification and Self-Esteem Among Native Dutch People. *Frontiers in Psychology, 9,* 721. https://doi.org/10.3389/fpsyg.2018.00721

Van Gordon, W., Shonin, E., Diouri, S., Garcia-Campayo, J., Kotera, Y. & Griffiths, M. (2018). Ontological addiction theory: Attachment to me, mine, and I. *Journal of Behavioral Addictions,* 7(4), 892-896. https://doi.org/10.1556/2006.7.2018.45

Watkins, M. (1992). From individualism to the interdependent self: Changing the paradigm of the self in psychotherapy. *Psychological Perspectives,* 27(1), 52-69. https://doi.org/10.1080/00332929208408110

Appendix A

	Buddhism	Stoicism	Existential Analysis
Considered to be	Enduring eastern religion	Ancient western philosophy	Psychotherapeutic paradigm
Daily practice	Mindfulness and compassion. Tranquility and insight meditations.	"Armamentarium" of reflective practices.	Self-experiencing in inner dialogue
Purpose of thinking	Cultivating virtue. Understanding the nature of thoughts.	Self-training in virtues	Understanding and deciding
Wellbeing concept	Attaining enlightenment is to overcome lust, greed, aversion, and hatred. Enlightenment destroys the delusion of a mechanistic world, and accepts impermanence, non-self, and suffering.	Completing the development of our rational character for the sake of eudaimonia. To live harmoniously as social creatures entails an attitude of loving humankind ("philanthropy") and identifying as a citizen of the cosmopolis.	Living with inner consent, being emotionally and spiritually free and spontaneous, saying Yes to Life within and sometimes despite circumstances.
View of self	Non-self is full due to co-arising or co-constitution of phenomena experienced dynamically. Inter-related processes give rise to the sense of "I" inseparable from the environment.	Virtuous self is cultivated through training. Training can supervene disposition. Four virtues are cardinal: wisdom, courage, temperance, and justice.	The deep *person (nous)* is unique and never sick, but trauma, development and circumstances can disrupt *ego* development leading to deficits, blockages, rigidities, inhibitions, incapacities. Innate and acquired personality governs coping style.

Table 1: *Summary of Key features in Buddhism, Stoicism and Länglean Existential Analysis*

	Buddhism	Stoicism	Existential Analysis
Emotionality concept	Pleasant and unpleasant sensations can come and go. Eight mundane concerns (e.g., material possessions, sensations, others' perceptions of us) give rise to delight and distress. Wise people experience both with nonattachment.	Emotions are judgements that can be subject to rationality. Rationality is virtue. Love of mankind is based in family love. Externals may be preferred or dispreferred. Fate can be met with equanimity.	Emotion shows us where life is. Consent is a sentiment based on inner harmonizing. Emotional blockages limit our experience, our capacity to feel what is valuable, and can stunt moral conscience's development.
Will concept	Volition is limited. The inter-relatedness of all phenomena means causality arises in systemic interactions and is not mechanistic.	Dichotomy of control: we are subject to situations, and we use our rationality to respond. Souls have the capacity to choose not to be affected by pain, whereas bodies cannot.	Will is the actualization of one's freedom and is generated by the ego on the basis of perception of reality, choice between felt values, personal decision, and resolution to make it real. If will follows the personally felt sense, it is authentic and leads to a life with inner consent. Then the act is responsible.
Nature of suffering	Inevitable	Inevitable	Inevitable
Relation to mortality	Death precedes rebirth. Attaining enlightenment breaks the cycle.	Death is accepted as part of Nature.	Death belongs in life.
Exemplar	Buddha	Sage	Authentically acting person

Table 1 cont: *Summary of Key features in Buddhism, Stoicism and Länglean Existential Analysis*

A Natural History of a Psychologist Career

Susan D. Raeburn

Abstract: *This chapter narrates the natural history of the longstanding career of a Northern California psychologist, Dr. Susan D. Raeburn. From childhood origins of the budding desire and occupational goal to study psychology to the long and winding road of achieving the goal with little practical or financial help, Dr. Raeburn shares the personal, professional, and, finally, political conclusions that she has come to live by and embody as a clinical psychologist for thirty-six years in professional practice. Micro and macro reflections on the state of the profession and mental health care policies will be suggested.*

Introduction

When I was in the eighth grade at Northridge Junior High in Los Angeles, California, my school counselor asked me what I wanted to be when I grew up. I said, "a psychologist." I loved reading metaphysics and biography, and already had a pretty heavy loading of emotional loss, displacement, and adverse childhood experiences. Nonetheless, I was a resilient and curious kid with the help of a beloved aunt who seemed to understand me and vice-versa.

A precocious friend had just taken me to see Fellini's *Juliet of the Spirits.* It was not particularly age-appropriate for either of us at fourteen but we loved it. At the end of that film, the Jungian psychologist character, a statuesque older American woman, walked Juliet through a dark and mysterious forest, helping her reflect on her life. It turns out she helped me reflect on mine in some blur of artistic vision, identification, and emotional depth. This was all very, very cool.

Who knew that I'd end up going to college for twelve years to get a PhD. Fortunately, you could work your way through school in those days without incurring enormous financial debt; it required considerable emotional grit and just took a hell of a lot longer.

What follows is a free-wheeling account of my experience of becoming a clinical psychologist. I have studied, lived through, observed, rejected, and utilized a range of clinical approaches - fads and fashions - during my many years of clinical practice. In case you're wondering: along with self-employment in private practice, I worked at Stanford University Medical Center for almost ten years and Kaiser Permanente, part-time, for twenty-four more years. I used to tell my pre- and post-doctoral trainees, "Whatever you think you know now, wait ten years, or twenty, or thirty…".

In sharing this story of my "long and winding road," it is my hope that I have learned something of value for both myself and others about being of service as a psychologist.

Undergraduate Years: 1968-1972

With a California State Scholarship and part-time employment, I started at California State Northridge and soon joined the student protests against the Vietnam War. I transferred to UCLA and my psychology studies continued with the icy cold behaviorism of B.F. Skinner in which anything that could not be "observed and measured" was discounted as not scientific and, therefore, not really that important. That got boring and turned me off from clinical psychology for a while.

The best class I took at UCLA was *Intergroup Conflict and Prejudice*. The famous sociologist, Melvin Seeman, explained the importance of equal status exposure in breaking down racial stereotypes and hatred. As the violence of the Watts Riots blew up in L.A., this social-psychological perspective was extremely helpful and has stayed with me ever since.

Master's Program: 1972-1974

Starting a master's program at San Francisco State, I studied social psychology. Like many women of my generation, I'd started reading feminist writers such as Betty Freidan, Anais Nin, Simone de Beauvoir and social psychologists like Sandra Bem who wrote on gender and sexuality. I anticipated becoming a researcher more than a clinician.

My narrow view of clinical psychology expanded. I heard guest lectures by clinical psychologists and learned about the relational humanism of Carl Rogers, a clearer view of Freud, and Morris Rosenberg's principles of nonviolent communication among others. I wrote a Thesis on *The Effects of Rosenberg's Communication Skills on Locus of Control of Reinforcement.*

I read Kurt Lewin who popularized Field Theory in the 1940's examining patterns of interaction between the individual and the environment. Systems theory appealed to me, and it seems even more relevant now as we see the intersectionality of gender, race, social class, and caste.

Other early influences included the anti-psychiatry psychiatrist R.D. Laing. He saw mental illness as an understandable response to an insane world and wrote that the 'normally' alienated person is assumed to be sane. Other forms of alienation that are different from the mainstream are those labeled by the majority as bad or mad. (1)

In a similar vein, Thomas Szasz argued that mental illness is often a stand-in for human problems of living and that except for a few identifiable brain diseases, there are no biological, chemical, or biopsy tests for verifying DSM diagnoses. He continued to oppose *coercive* involuntary treatment but continued to practice psychiatry. (2)

These exposures facilitated the return of my path to clinical psychology as various aspects of meaning and heart evolved into a more compelling picture for me. However, this was not right away. I was sick of being in school and being broke. I took a four-year break before returning to school to get a PhD.

Worlds of Work: 1974-1978

The job market for a young woman with a newly minted master's degree in social psychology and no secretarial skills was not exactly the Land of Milk and Honey in 1974. *Remind me why I never took typing in high school?*

Nonetheless, I made the most of it until something interesting appeared and got things going professionally. By intention, I'd never worked in a corporate environment. Nevertheless, I became the mail girl for a major public accounting firm in the financial district of San Francisco. I'd industriously enter the skyscraper downtown and push the mail cart around three floors of only male accountants, all of whom also had master's degrees but made three times more money than me.

It was intellectually stultifying and personally humiliating. What really helped during this six-month period was listening to Jimmy Cliff's iconic Reggae songs "Sitting in Limbo" and "You Can Get It If You Really Want" which became my theme songs—an early lesson in what I would now call stress management and resilience! In the meantime, I continued to apply for any jobs that I felt could go on a professional resume. There was plenty more to it but that's all you guys get to hear.

The tide finally started shifting. I landed a real job in the Mayor's Office as a Program Evaluator for the San Francisco Model Cities Agency under the Department of Housing and Urban Development (HUD).

This federal poverty program was already in its last two years of funding; however, what I lost in long-term job security I gained in increased salary, an interesting multicultural work environment, freedom to do my job as I saw fit, and getting to work closely with a wonderful colleague, Barbara Smith, who is still a lifelong friend.

The Model Cities Program was mandated to hire people from the "Model Neighborhoods" in San Francisco – the Mission, a Latino enclave, and Bayview Hunters Point (considered a Black ghetto at that time). In a sign of those very different times, I was sort of a reverse Affirmative Action hire in that the Agency needed an academic type who could write. I was so relieved to get a real job and enter the vibrant mix of culture that existed there. The transplanted Jamaican staff turned me on to great reggae artists like Augustas Pablo and Linton Kwesi Johnson.

Unbeknownst to my new boss, I'd never actually done a program evaluation in my life. I had, however, learned some relevant concepts and buzzwords as a teaching assistant in a program evaluation class at SF State to ace the essay I was required to write. Eventually, I learned how to evaluate programs as Barbara and I modeled our approach after the excellent Chicago Model Cities Program. We volunteered and did the final program evaluation for the agency. God knows no one else there wanted to do that much work.

We witnessed many aspects of San Francisco history interviewing people in early stages of their careers (e.g., Harvey Milk, Dianne Feinstein). Mayor George Moscone eventually wrote me a letter of recommendation to grad school. One of my fellow program evaluators really wanted to be an actor. Barbara and I were supportive fans and made sure to go to his student plays at the American Conservatory Theatre (ACT). Eventually, our colleague, Danny Glover, became a famous actor. The last time I saw him I shared that I still have his chicken curry recipe from one of the agency potlucks.

Barbara went on to the San Francisco Housing Authority. Years later, she became the Director. I became the Assistant Director of Program Evaluation for Alameda County Mental Health in Oakland. I learned about the politics of funding for mental health and social services which was fundamental in setting the stage for my return to school with a clearer focus on becoming a clinical psychologist.

In 1978, Proposition 13 was passed by the voters of California. Property owners were happy to have their property taxes cut, but the funding for county services was cut and I was laid off - just in time to collect unemployment insurance and start my PhD program.

Worlds of Work, PhD Program, Internships, and Licensure: 1978-1987

My interest in what we would now describe as *intersectionality* led me to the program in Social-Clinical Psychology at the Wright Institute in Berkeley. Co-founded by Mervin Freeman and Nevitt Sanford (who co-wrote *The Authoritarian Personality* with Theodor Adorno), The Wright was known for its social activism. They offered an organizational psychology program, but I entered the psychoanalytically influenced Social-Clinical PhD curriculum.

We studied British theories of object-relations and psychoanalytic approaches highlighting unconscious processes (now understood as the powerful *implicit memory* system). Some of the more rigid psychoanalytic tenets at that time were later discounted by many of us as not that therapeutic. For example, viewing the therapist as a "blank screen" — in which the less said by the therapist, the greater the client would meaningfully project onto the therapist for analysis (as though the therapists didn't have some unintegrated unconscious projections of their own).

Years later, more than one client reluctantly came to therapy having been turned off by a rigidly psychoanalytic therapist who came across as cold, hostile, and unhelpful. This non-relational "one, not two-person" therapy approach has since been de-emphasized as the field of psychology learned more about the centrality of attachment, relationship, and somatic processes.

What a relief many of us felt when first hearing about the work of "Self in Relation" psychologists such as Jean Baker Miller, Janet Surrey, and Carol Gilligan at The Stone Center for Developmental Studies at Wellesley College. Eric Fromm is seen as an early inspiration of this relational perspective although the Stone Center writers incorporated more of a clear analysis of gender and culture.

Various approaches were considered at the Wright Institute during those years and students chose their allegiances accordingly. The French philosopher Michael Foucault was popular as he saw mental illness as a socially constructed tool of state power. Others rallied around the work of Lacan, Klein, and Kernberg. Christopher Lasch's bestseller, *The Culture of Narcissism,* was popular. Little did we know how that idea would loom even larger in the era of Donald Trump.

I embraced Heinz Kohut's relational psychoanalytic approach, "self-psychology." Kohut emphasized the repairing of the inevitable interpersonal breaches through empathic attunement, thus allowing the client to develop a healthy internalized sense of self in the transference. His theories continue to inform my work with clients in the development of the self, attachment, and affect regulation.

British psychologist/psychiatrist John Bowlby's theories on attachment styles were similarly influential to me. Researchers such as Ainsworth, Main, and Solomon helped Bowlby's theories re-emerge fully to influence the practice of psychology. This theoretical shift was further strengthened by UCLA neuropsychologist, Allan Schore, who published two seminal books on the biological underpinnings of early childhood development including attachment processes and trauma.

I began to clarify my interests in working with artists and musicians. I wrote a paper for a Group Process class titled "The Band as a Small Group and the Audience as a Large Group." For General Systems Theory, I wrote "The Popular Music Industry as an Open System." I met with music industry professionals such as the concert promoter, Bill Graham, and San Francisco Chronicle's Music Critic, Joel Selvin, to help ground my understanding of the industry. I wrote a dissertation on *Occupational Stress and Coping in Professional Rock Musicians*.

And, yes, I continued to work my way through those last five years of the PhD program. After getting laid off with Prop 13, I happily existed on unemployment insurance for the first year at the Wright Institute—a true gift of being able to be a full-time student. After that, I was, fortunately, re-hired as a Program Specialist for Alameda County Public Health.

While juggling class schedules at the Wright Institute, I worked full-time writing grants for Maternal and Child Health (MCH) and Vietnam Refugees, initially under Jimmy Carter and, later, during the Reagan administration. The grant requirements for MCH altered greatly when Reagan ran the show, much to the detriment of women and children, in my opinion.

I also staffed the Adult Day Healthcare Council (ADHC) with many amazing "Gray Panther" social activists. ADHC was geared towards keeping seniors out of nursing homes whenever possible by developing social daycare programs and keeping for-profit businesses out of the enterprise.

One of the federal grants positively changed my life and super-charged my psychology career. Through the efforts of my colleague, Barry Handon, M.D., MPH, Alameda County got funded by the Center for Disease Control (CDC) to implement a cutting-edge Health Education and Risk Reduction program. We called it the Lifestyle Enhancement Program. I became a "Trainer-of-Trainers" for an eight-week stress management course designed by our grant consultant, W. Stewart Agras, M.D. from the Department of Psychiatry and Behavioral Health Services at Stanford University Medical Center. My work at the County started to genuinely interface with being a graduate student in psychology.

I learned to teach stress management practices such as the *body scan*, self-monitoring, and the challenging of "stress-producing" beliefs. Not only did these practices pre-date the current era of mindfulness meditation made popular by Jon Kabat-Zinn at Mass General in Behavioral Medicine, but they introduced me to cognitive psychology with an updated and more humane version of behavioral practices in clinical psychology.

Best of all, I became a pre- and post-doctoral fellow at Stanford Medical Center with Stewart Agras. I was trained in cognitive-behavioral therapy. I remained at Stanford for many more years as a staff psychologist treating anxiety and eating disorders as well as participated in NIMH controlled trials on bulimia and anorexia. My colleagues in the Behavioral Medicine Clinic joked that we "talked about the transference behind Dr. Agras' back." I got licensed as a California clinical psychologist in 1987.

After the death of a close cousin from his cocaine addiction, I also started working in the Alcohol and Drug Treatment Center at Stanford. Between my family history of intergenerational alcoholism and my ongoing interest in working with musicians and artists, it was meaningful to me to learn about recovery from addictions.

After nine years of commuting from Oakland to Palo Alto, I needed to work closer to home. I'd established a successful half-time private practice in

Berkeley, but I didn't want to rely fully on self-employment. I appreciated having the health benefits and the security of a paid gig.

The universe helped me out in that two psychologist friends were working at Kaiser Permanente-Walnut Creek in the Chemical Dependency Services Program and told me that a half-time job was opening up. I got the job and worked at Kaiser running addiction recovery groups and supervising pre-doctoral interns for the next twenty-four years. I was ready to retire from Kaiser and did just that in 2016.

While continuing two days a week of private practice with mostly long-term clients, I've been enjoying a five-day work weekend doing some writing projects and conference talks ever since.

Close to My Heart: Performing Arts Medicine and Psychology

It turned out that my dissertation was the first American academic study of its kind. Years later, I connected with Dr. Geoff Wills who had done a larger study in the UK right around the same time. In 1986, I connected with a group of physicians and educators who worked with musicians and dancers belonging to a relatively new organization, the Performing Arts Medicine Association (PAMA).

PAMA was founded in 1983 by Alice Brandfonbrener, M.D. at Northwestern University in Chicago and Richard Lederman, M.D. at the Cleveland Clinic in Ohio. I started publishing articles in the PAMA journal, *Medical Problems of Performing Artists*, in 1987 and eventually joined its editorial board. Although PAMA members in the early years seemed to be working exclusively with classical musicians and ballet rather than popular musicians or modern dancers, I was delighted to have found some of my "professional tribe."

That tribe has recently grown to include an international group of clinicians, many of whom initially worked in the music industry. Tamsin Embleton, a British tour manager-turned-psychotherapist, started the Music Industry Therapist Collective (MITC). She developed a groundbreaking book, *Touring and Mental Health: The Music Industry*

Manual, for which I contributed a couple of chapters. Various other organizations (e.g., the SIMS Foundation, the New Orleans Musicians Clinic, MusiCares, The Actors Fund, Backline, Amber Health) have developed services in support of musician and tour crew mental health. Many others have come and gone due to lack of funding.

What Helps Heal and What Does Not

Although I won't be solving the nature-nurture dilemma here, I will share how I have come to think about it as I try to address the ambitious tasks assigned for this volume.

The tasks were as follows:

- To critique the biomedical model of mental health and practice of psychiatric diagnosing
- To provide practical and implementable alternatives to psychiatric diagnosing
- To present micro and macro and systems-level alternatives to DSM and ICD diagnosing.

I was encouraged by recent developments in the field of psychology as represented by the American Psychological Association (APA), of which I remain a member (except for the dark years during which I protested the APA's alignment with the Bush Administration over allowing the participation of psychologists in torture practices at Guantanamo).

Current APA leaders have acknowledged the need to increase emphasis on *primary prevention* at individual and societal systems levels. In a recent article from the American Psychological Association, Isha Metzger, PhD wrote: "People can't focus on their mental health when they have larger social and structural issues to contend with" The article further describes research and organizational efforts to address racism and discrimination to improve mental, behavioral and physical health on a broader scale, thus *acknowledging the social determinants of health*. The article acknowledges that "a growing public conversation around burnout, stress, and self-care post-pandemic is also influencing the field." (3, p. 92).

Working Assumptions of Doing Psychotherapy: Micro-Level Considerations

The cultural anthropologist, William P. Delaney, articulated his view of unhelpful ethnographic practices that resonates with unhelpful diagnostic approaches to psychotherapy.

He wrote: "I define ethnographic cynicism as a failure to... gather good field data in a disciplined fashion. It stops respecting the integrity of the subject matter and enlists field data into the service of ideological and theoretical biases; this can be done unconsciously. It succumbs to the romance of ideas and concepts over the more modest, disciplined description of events and persons." (4)

DSM categories skew negative towards pathology, and the equivalent "ethnographic cynicism" occurs when psychologists fall lazy prey to the pathologizing bent of DSM-V categorizations without observing their client in a more nuanced way over time. The rigid and self-serving short-term focus of managed care companies on "medical necessity" further establishes and maintains this practice.

Here are the principles that I endorse in the practice of effective psychotherapy:

- Psychotherapy starts with an open-hearted observation of the client as a whole person who is seeking your help in reducing suffering and clarifying its causes. Observation, over time, must precede premature and/or glib diagnostic assumptions to minimize the therapist's own anxiety. Therapists require patience and a flexible tolerance of uncertainty and ambiguity as the client's diagnostic and interpersonal picture comes into clearer focus over time.
- Therapy is a "two-person" process in which *both* participants have unconscious elements and attachment needs. It is the therapist's responsibility to develop mature self-awareness and authenticity which, then, makes accurate attunement to the client possible. This

includes owning and correcting empathic failures on the part of the therapist, an experience that many clients have never experienced in their family-of-origin.

- DSM-V continues the tradition of overemphasizing pathology to the detriment of psychological health and resilience. However, sometimes psychotherapy does require a diagnostic DSM-V code so clients can get paid by their insurance company. In that case, clients need to be informed and understand the result of what may show up in his/her medical record.

- Sometimes, psychotherapy includes a referral to a psychiatrist for psychiatric medication. I've consistently maintained a conservative approach to psychiatric medications and have never considered them as a first resort given issues of possible adverse side effects, dependence, potential addiction, ineffectiveness, and stigma.

- It remains important to distinguish difficult psychological states from brain-based disorders. In a recent conversation with Dr. Rick Hanson, Dr. Chris Palmer, assistant professor of psychiatry at Harvard Medical School, discussed his work on severe conditions like schizophrenia and psychiatry's current challenges with treatment-resistant conditions. He said: *"Nobody in their right mind should consider PTSD-resulting from ongoing bullying for example as a brain disorder or chemical imbalance. And yet that is the way DSM describes it, and unfortunately that's the way some clinicians will treat it: You've got PTSD? Here's a pill."* (5)

Theoretical Considerations

My theoretical investments in psychology now include a select combination of Rogers' humanism, Jung's shadow work, Kohut's focus on repair of empathic failures, Bowlby's attachment theories, somatic therapies (i.e., Levine's, Porges', and Van der Kolk's), and systems' approaches in the form of Schwartz's Internal Family Systems. As psychology has increasingly secularized Buddhist principles, the mindfulness teachings of Jon Kabat-Zinn, Linehan's Dialectical Behavior Therapy (DBT), and Hayes' Acceptance and Commitment Therapy (ACT) have been helpful to me and my clients. Dan Siegel's emphasis on increasing *flexibility and integration* has become a foundation of my practice, not to mention my personal life.

If a client presents with an active behavioral symptom such as bulimia, self-injurious behavior, panic attacks, or active chemical or behavioral addictions, I get very symptom-focused and focus on cognitive-behavioral techniques to reduce harm. As the *therapeutic alliance* develops and the presenting symptoms begin to resolve over time, my focus shifts and deepens accordingly.

Working Assumptions of Doing Psychotherapy: Macro-Level Considerations

I have witnessed the increasing overreliance on the medical model in psychiatry (and often in psychology) over the last several decades; that is, where the *bio* part of the more inclusive *bio-psycho-social* model (that I do endorse) gets inflated. This appears to be a product of the outsized influence of pharmaceutical companies and their lobbyists along with a lack of access and adequate funding to more costly treatments (such as short and, especially, long-term psychotherapy). The hyper-capitalism of the larger systems continues to promote a self-serving focus on *individual* responsibility when the surrounding support *systems for primary prevention* are broken and need to be rehabilitated.

The work of psychologists and psychiatrists, such as Bruce Alexander and Gabor Maté, are relevant to the conversation. Best-known for his "Rat Lab" studies highlighting the power of healthy "enriched" environments in the 1970's, Canadian psychologist and researcher, Bruce Alexander, wrote an enlightening and encyclopedic book on the often-tragic impact on people of the neoliberal, hyper-capitalist systems in which mental healthcare remains embedded. Likewise, Gabor Maté has written extensively on the toxic effects of trauma.

Societal Priorities

Regarding the societal aspects of the mental health care system, I reflect on John F. Kennedy's progressive call for the replacement of state psychiatric hospitals with community care services in 1963. He envisioned building 1,500 outpatient mental health services to offer them community vs. institutional care. (6) His nephew, Robert Kennedy Jr., recently suggested that federal taxes from the legalization of marijuana could be used in the service of establishing community recovery centers in disenfranchised sections of the US with high rates of addiction. This makes a lot of sense to me.

The Lanterman-Petris Act was signed into law in 1967 in California and went into full effect in 1972. It was supposed to "provide prompt psychiatric evaluation and treatment of persons with serious mental disorders or impaired by chronic alcoholism" and "guarantee and protect public safety." That never happened. (7)

Ronald Reagan closed the state hospitals for the "severely mentally ill" in 1967, but without fulfilling the original promise of funding community-based services for those thoroughly displaced. In 1972, that promise was fully decimated by Reagan in California. Explain that to the residents and business owners in San Francisco's Civic Center and Tenderloin neighborhoods where the homelessness and Fentanyl crisis remains in full swing today.

How does this interact with my practice of being a psychologist? For starters, it seems to have landed in the continuing ascension of hyper-capitalism and neoliberalism since the 70's which now painfully interact with increased global anxieties around climate change, mass migration, extremes of income inequality, political polarization, and with worsening statistics on mental health and longevity across many age-groups in the U.S.

We are living the painful and ongoing after-effects of these neo-liberal policies in which the highest-earning 20% of families in the U.S. made more than the half of all U.S. income in 2018 (8). Other reports are even more poignant: in the San Francisco Bay Area and Oakland, where I live, estimates of the homeless population now clock in at 38,000 individuals on any given night, an increase of 35 % since 2019. (9)

Where Do We Need to Go?

In my years of private practice, I've jumped on and off "managed care" insurance agreements that became intrusive to me and to my clients. I've charged wealthier clients more and starving artist clients less. My pro-bono work has mostly been around writing mental health stuff for free, presenting it at conferences at my own expense. Now "semi-retired," I have tried to "do good in the world," although I am not a political activist and am more likely to throw money at trustworthy progressive causes (e.g., the work of the progressive organization *Move On* and Robert Reich's *Inequality Media*).

Unions need to be reinvigorated. I repeatedly walked the picket line as a Kaiser Permanente psychologist in the National Union of Healthcare Workers (NUHW), protesting the limitations of Kaiser's mental health services. As a self-employed therapist, I like to quip that I can only walk a picket line now against myself.

Non-profit organizations need more federal and state funding for community mental health and housing. This is painfully overdue given what is happening in our streets. In spite of the lack of adequate funding for care, there are many, many committed therapists working in the trenches of community mental health and non-profit organizations across the country.

Social Connection and Self-help Models of Recovery

The World Health Organization (WHO) has declared that social isolation and loneliness is a significant health risk factor for physical and mental health. Having worked with hundreds of clients with eating disorders, chemical dependency, and other behavioral "process" addictions over the years, I remain actively impressed with the workings of FREE self-help organizations such as Alcoholics Anonymous, Adult Children of Alcoholics (ACOA), and many others.

I believe that this model of free self-help groups based on honest social connection could be applied to many other mental health and behavioral problems.

Reducing Stigma

We have increasingly seen public figures disclose their personal mental health struggles and journeys of recovery. This development clearly helps reduce stigma for others. A US Senator talked openly about his hospitalization for depression; a presidential candidate self-disclosed that he has been sober for decades while remaining actively engaged in a 12-Step program. I admire this kind of individual and collective courage, especially given this era of increased personal risk of harm in our polarized climate.

Conclusion

How individuals manage stress and heal mental health challenges is invariably impacted by the health or dysfunction of the environments around them. In his book on resilience, Stephen Southwick states that healthy adaptation to stress depends not only on the individual but also on the resources of family, friends, various organizations, and on the characteristics of specific cultures, communities, societies, and governments - all of which may be more or less resilient. (10)

Healing personal and family trauma and supporting political action at the local, state, and federal levels to elect humanistic and enlightened brokers seem to be our greatest path forward for meaningful change. I deeply hope that MLK is correct that the *arc of the moral universe is long but it bends toward justice*. It would be especially encouraging if that arc gets going in the right direction while I'm still here to see it. (11)

References

1. Laing, R.D. *The Politics of Experience and the Bird of Paradise.* Harmondsworth: Penguin, 1967.

2. Szasz, Thomas S., *The Myth of Mental Illness: Foundations of a Theory of Personal Conduct,* Harpers Paperback, 2010.

3. Weir, Kirsten, "Rebranding the Field: The Big Tent of Behavioral Health," APA Monitor on Psychology, January - February, 2023, p. 92.

4. Delaney, William P., "Ethnographic Nihilism", Academia.edu, independent.academia.edu/williamdelaney2. p. 1. September, 2023.

5. Rick Hanson, PhD, Being Well Podcast: "Metabolism, Brain Energy, and Mental Health with Dr. Chris Palmer," September 1, 2023.

6. Prionas, Schuyler Hudak, "How California Can Carry JFK's Torch with Mental Health Legislation." San Francisco Examiner, Sept. 23, 2023.

7. Davis, K., McDonald, J. "In California, jails are now the mental health centers of last resort." The San Diego Union-Tribune, Sept. 20, 2019.

8. Schaeffer, Katharine, "Six Facts about income inequality in the U.S." Pew Research Center. February 7, 2020. https://www.pewresearch.org.

9. Anthony, Kate, Modi, Kunal, Rajgopal, Yu, Gordon. "Homelessness in the San Francisco Bay Area: The crisis and a path forward." McKinsey & Company, Social Sector, July 11, 2019/Article.

10. Southwick, S. M. and Charney, D. S. (2018). *Resilience*, 2nd edition. Cambridge: Cambridge University Press. p. 9.

11. Ellis, Deborah, "The Arc of the Moral Universe is Long, But it Bends Towards Justice." https://obamawhitehousearchives.gov/ blog/2011/10/21/arc-moral-universe-long-it-bends-toward-justice# The White House President Barack Obama, October 21, 2011.

Contributors

Sofia Adam holds a doctorate degree from the Department of Social Administration and Political Science of the Democritus University of Thrace. She is an Assistant Professor in the subject of Local Development and Social Policy at the Department of Social Policy of Democritus University of Thrace.

Paul Blackburn, PhD started his professional life as a secondary school teacher in an area of socio-economic disadvantage, before coming to understand that he was far more concerned with the context of the young people's lives than trying to teach them French. With a background in systemic family therapy, Paul has worked in UK mental health services for 40 years, leading on developments in his local area for young people experiencing what the system calls 'psychosis'. Over the past two years, he has been involved in the formation of the Emotions are not Illnesses (ERNI) declaration and movement: https://www.ernimovement.com/

Mary Boyle, PhD is Emeritus Professor of Clinical Psychology at the University of East London, UK, where she was Head of the Doctoral Programme in Clinical Psychology. She has also worked in adult mental health and women's health in the NHS. She is the author of *Schizophrenia: A Scientific Delusion?* and *Rethinking Abortion: Psychology, Gender Power and the Law* (Routledge) and many articles and chapters on women's health and on problems of psychiatric diagnostic models. With Dr Lucy Johnstone, she is co-author of *A Straight Talking Introduction to the Power Threat Meaning Framework: An Alternative to Psychiatric Diagnosis* (PCCS Books).

G. Kenneth Bradford, PhD is currently an independent scholar, Dharma teacher and contemplative yogin integrating Buddhist and Existential-Phenomenological thought and practice. Formerly, he was licensed as a clinical psychologist practicing psychotherapy in the San Francisco Bay Area, and Adjunct Professor at John F. Kennedy University and California Institute of Integral Studies. Publications include *Opening Yourself: The Psychology and Yoga of Self-liberation* (2021); *The I of the Other: Mindfulness-Based Diagnosis & the Question of Sanity* (2013); and *Listening from the Heart* *of Silence: Nondual Wisdom and Psychotherapy, Vol. 2* (2007, with John Prendergast); as well as numerous peer-reviewed articles intertwining psychology and spirituality, including on "Radical Authenticity," "Non-self Psychology" & "On the Essence of Freedom." He can be reached via his website: https://authenticpresence.net/.

Josh Bylotas is a licensed clinical social worker specializing in clinical practice with military and veteran populations. His practice interests include suicide prevention and cognitive-behavioral therapies. Josh is currently a doctoral student at Colorado State University researching suicide risk and protective factors.

Arnoldo Cantú is a licensed clinical social worker with experience in school social work, community behavioral health, and currently working in private practice. His interests consist of working with children, adolescents, their families, and adults in a clinical capacity. Cantú was born in Mexico and considers Texas home, having grown up in the Rio Grande Valley. He is currently a doctoral student at Colorado State University with an interest in researching conceptual and practical alternatives to the DSM.

Professor Timothy Carey is the Chair, Country Health Research at Curtin University. Tim is a researcher-clinician with a PhD in Clinical Psychology, an MSc in Statistics, a Postgraduate Certificate in Biostatistics, and tertiary qualifications in primary, preschool, and special education. He is a senior Australian academic and Fulbright Scholar who has combined clinical practice with research and university teaching and training throughout his career. He has worked in rural and underserved communities in both Scotland and remote Australia and as an academic in Australia, the US, and Rwanda. He has over 175 publications and has presented his work at conferences and other scientific meetings both nationally and internationally. His In Control blog on Psychology Today has had over 1.48 million views. He is one of the world's leading scholars in the science of control and its application to wellbeing and harmonious social living.

Sarah Clayton, MA Psychology (Hons), MLitt is a writer who thrives in the realms of both non-fiction and crime fiction. Her work, "The Write Wild

Method" stands as a testament to her dedication to nurturing writers and sparking creativity via an individual's relationship with the natural world. In her non-fiction writings, Sarah delves deep into the profound and transformative potential of the human-nature connection. With a keen focus on existential anxiety, she illustrates how a profound relationship with nature has the remarkable power to heal and transform individuals, offering solace and meaning. As a seasoned writing mentor and creativity coach, Sarah aims to guide aspiring writers towards growth and success.

Jonah Cohen is a psychologist at Massachusetts General Hospital (MGH) and is an Assistant Professor at Harvard Medical School. At MGH, Jonah is the associate director for the Center for Anxiety and Traumatic Stress Disorders and an assistant director of Psychology Training. He also is a candidate at Boston Psychoanalytic Society and Institute. His clinical and research interests focus on the integration of theoretical orientations for complex clinical presentations.

Rachel Cooper is Professor of History and Philosophy of Science at Lancaster University, UK. She is the author of *Classifying Madness* (Springer, 2005), *Psychiatry and Philosophy of Science* (Routledge, 2007), and *Diagnosing the Diagnostic and Statistical Manual of Mental Disorders* (Karnac, 2014).

Gemma Dent is in the process of completing a doctorate in clinical psychology. As the project coordinator for the ERNI movement, she has been instrumental in connecting with like-minded others who are committed to rethinking current ideology and promoting system change within mental health services. https://www.ernimovement.com/

Todd DuBose is a Distinguished Full Professor at The Chicago School of Professional Psychology. He is also a licensed psychologist with over thirty-five years of clinical experience, nine of those years as a former chaplain at the legendary Bellevue Hospital in New York City and has over twenty years of experience as a teacher, supervisor, and consultant in local, national and international venues, including presentations and teaching in over twelve countries. He holds advanced degrees in the integration of continental philosophy of religion and human science clinical psychology. He is committed to the public-scholar, engaged practitioner model of scholarship and praxis and is very active in addressing community violence, food insecurity and at-risk youth, and advocating for critical-existential-hermeneutical-phenomenological alternatives of care. He is on the board of The International Society for Ethical Psychology and Psychiatry (ISEPP).

Jay S. Efran is Professor Emeritus of Psychology at Temple University. He is the recipient of the Pennsylvania Psychological Association's 2009 award for Distinguished Contributions to the Science and Profession of Psychology, the 2006 Lifetime Achievement Award of the Constructivist Psychology Network, and teaching excellence awards from both the University of Rochester and Temple University. At Temple, he served as director of clinical training and director of the Psychological Services Center. He is a Fellow of the American Psychological Association and the American Group Psychotherapy Association.

Laura Faith is currently a Psychologist at the Richard L. Roudebush VA Medical Center in Indianapolis, IN. She received her Ph.D. in clinical psychology from The University of Missouri in Kansas City (UMKC) where she received specialized training in research and treatments for individuals with psychosis. She trained with Paul Lysaker to learn the metacognitive framework for individuals with psychosis and Metacognitive Reflection and Insight Therapy (MERIT) during internship and post-doctoral training. Currently, she uses MERIT with individuals receiving outpatient care for serious mental illnesses.

Justin Garson is a philosopher and historian of science at Hunter College and The Graduate Center, City University of New York. He's the author of *Madness: A Philosophical Exploration* (Oxford, 2022), *The Biological Mind: Second Edition* (Routledge, 2022), and the forthcoming *The Madness Pill: The Quest to Create Insanity and One Doctor's Discovery that Transformed Psychiatry* (St. Martin's Press). He also contributes to Psychology-Today.com, Aeon and MadInAmerica.com on changing paradigms of mental illness.

Robert Griffiths is Lecturer in Mental Health at the University of Manchester and also holds an honorary position at Greater Manchester Mental Health NHS Foundation Trust as Director of the Mental Health Nursing Research Unit. He has worked clinically in Assertive Outreach and Early Intervention in Psychosis mental health services. Robert is a former National Institute of Health Research (NIHR) Clinical Doctoral Research Fellow (2016-2019). His current research interests include the development of clinical applications of a theory of human behaviour called Perceptual Control Theory and evaluating the use of Method of Levels – a transdiagnostic approach to psychological therapy – for people reporting psychosis.

Richard Hallam worked as a clinical psychologist, researcher, and lecturer until 2006, combining work in the British National Health Service with teaching on the clinical doctoral programs at the University of East London and at University College London. His research interests have included theory in CBT, anxiety problems, tinnitus and hearing impairment, concept of self, and human evolution. Since 2006, he has worked independently as a therapist, authored several books, and self-published under the imprint Polpresa Press.

Kate Hammer is an existential therapist and coaching psychologist based in Central London (UK) with a thriving private practice online. Trained in existential analysis and logotherapy by Alfried Längle, the successor of Viktor Frankl, Kate also sees clients in-person for counselling and therapy. Client themes include anxiety, grief, stasis, worthlessness, non-belonging, racial trauma, gender questioning, uncoupling, cynicism and meaninglessness. Kate is a member of the Race Reflections community. Pro bono work has included Psychosis Therapy Project and piloting group coaching in the community with a local mental health agency.

Jay Joseph, Psy.D. is a clinical psychologist practicing in the San Francisco Bay Area. He has analyzed genetic research in the social and behavioral sciences since the late 1990s and is critical of medical models of human psychological distress and dysfunction. He is the author of four books, most recently *Schizophrenia and Genetics: The End of an Illusion* (2023). A complete list of his articles and book chapters is on his website:

https://jayjoseph.net/publications/. Many of his online articles can be found at the Mad in America website: https://www.madinamerica.com/author/jjoseph/

Sarah Knutson is an ex-lawyer, ex-therapist, survivor-activist. Past experience includes work with Intentional Peer Support, Mad in America and organizing (pre-covid) online peer support for the psychiatric survivor community around a variety of realities that could not be safely named or discussed in mainstream clinical circles. Sarah is currently active with All Brains Belong in Montpelier, VT and working on a critical psychiatry book about the broader stress/ survival/ diversity paradigm.

Athanasios Koutsoklenis holds a doctorate degree from the Department of Educational and Social Policy of the University of Macedonia. He is an Assistant Professor in the subject of Inclusive Education at the Department of Elementary Education of Democritus University of Thrace.

Alfried Laengle, M.D., Ph.D. (psychology), born 1951 in Austria, founder (1983) and long-term president of the International Society for Logotherapy and Existential Analysis (Vienna), scholar and collaborator of Viktor Frankl. Professor at the Moscow's HSE-university and Vienna's Sigmund Freud University. 400 publications, two honorary doctorates, six honorary professor degrees, 2 decorations of the Republic of Austria. www.laengle.info

Don Laird is an adjunct instructor at Carlow University where he developed a graduate-level course titled "Applied Existential and Dynamic Approaches to Psychotherapy," which he also teaches. He has written papers and presented lectures on a variety of subjects including the application of existential and contemplative therapies, existential positive psychology, existential coaching, creativity, and existential themes in the works of Otto Rank, Edward Hopper, Ingmar Bergman, and Charles Dickens. Additionally, Don is in private practice at eTalkTherapy, LLC and is the Chair of Professional Development and Education for the International Network of Personal Meaning.

Eric Maisel, Ph.D., is the author of 50+ books, among them *The Future of Mental Health, Rethinking Depression, Humane Helping, Redesign Your Mind*, and *The Van Gogh Blues*. He writes the "Rethinking Mental Health" blog for *Psychology Today*, with 3,000,000+ views, and is the developer of, and lead editor for, the Ethics International Press Critical Psychology and Critical Psychiatry series.

Dr Ian Marsh is a Reader in the School of Allied and Public Health at Canterbury Christ Church University. Ian's main research interests are in critical approaches to suicide and suicide prevention. He is currently involved in research on online harms for UK Samaritans, and on suicide in public places for the railway industry, Highways England, and at coastal locations. He is academic lead for the Kent and Medway Suicide Prevention Group, is the Suicide-Safer Universities project lead in Canterbury and has worked with Universities UK on developing suicide-safer approaches. Ian was a co-founder of the Critical Suicide Studies Network.

Niall McLaren is a retired psychiatrist and author who graduated in medicine from the University of Western Australia in 1970, and in psychiatry in 1977. Since then, he has worked at the rough end of psychiatry, including six years in the remote Kimberley Region of WA. In 1982, he began studying philosophy and continued clinical work while publishing on critical theory in psychiatry, which has often brought conflict with mainstream psychiatry. He has now published nine monographs in this field, as well as numerous peer-reviewed papers, chapters and articles, and has lectured at international conferences and at major universities overseas.

Aubrie Musselman is currently a psychologist at the Travis W. Atkins VA Clinic within the Montana VA Health Care System. She received her doctorate in clinical psychology from Indiana State University where her research focused on evaluating the psychometric properties of MMPI scales measuring the schizophrenia construct. She completed her practicum training working therapeutically with individuals diagnosed with psychotic disorders under the supervision of Dr. Paul Lysaker and completed her predoctoral internship with the Montana VAHCS.

Craig Newnes is a Consultant Critical Psychologist, editor and author. He has published numerous book chapters and academic articles and is Editor of *The Journal of Critical Psychology, Counselling and Psychotherapy*. He was, for 19 years, the editor of *Clinical Psychology Forum*, the in-house practice journal of the Division of Clinical Psychology of The British Psychological Society and Director of Psychological Therapies for Shropshire's Community and Mental Health Services Trust. He has edited and authored over twenty books. For PCCS Books he authored *Clinical Psychology: A critical examination* (2014) as part of the Critical Examination series for which he was also Commissioning Editor and *Children in Society: Politics, policies and interventions* (2015). For Palgrave he authored *Inscription, Diagnosis, Deception and the Mental Health Industry: How Psy governs us all* (2016) and, for Routledge, he edited *Racism in Psychology* (2021) and, with Laura Golding, *Teaching Critical Psychology* (2018). In 2023, *Withdrawal from Prescribed Psychotropic Drugs*, co-edited with Peter Lehmann, was published by Egalitarian Publishing.

Ian Parker is a psychoanalyst and Marxist working in Manchester, UK, part of the editorial collective of *Asylum: Magazine for Radical Mental Health*. He is co-founder and co-director (with Erica Burman) of the Discourse Unit and Managing Editor of *Annual Review of Critical Psychology*.

Sarah E. Queller is the clinical psychologist and program coordinator for the psychiatric inpatient unit at the Richard L. Roudebush VAMC in Indianapolis, Indiana. She earned a B.A. in English from Kenyon College, an M.A. in forensic psychology from George Washington University, and a Psy.D. in clinical psychology from the University of Indianapolis. In her current position, she adapts Metacognitive Reflection and Insight Therapy (MERIT)'s recovery-oriented, metacognitive framework for meaning-making in an acute psychiatric setting.

Dr. Susan Raeburn is a clinical psychologist in Oakland, CA, largely working with performing artists. She attended U.C.L.A., San Francisco State University, and the Wright Institute, Berkeley. She was a staff psychologist at Stanford University Medical Center and at Kaiser Permanente. Susan has published peer-reviewed articles on eating disorders, addictions, and musician mental health. With Eric Maisel, she co-authored *Creative Recovery* (2008). She contributed chapters to *Touring and Mental Health: The Music Industry Manual* (2023). Susan has been active at music industry conferences and the Performing Arts Medicine Association where she is on the Editorial Board of their journal. She is a member of the Music Industry Therapist Collective, an international group of therapists with music industry experience.

Jonathan D. Raskin, Ph.D. is professor and chair in the Department of Psychology at the State University of New York at New Paltz. Dr. Raskin has published extensively on constructivist approaches to psychology and psychotherapy. He has also studied psychologist attitudes to the DSM and its alternatives. Dr. Raskin served as the 2020-21 president of the Society for Humanistic Psychology (Division 32 of the American Psychological Association). In addition to many journal articles and book chapters, Dr. Raskin is author of *Psychopathology and Mental Distress: Contrasting Perspectives* (2nd ed.), managing editor of the *Journal of Constructivist Psychology,* and a licensed psychologist with an active private practice.

Elizabeth Root, MSW, MS Ed. is a retired clinical social worker who treated children and families for 19 years in the public sector in Central New York. She currently lives in Trumansburg, NY in the heart of the Finger Lakes.

Jeffrey Rubin grew up in Brooklyn and received his PhD from the University of Minnesota. In his earlier life, he worked in clinical settings, schools, and a juvenile correctional facility. He has published research-based articles in *Professional Psychology: Research and Practice, The American Psychologist, Counseling and Values,* and *The Journal of Humanistic Psychology.* More recently, he authored three novels, *A Hero Grows in Brooklyn, Fights in the Streets, Tears in the Sand,* and *Love, Sex, and Respect.* Currently, he writes a blog titled *From Insults to Respect* that features suggestions for working through conflict, dealing with anger, and supporting respectful relationships.

Dr. Chuck Ruby is a licensed psychologist. He is the Executive Director of the International Society for Ethical Psychology and Psychiatry (ISEPP) and the General Manager of The Pinnacle Center. He was trained at Florida State University, receiving his Ph.D. in psychology in 1995. Dr. Ruby is a retired Lieutenant Colonel with the Air Force Office of Special Investigations. He is the author of *Smoke and Mirrors: How You Are Being Fooled About Mental Illness - An Insider's Warning to Consumers*.

Dr William Van Gordon is a Chartered Psychologist and Associate Professor of Contemplative Psychology at the University of Derby (UK), where he also Chairs the School of Psychology Research Committee. He is internationally recognised for advancing the Contemplative Psychology research agenda, to which he has contributed over 100 peer-reviewed papers. William writes a regular blog on Contemplative Psychology for Psychology Today (https://www.psychologytoday.com/gb/contributors/william-van-gordon-phd) and is author of *The Way of the Mindful Warrior* (https://a.co/d/aHdVnsf).

Jo Watson is a psychotherapist, supervisor, trainer and activist. She has worked for the last 25 years with people who have experienced trauma and adversity. Jo is the founder of the Facebook group 'Drop The Disorder!' and adisorder4everyone.com (AD4E) that hosts events that challenge the culture of 'diagnosis and disorder' and the medicalisation of emotional distress and a founding member of madintheuk.com. She is the editor of the PCCS books Drop the Disorder! - Challenging the Culture of Psychiatric Diagnosis, and We are the Change-Makers; Poems supporting Drop the Disorder.

Courtney N. Wiesepape is a psychologist at the Austin VA Clinic within the Central Texas Health Care system. She received her doctorate in clinical psychology from Indiana State University where she studied the identification and assessment of schizotypy and schizophrenia spectrum disorders. She trained with Dr. Paul H. Lysaker during internship and post-doctoral years, focusing on the treatment and research of psychotic disorders through the lens of a metacognitive model. In practice, she utilizes metacognitively oriented psychotherapy with an emphasis on recovery and meaning making.

Paul T. P. Wong is Professor Emeritus of Trent University, a Fellow of APA, APS, and CPA, and the founding President of the International Network on Personal Meaning. As a servant leader, he has been a pastor, founding director of the graduate program of counselling psychology of Trinity Western University, and Head of Social Sciences of Tyndale University. A prolific writer, he has published eight books and 300+ journal articles and chapters. He is world-renowned for his research on the new science of suffering, indigenous psychology, servant leadership, quest for meaning, self-transcendence, death acceptance, successful aging, and palliative care.